The Physiological Management of Diabetes in Children

The Physiological Management of Diabetes in Children

Robert L. Jackson, M.D.
Professor of Pediatrics, University of Kansas School of Medicine, Kansas City; *Emeritus Professor of Child Health,* University of Missouri, Columbia

Richard A. Guthrie, M.D.
Professor of Pediatrics, University of Kansas School of Medicine, Wichita; *Director,* Kansas Regional Diabetes Center, Wichita

With a Foreword by

Jay Skyler

Former Editor of *Diabetes Care*

MEDICAL EXAMINATION PUBLISHING CO.

Jackson, Robert L. (date)
The physiological management of diabetes in children.

Includes bibliographies and index.
1. Diabetes in children. I. Guthrie, Richard A. (date). II. Title. [DNLM: 1. Diabetes Mellitus, Insulin-Dependent -- therapy. WK 815 J13p]
RJ420.D5J33 1985 618.92'462 85-15505
ISBN 0-87488-308-3

52 Vanderbilt Ave.
New York, N.Y.

Dedicated to the parents of the child with diabetes. You have been our best teachers.

Contents

Contributors

MARTHA U. BARNARD, R.N., *Faculty Clinician,* University of Kansas College of Health Sciences, Hospital School of Medicine, and School of Nursing, Department of Pediatrics, Department of Endocrinology, Kansas Regional Diabetes Center

MARIA TERESA GARCIA-OTERO CLABOTS, M.D., *Instructor,* Pediatric Endocrinology, University of Kansas College of Health Sciences and Hospital

DIANA GUTHRIE, R.N., Ph.D., *Associate Professor; Diabetes Nurse Specialist,* Kansas Regional Diabetes Center of the University of Kansas School of Medicine at Wichita

RICHARD A. GUTHRIE, M.D., *Professor of Pediatrics,* University of Kansas School of Medicine, Wichita; *Director,* Kansas Regional Diabetes Center, Wichita

ROBERT L. JACKSON, M.D., *Professor of Pediatrics,* University of Kansas School of Medicine, Kansas City; *Emeritus Professor,* Child Health, University of Missouri, Columbia

RACHEL G. JORGENSEN, R.N., M.N., *Diabetes Nurse Coordinator,* University of Kansas Regional Diabetes Center, Kansas City Campus, University of Kansas College of Health Sciences and Hospital

WAYNE V. MOORE, M.D., Ph.D., *Professor of Pediatrics,* University of Kansas Medical Center

DEBORAH K. OLSON, R.D., *Courtesy Teaching Associate,* University of Kansas Medical Center College of Health Sciences and Hospital

LIBBIE J. RUSSO, M.D., *Assistant Professor of Pediatrics,* Section of Endocrinology, University of Kansas Medical Center

Foreword

This book describes a management approach to childhood diabetes evolved over nearly five decades by Dr. Robert Jackson. Together with his most noted disciple, Dr. Richard Guthrie, Bob Jackson has articulated in this book the details of a management scheme which has been both highly successful and highly controversial. It is a scheme which has come more and more to be emulated by diabetologists across the world, in terms of the principles of management if not the details.

The premise on which Jackson and Guthrie base their management program is that normal physiology should be and can be mimicked in the management of childhood diabetes. The successful implementation of this premise requires an expenditure of effort - on the part of patients, their families, and the health professionals caring for them - that is substantially greater than that commonly employed in the management of childhood diabetes. Thus, the approach has been fraught with difficulty when it has been attempted to be duplicated by others. Often, the ego strength of the physicians attempting to emulate the Jackson/Guthrie formula has been such that rather than admit their inability to achieve success with the approach, they have attacked the premises upon which it is based. This is more of a commentary on the tremendous expenditure of time and effort necessary to achieve success than it is on either the abilities of the health professionals and patients involved or on the system itself. Yet, over the past decade, the growth of such techniques as patient self-monitoring of blood glucose (SMBG); the use of multiple component insulin regimens; and a growing appreciation of the relationship between hyperglycemia and the frequency, severity, and progression of the microvascular and neurological complications of diabetes have all led to increased use of management programs aimed at normal physiology - a target of near normalization of glycemia and of glycosylated hemoglobin as an index of overall glucose control. With the awareness that meticulous glucose control could be attained in at least some of their patients with appropriate motivation, patient education, and effort expended, many experts and physicians have found renewed interest in the Jackson/Guthrie approach and vindication of this effort. This has led many practitioners and experts to ask Bob Jackson and Dick Guthrie to enunciate the details of their management scheme. To that end, they consented and have written this book. It is now incumbent upon us as diabetologists and practitioners to critically evaluate the details of the management scheme, and in our daily practices apply those that prove worthwhile to our patients.

It seems to me worthwhile to place this work and its authors in an historical perspective. The history of pediatric diabetology in the United States warrants examination in this context. Prior to the isolation of insulin in the early 1920s, patients with childhood diabetes traversed a relentlessly progressive course to starvation, wasting, and death from ketoacidosis. Insulin offered the opportunity for life. As it would turn out, however, insulin would also offer the opportunity for individuals to live long enough to suffer the devastating chronic complications of diabetes, including retinopathy and blindness, nephropathy and kidney failure, neuropathy, and accelerated atherosclerosis. When first made available, insulin usage was principally by prevailing diabetes experts who were grounded in adult rather than childhood medicine. Indeed, many of the most noted authorities on childhood diabetes throughout this century have been and continue to be physicians principally trained in adult rather than childhood medicine, but who have become experts on childhood diabetes. The reasons for this are several. Perhaps the most important is that pediatric diabetology had trouble finding a niche in conventional pediatric circles. The father of pediatric endocrinology, Dr. Lawson Wilkins of Johns Hopkins Medical School and the Harriet Lane Home, declared that diabetes was not an endocrine disease. This led to the rejection of diabetes by him and most of the individuals whom he trained and who remain the leaders of pediatric endocrinology even today. In fact, those pediatric endocrinologists trained by Lawson Wilkins who had an affinity for diabetes were long considered "black sheep" of the Wilkins family. Yet, these individuals have evolved into some of the most noted leaders in diabetes in this country.

Overtly rejected by the endocrinologists, diabetes was forced to take root in other arenas. Like any refugee, diabetes found itself winding up in what today might seem to be apparently strange places. Because glycosuria and polyuria were predominant symptoms, in some institutions the nephrologists became the diabetes experts and managed this disease. Even today, there is a lineage of pediatric diabetes which traces itself to the heritage of nephrology and a number of medical schools have divisions of "pediatric nephrology and diabetology." In other institutions, the diabetes was managed by the experts in genetic and metabolic diseases. Indeed, diabetes is both a disease with genetic predisposition and certainly a disorderea metabolism. But it is not generally considered one of the "classical" inborn errors of metabolism in the sense of Archibald Garrod. In still other institutions, pediatric nutritionists assumed the role of diabetes expert, based on the need for dietary management as a cornerstone of diabetes therapy. It was from a tradition of nutrition, at the renowned University of Iowa Nutritional Center, that Bob Jackson evolved as a diabetologist. He was motivated by a desire to emulate normal pediatric nutrition, growth, and development in the management of childhood diabetes.

Another problem that has plagued childhood diabetes is the pattern of health care delivery in the United States. Since diabetes is the second most common chronic disease of childhood (second only to asthma), many primary care pediatricians desire to provide continuing care for their patients. Given (1) the fact that, until recently, most diabetes experts had populated only medical schools, and (2) the difficulty in identifying who were the diabetes experts in many of those medical schools (vita supra), it is not surprising that the management of childhood diabetes often remains in the purview of the primary care pediatrician. It is my contention that the primary care pediatrician generally is unable to provide optimal diabetes management. This is generally no fault of the primary care giver, but rather a commentary on the intensive team effort required for optimal diabetes management. There are simply too few patients with diabetes in the average primary care practice to warrant the creation of a diabetes team (nurse educator, dietitian, psychological social worker, youth counselor), or to warrant the practitioner him- or herself taking the requisite time from an otherwise busy practice to become an expert in contemporary diabetes management. Moreover, the practitioner is lulled into a false sense of security based on the fact that it is relatively easy to keep the patient out of ketoacidosis, attending school, and feeling generally well. Because the chronic complications of diabetes enumerated above do not make their appearance until after 15 or 20 years duration of the disease, the patients by then are no longer cared for by the pediatrician, who thus has no direct appreciation of the impact of his or her efforts. Moreover, most doctors are reluctant to "inflict pain" on their patients by prescribing more than one injection, or "inflict psychological harm" on their patients by prescribing a detailed nutritional plan. Yet, this is a deception. Children with diabetes can have a *more flexible life style* - more akin to their contemporaries - without sabotaging their diabetes management, by taking insulin in a physiologic distribution and by paying careful attention to nutritional planning.

In this volume, Robert Jackson and Richard Guthrie outline an approach to childhood diabetes that has proved successful in their hands and those of others. It is an approach worthy of careful examination and scrutiny by anyone interested in childhood diabetes.

Jay S. Skyler, M.D.

Acknowledgments

The treatment described in this book gradually evolved over the past half century. The authors are indebted to countless former associates who participated in successive modifications as our basic and applied knowledge increased, and as technical advances became available. With the kind permission of *Upjohn Co.,* the book incorporates some material published previously in *Current Concepts,* 1975. Wayne V. Moore, M.D., Ph.D., Director of Pediatric Endocrinology (KUMC) and M. Teresa Garcia-Otero Clabots, M.D., Assistant Professor of Pediatric Endocrinology (KUMC) contributed Section B, Chapter 6 (Pathology and Management of Ketoacidosis); Libbie J. Russo, M.D., Assistant Professor, Pediatric Endocrinology (KUMC) contributed to Section F, Chapter 6 (Diabetes and Exercise) and also helped with editing other chapters; Debbie Olson, R.D. (KUMC) participated in writing Section E, Chapter 6 (Nutritional Management); Diana Guthrie, R.N., M.S.P.H., Ph.D. (KUMC - Wichita) participated in writing Section A, Chapter 9 (Psychosocial Problems); Martha U. Barnard, R.N., Ph.D. (KUMC) participated in writing Section B, Chapter 9 (Compliance); Rachel G. Jorgensen, R.N., M.N. (KUMC) contributed to the writing of Chapter 12 (Recent Advances in Diabetic Therapy).

In addition, the authors wish to thank Dr. Jay Skyler for encouraging them to undertake this project, for writing the Foreword and for sharing with us his hopes for the future. Credit also must be given to the parents of children with diabetes for many practical innovations to simplify home care, and also to Jim Fisher, Deborah Cone, and Beth Hall for their secretarial assistance in preparing the manuscript.

notice

The authors and the publisher of this book have made every effort to ensure that all therapeutic modalities that are recommended are in accordance with accepted standards at the time of publication.

The drugs specified within this book may not have specific approval by the Food and Drug Administration in regard to the indications and dosages that are recommended by the authors. The manufacturer's package insert is the best source of current prescribing information.

Chapter 1

INTRODUCTION

Robert L. Jackson, M.D.

It has become increasingly evident that diabetes mellitus comprises a diverse spectrum of conditions which cause hyperglycemia. Diabetes, like other descriptive words such as anemia or arthritis, simply denotes a clinical syndrome. In recent years, this syndrome has been divided into two major forms based on insulin production ability and peripheral insulin sensitivity. It is now well recognized that diabetes in children and young adults is very different from diabetes in middle-aged or elderly patients and requires special consideration. The majority of children and young adults are undernourished when insulin-dependent (type I) diabetes is first discovered, and the onset of symptoms and signs is relatively sudden. By contrast, most older patients with insulin-resistant (type II) diabetes are obese, and the onset of the disease is insidious.

Diabetes in children is more severe than it is in adults, and nutritional requirements are relatively greater and constantly changing. Infections are more prevalent and severe, especially during the preschool years, as children are exposed to infections more frequently and are immunologically less mature. Exercise is more erratic and the emotional pattern is less predictable, especially during adolescence.

The term insulin-deficient or insulin-dependent (type I) is now applied to the juvenile type of diabetes because endogenous insulin is decreased or absent. Insulin-dependent diabetes also is referred to as growth-onset diabetes because the onset of symptoms and signs frequently occurs during the prepubertal growth spurt. Children with type I diabetes continue to be insulin-dependent during adult life, but the insulin and food requirements become less variable after growth is completed.

Most physicians recognize the necessity of knowing how to treat the life-threatening complications of diabetes. Nonetheless, the difficulties encountered in the long-term management of diabetes in the child and adolescent are so numerous that too often the disease is treated inadequately. *It is dangerously easy for doctors to undertake the management of a child with diabetes in such a way as to satisfy the parents and the child.* However, it is of vital importance for the child with diabetes to have expert care. As soon as possible after the diagnosis is confirmed and emergency treatment of ketoacidosis makes it safe, the child should be transferred to a diabetic center for specialized care.

Early physiologic insulin replacement is needed to restore health, permit normal growth and maturation, and hopefully prevent the development of both short- and long-term complications. The center should have the personnel and pediatric facilities necessary to provide optimal medical care of the child and also to provide emotional support and education of the family. The health team should include a pediatrician, nurse, dietitian, and social worker with special training and experience in evaluating families and in managing children with diabetes. An educational program and recreational outlets should be available in the pediatric division, so the child may continue with school and have daily, closely supervised physical activity during metabolic recovery. These facilities are necessary not only for the overall well-being of the child but also to make it possible for the physician to regulate the rapidly decreasing insulin requirement during the period of metabolic recovery.

Advances in nutritional knowledge, refinements in the treatment of acute complications such as acidosis and coma, introduction of refined and prolonged-acting insulin preparations, and the discovery of antibacterial agents with which to combat intercurrent infections have made it possible to attain and maintain a high degree of control of the disease. The task is not easy. It requires understanding, judgment, self-discipline, and acceptance of the concept of maintaining optimum health. The health status and life expectancy of the child with diabetes mellitus are thereby greatly increased.

In the past, to decrease the likelihood of insulin reactions and to simplify the management of children with diabetes, most physicians elected to encourage good nutritional habits and to give as few injections of insulin as possible to control the symptoms and signs of the disease. No attempt was made to completely control glycosuria even during the remission period. However, in recent years an ever-increasing number of young adults with onset of diabetes in childhood are being recognized to have microvascular complications. The insidious development of these serious complications in early adult life indicates to us that, too often, the disease is managed inadequately. Additional well-controlled studies are needed to further elucidate the interrelationship of the degree of metabolic control to the development of these serious vascular changes. Many internists and ophthalmologists who care for these young adults have become convinced that a higher degree of control is desirable in an attempt to delay or prevent the vascular changes. On the other hand, some pediatricians and family physicians remain skeptical. In children, overt vascular changes develop slowly over many years and are not detectable clinically until early or midadult life.

In our opinion, most children with diabetes receive delayed and inadequate treatment at the time of onset of symptoms. Too often children are managed as if they were small adults. If the diagnosis is made before the onset of ketoacidosis, precious time often is lost by observing the response of the children to nothing more than a modified dietary plan. After a few days when the dietary management is found ineffective, some of the children are then submitted to an ineffective therapeutic trial with an oral hypoglycemic agent. Many studies indicate that oral hypoglycemic agents such as sulfonylureas are not effective for the treatment of children with diabetes. In these cases, insulin therapy may not be begun until all forms of treatment are found to be ineffective. At that time, once-daily doses of an intermediate-type insulin usually have been prescribed. Because most diabetic children continue to produce varying amounts of endogenous insulin during the early weeks or even months after onset of the disease, they usually will have a good response to an improved dietary program and once-daily injections of an intermediate-type insulin. Nevertheless, we have found that to approximate physiologic control (essentially normal diurnal blood glucose levels) children need carefully structured food intake and at least twice-daily injections of insulin. Our experience also indicates that the insulin deficiency in children who receive delayed or suboptimal treatment quite rapidly progresses and usually is complete within a few months. Typically, the once-daily morning dose of insulin is gradually increased in an attempt to control the recurrence of nocturia and the increasing glycosuria in the prebreakfast urine specimens. The result is that the children, from overinsulinization during the day, begin to experience hypoglycemic episodes of varying intensities, usually during the late morning or early afternoon. They then are considered to have so-called brittle diabetes, sometimes with the added possibility of a convulsive disorder. It is not until this time, when the condition has deteriorated to total diabetes, that many children are first referred for specialized care.

We recommend that *every child with diabetes receive physiologic insulin replacement as soon as the diagnosis is confirmed.* In our experience, the exogenous insulin requirement varies, depending upon how early the diagnosis is made and how soon and how physiologically the insulin is given. The earlier the diagnosis is made, the lower the amount of insulin required and the easier it will be to attain and maintain a high degree of control with decreased risk of hypoglycemia. The optimal management of this early phase of diabetes is discussed in detail in Chapter 6.

In addition to expert medical care, the parents and children need to receive intensive education over a period of weeks from a health team consisting of a physician, nurse, and dietitian who have time and are experienced in teaching home management of children with diabetes. Detailed social information also needs to be obtained by an experienced social worker to evaluate the family and community resources and also to provide emotional support for the parents. We wish to stress that the combined efforts of an experienced health team are necessary to prepare the family to continue the regimen after they return home. If the children are to make good adjustments, not only the family but also the community need to be educated through whatever local resources are available or can be developed.

It is imperative that the parents and children understand clearly the plan of treatment, including the need for insulin, as soon as possible and that they face the reality of the situation. Responsibility for management rests with the parents; the physician should instruct and help qualify them. As soon as the children are old enough, they should be similarly trained. The parents need to know about the nature of the disease, the theory of management, and the recognition and treatment of complications. During the early months after onset, the parents should receive as much information as they can understand and as the health care team can impart.

It is necessary and important to instruct both parents and have each participate in the care of the child. Although the children should gradually assume more responsibility for their own care, it is undesirable and unrealistic to expect children, even adolescents, to assume primary responsibility for their own care. The psychosocial and educational aspects of diabetic management will be further delineated in Chapters 7 and 9.

This book is designed to impart to physicians, medical students, and other health care professionals the benefit of over 50 years of accumulated experience in managing children with diabetes mellitus. The children and their parents have been our best teachers. We hope, that by recording what we have gradually learned by close observation of the children and by teaching the parents how to apply new scientific information, we may improve the quality of life and longevity of children who have or may acquire diabetes. The book is not intended to be an in-depth scientific treatise on diabetes or an attempt to make diabetologists of pediatricians and family physicians but to assist in their role of providing optimal management of children under their care.

Chapter 2

HISTORICAL BACKGROUND

Robert L. Jackson, M.D.

Before the discovery of insulin in 1922, children with diabetes became severely undernourished and were doomed to a brief and miserable existence. Restricted intake of calories, especially carbohydrate foods, and moderate increased physical activity offered the only known means of therapeutic control, which merely postponed a fatal attack of acidosis. During the first years after insulin became available, when a restricted diet and one or two doses of regular insulin were given, children were spared an early death but diabetic dwarfism became a common problem.

In 1934, the senior author began his postgraduate training in the Pediatric Department at the State University of Iowa. At that time, Drs. P. C. Jeans and G. Stearns were doing metabolic studies designed to determine the nutritional requirements of infants and children during growth and maturation. The inadequacy of the restricted diets being advocated for children with diabetes was obvious. Consequently, a prospective study of children with diabetes was undertaken with J. D. Boyd to determine if providing optimal nutritional management as well as maintaining a high degree of metabolic control would alter the clinical course of the disease. The clinical and research facilities of the State University of Iowa Hospital provided an unusual opportunity to study and observe the clinical course of chronic disorders such as diabetes. Without added expense to the family, members of the faculty were able to admit and retain patients in the university hospital for research studies. A statewide ambulance service also made it possible to have the patients returned to the hospital for reappraisal or for readmission as often as the staff desired or as their condition required. In the state of Iowa, we also arranged for diabetic children to be eligible for assistance through the State Crippled Children's Division. The program was directed toward case finding, provision of suitable medical and hospital care, correction of related disturbances of health, arrangement for suitable follow-up services, and interpretation of the problems involved to the individuals and agencies concerned with the child's welfare. This service was administered through the Pediatric Department of the College of Medicine. Assistance for children with diabetes mellitus in accordance with their individual needs was coordinated through the local physician. Upon request from any physician, a field worker (nurse or medical social worker from our diabetic clinic) called at the doctor's office for advice and information. The child's medical condition was then interpreted by our field workers to teachers and other members of the family and community.

In 1940, under the title, *Stabilization of the Diabetic Child,* we published our observations relative to the uniformity of the clinical response of children with recent onset of diabetes to physiologic insulin replacement during metabolic recovery. The children were given three equal caloric meals designed to provide all known essential nutrients with adequate calories to correct their undernutrition. Regular insulin (the only form of insulin then available) was given 30 min before each meal. However, to control nocturnal glycosuria and attain essentially normal diurnal blood glucose levels, we found it necessary to give an additional small dose of insulin during the night. As a definitive objective for metabolic control, we determined the range of diurnal fluctuations of blood glucose levels in normal children receiving comparable food intake and physical activity as designed for the children with diabetes.

By close observation of the children in the hospital, we gradually learned that, in addition to giving accurate doses of insulin and close supervision and timing of the meals, it also was necessary to provide emotional support for the parents and the child, as well as to maintain a relatively constant physical activity pattern for the child throughout each day.

In children with recent onset of diabetes we also gradually learned by trial and error that after the first few days of rapid clinical improvement when the insulin and nutritional requirements are high and rapidly changing, it was possible to avoid hypoglycemia, control glycosuria, and maintain essentially normal diurnal blood glucose levels if we reduced daily each of the four daily doses of insulin (by about 7%) or increased the caloric intake of each meal (by about 10%) for a period of 2-3 weeks. During this time, the child rapidly regained expected weight for actual height. After this time of rapid nutritional repletion and improved physical fitness, which we called the period of metabolic recovery, the daily insulin requirement remained relatively constant and usually varied from 0.2 to 0.4 U/kg/day. The average percentage of insulin required for utilization of three equal caloric meals was 35% 30 min before breakfast at about 7:00 a.m., 22% 30 min before lunch at about 12:00 noon, 28% 30 min before the evening meal at about 5:30 p.m. and 15% at about 1:00 a.m.

Repeated attempts to further reduce or to discontinue insulin replacement while receiving an optimal nutritional intake always resulted in hyperglycemia and prompt recurrence of glycosuria, except in a few postpubescent girls who remained aglycosuric for varying periods of time but eventually became insulin-dependent. However, we did observe that if the children with recent onset of diabetes continued to receive four small doses of insulin daily and a structured meal plan, it was possible to maintain complete control of glycosuria and that the relatively low insulin requirement (< 0.5 U/kg/day) persisted for many months. We called this early period of partial remission the honeymoon period (see Chapter 5B).

In 1944, Brush reported a similar study (2). Early in the development of his regimen of management, insulin reactions were considered as favorable indications of improvement. Later, as more predictable patterns of response emerged, efforts were directed toward avoiding hypoglycemic episodes. Brush summarized his findings as follows: "Children with diabetes mellitus who have not had previous treatment are capable of recovering an appreciable capacity to regulate the level of blood sugar regardless of the severity of the symptoms when treatment is commenced, provided the therapeutic regimen is directed toward the administration of insulin in such amounts as temporarily to relieve the islet apparatus of any contribution to the total insulin needed by the organism."

In the first issue of the Proceedings of the American Diabetes Association (1941) under the title, *Avoidance of Degenerative Lesions in Diabetes Mellitus* (3), we stated,

> "Maintenance of life is not sufficient in itself as a goal in the treatment of diabetes mellitus. Insulin has made it easy for the patient with diabetes to survive. Therapy with insulin has such a broad zone of safety that its use tends to encourage a policy of "laissez faire" on the part of the physician and of the patient. Degenerative changes frequently develop in adult diabetic patients who have been led to think that the management of their disease has been adequate. Because of this fact, confusion has arisen as to the essential cause of the sequelae of diabetes mellitus; are they inherent in the disease itself, or do they reflect inadequacies in the level of control maintained throughout short or long term intervals of the diabetic patient's life? To make an adequate appraisal of the part played by the disease itself as distinguished from conditions imposed by its non-control, it is necessary that test subjects live under a regimen which is as free from *unphysiologic* conditions as circumstances will permit. One must bear in mind that impaired handling of sugar in the diabetic subject leads to certain perversions of the composition of body fluids, only one of which is the elevation of the level of glucose in the blood and resultant glycosuria. *A physiologic level of control is one which would avoid any degree of hyper- or hypoglycemia or glycosuria, and which would conserve the sugar*

handling function in maximal degrees. Presumably if one could accomplish this, all conceivable disturbances of the body due to diabetes would be avoided. Through suitable nutritional guidance and the proper administration of insulin *one can work toward an approximation of that state.* Ideal control must be quantitatively as well as qualitatively adequate in all regards, if it is to serve its designed purpose. This implies not only that the food intake must be adapted to the control of the diabetic state, but also it must be fully adequate for optimum nutrition if a *physiologic* status is to be our goal. Further, the regimen of management must be dynamic; it must be subject to continued re-evaluation and adjustment, and must be projected into the patient's future life so that lapses in control will be avoided in so far as possible. When dealing with the child subject, the state of childhood must be met suitably through the course of management. To make all these things possible, one must have the continued and unremittent cooperation of the patient, members of his household, and those in his community who in any way are concerned with his pattern of life. Adequate physical and financial facilities must be assured for the maintenance of the prescribed regimen. No one cognizant of the problems of diabetic care will question the desirability of any of the requisites specified, yet all will realize the unlikelihood that they will be met or even approached by the great majority of patients. Even under the best of auspices, diabetic control will fall considerably short of that outlined, and of that which the physician would recommend. In the patients under the most exacting regimen, intervals of excellent control frequently will be interspersed with others characterized by inadequacy. For long intervals patients may seem none the worse for poor control. Even though they may not appear to suffer from the compromised level of management which they have adopted, this does not justify anyone to conclude that they are not being affected adversely by the inadequacies of that compromise as compared with a more *physiologic level of control.* The effects of poor control of diabetes are cumulative, and terminate in serious complications or sequelae which lead to impaired function or to death. In studying the factors which lead to the development of degenerative changes in the diabetic patient, there are outstanding advantages in using the child with diabetes as a test subject. Conclusions derived from the child's condition should be applicable to the adult, because the pattern of the metabolic disturbance is not conditioned by the age of the subject. Moreover, confusion may be avoided in view of the fact that children do not exhibit degenerative changes which are commonplace during the period of postmaturity. Furthermore, the exaggerated response of the child's organism to abnormal metabolic conditions makes it easier to detect adverse states with him than with the adult subject. In the diabetic child we may be justified in concluding that abnormalities of function or of structure which arise must be related to his regimen of living, to his disease, or to the interplay between the two."

In 1938 under the title, *Dangers in the Use of Protamine Zinc Insulin* (4), we reported that the duration of action of protamine zinc insulin (PZI) exceeded 24 hr, which resulted in unpredictable cumulative action from day to day. In contrast to the infrequent and relatively mild insulin reactions observed in children receiving four injections of regular insulin, severe prolonged hypoglycemia was observed to develop insidiously in some children receiving PZI with or without injections of regular insulin. The hypoglycemic state in a few children was associated with unconsciousness and convulsions and required intravenous administration of glucose. Consequently, in order to use PZI and avoid serious insulin reactions, it would be necessary to sacrifice the level of metabolic control. We were unwilling to make this compromise and continued the regimen of four injections of regular insulin daily.

The relative amounts of carbohydrate and fat best suited for patients with diabetes had been of interest to many investigators and perplexed physicians for centuries prior to the availability of insulin. In 1942 (5), we did a study to determine if it was desirable or necessary to control the relative amounts of carbohydrate and fat in the meals of children with diabetes receiving physiologic insulin replacement. We found that the relative amount of fat and complex carbohydrate in the meals made no difference in the diurnal blood glucose level. We concluded that *in the treatment of the child with stabilized diabetes, emphasis should be directed toward having nutritionally complete food intake similar to the natural eating habits of the family and quantified primarily from the standpoint of calories.* If these criteria were satisfied, no special attention needed to be given to the fatty acid/dextrose contents of the meals. However, it was desirable to regulate the amount and rate of ingestion of simple sugars and fiber to avoid postprandial hyperglycemia. For example, eating an orange was preferable to drinking orange juice.

The early clinical reports in the 1940s on globin insulin, which showed that the duration of its action was definitely less than 24 hr and that the major effect had subsided by 14–16 hr, suggested the possibility of using this type of insulin for the treatment of children with diabetes. We modified our regimen of therapy on the basis of a study we published in 1945 (6). During the control period the subjects received three equicaloric meals. As previously described, regular insulin was administered 30 min before each meal and once during the night (usually at 1:00 a.m.). The distribution of the day's dose among four injections approximated 35, 22, 28, and 15% respectively. During one experimental period the same quantity of regular insulin was given at the same time before the morning, noon, and evening meals and the remaining 15% of the day's requirement was given as globin insulin with zinc 30 min before the evening meal in place of the 1:00 a.m. dose of regular insulin. This plan proved unsatisfactory because hypoglycemia developed between 8:00 and 10:00 p.m., with a gradual rise in the level of blood sugar during the night, so that the level of the fasting blood sugar was high (150–180 mg%). The patients gradually lost their physiologic level of control, and the morning urine specimen began showing traces of sugar. The response was similar to that obtained when three doses of regular insulin were used. Consequently, in another experimental period the regimen was modified by administering, 30 min before the evening meal, an amount of globin insulin with zinc equal to the total amount of regular insulin given before the evening meal and during the night (43% of the total 24-hr requirement). This plan was fairly satisfactory and the patients remained under good control. However, the urine occasionally contained a trace of sugar after the evening meal, and the blood sugar values were low in the early morning. In the next experimental period, regular insulin was administered 30 min before the morning and noon meals; the evening and night doses of the previous regimen (43% of the total) were combined and given as globin insulin with zinc 1 hr before the evening meal. This modification corrected the slight hyperglycemia and mild glycosuria after the evening meal, but the blood sugar values became low between 8:00 and 10:00 p.m. In the last experimental period, the size of the evening meal was decreased slightly, and a small snack was given later, during the early part of the evening. A number of variations of snacks were tried, and it was found that the most satisfactory plan was to give half of the milk from the evening meal as a snack 3 hr after the evening meal. Using this plan, we were again able to attain normal diurnal blood glucose levels.

It is of special interest to note that most of the parents of the children under care in our clinic were somewhat hesitant about changing to the new regimen and eliminating the night dose of regular insulin because they were so secure in caring for their children. However, all of the parents of the children later reported that they considered it a definite help to be able to go to bed at night without the responsibility of awakening the child in the middle of the night for a small dose of insulin. Some of the parents also believed that their children rested better.

From the study we concluded that it is possible and practical to keep diabetic children aglycosuric, except for very occasional traces of sugar in the urine, and free from clinically significant insulin reactions. This level of control can be obtained by the administration of four doses of regular insulin or by two doses of regular insulin and one dose of globin insulin with zinc and a structured meal plan. The study also provided objective evidence that parents do not object to multiple daily insulin injections if it is for the improved health of their child.

Exercise was known to be an important factor in the treatment of diabetes long before the availability of insulin. After the discovery of insulin, exercise as a factor influencing metabolic control received little attention until recent years. However, in our clinic where the objective of treatment was to maintain physiologic control, the effects of variations in physical activity became very apparent. Consequently, in 1948 we studied the effect of physical activity on the blood glucose levels of hospitalized diabetic children in varying degrees of metabolic control (7). No significant alterations in blood glucose levels were revealed after short periods of moderately intensive physical activity in physically fit diabetic children in good metabolic control. However, diabetic children during metabolic recovery had relatively rapid lowering of their blood glucose levels after short periods of moderately intensive physical activity due to their depleted nutritional stores. The home records of the children under our care also confirmed our hospital experimental study that short periods of moderate exercise, such as gymnasium classes and farm or household chores, were well tolerated by well-nourished children in good metabolic control, whereas prolonged periods (1-2 hr) of very strenuous exercise, such as football, basketball, or vigorous swimming, required compensatory measures to avoid insulin reactions. Early in our experience we advised lowering the dose of insulin before periods of strenuous activity. This method gave the apparent advantage of lowering the insulin requirement, but it resulted in hungry children with loss of body weight. We rapidly learned that it was much more physiologic and acceptable to increase and decrease the amount and kinds of foods ingested to compensate for variation in physical activity. After recognizing the importance of physical activity as a factor in diabetic management, insulin reactions were very infrequently encountered and usually were mild and easily managed if they did occur. This phase of management is discussed in detail in Chapter 6F.

Because of the improved health of the children and acceptance of our treatment plan by most of the parents, we never felt justified in observing a control group of children with diabetes receiving conventional management designed to keep the children as asymptomatic as possible but permitting varying degrees of glycosuria to avoid insulin reactions. Children receiving physiologic management practically never required rehospitalization and were growing and maturing at a normal rate. We also observed and documented that the self-discipline upon which physiologic control depends actually served to make the children psychologically better adjusted. In 1977, the psychiatric status of 40 diabetic youths in good control and 40 diabetic youths in poor control under observation in our clinic was compared with the psychiatric status of a matched nondiabetic control group selected from a family practice clinic (8). The number of youths with psychiatric diagnoses, interpersonal conflicts, and noninterpersonal conflicts was determined from a semistructured psychiatric interview done by John F. Simonds, M.D., Associate Professor of Child Psychiatry. The good control diabetic group had significantly fewer youths with both types of conflicts when compared with the control group and the poor control diabetic group. However, psychiatric diagnoses were made with equal frequency in all three groups. Results of a parent questionnaire concerning a youth's behavior problems revealed significant differences only for two items, anxiety and depression, which were more frequent problems for diabetic youths in poor control. The good control diabetic group seemed to be in the best mental health, and their families were less prone to divorce. Youths in poor diabetic control were not very different psychologically from the nondiabetic control group except for the parents' report of more frequent anxiety and depression. It was speculated that these youths were more anxious because of the progression of the diabetic condition, which became less predictable as the control worsened. The percentage of psychiatric diagnoses in the investigator's groups was low in contrast to other studies reported in the literature.

Early in 1973, neutral regular insulin became available. The availability of neutral regular insulin made it possible to premix NPH (Neutral Protamine Hagedorn) and regular insulins. In more recent years, we have been using mixtures of NPH and regular insulin in the treatment of most younger children with diabetes. Our basic and most common regimen for school-age children consists of a mixture of two parts NPH and one part regular insulin. Two-thirds of the total daily insulin dosage usually is given 30 min before an early morning breakfast, and the remaining one-third of the same mixture is given about 30 min before a late afternoon or early evening meal, as described in detail in Chapter 6.

Recent advances in research are encouraging. We are learning much more about human genetics, as well as the various environmental factors that influence the course of diabetes. Until more knowledge about genetics and the pathophysiology of the disease is available, good control is the only known means of delaying or averting degenerative changes associated with unphysiologic control.

REFERENCES

1. Jackson, R. L., Boyd, J., and Smith, T. E.: Stabilization of the diabetic child. *Am. J. Dis. Child.* 59:332-341, 1940.

2. Brush, J. M.: Initial stabilization of the diabetic child. *Am. J. Dis. Child.* 67:429-442, 1944.

3. Boyd, J. D., Jackson, R. L., and Allen J. H.: Avoidance of degeneration lesions in diabetes mellitus. *Proc. Am. Diabetes Assoc.* 1:99-110, 1941.

4. Jackson, R. L., and Boyd, J. D.: Dangers in the use of protamine zinc insulin. *J. Iowa St. Med. Soc.* 1:3-7, 1938.

5. Jackson, R. L., and Kenefick, J.: Dietary rations for the child with diabetes mellitus. *Am. J. Dis. Child.* 64: 807, 1942.

6. Jackson, R. L., and McIntosh, C. B.: Treatment of the diabetic child with reference to the use of globin insulin. *Am. J. Dis. Child.* 70:307-313, 1945.

7. Jackson, R. L., and Kelly, H. G.: A study of physical activity in juvenile diabetic patients. *J. Ped.* 33:155, 1948.

8. Simonds, J. F.: Psychiatric status of diabetes youth matched with a control group. *Diabetes* 26:921-925, 1977.

Chapter 3

PREVALENCE, ETIOLOGY, AND GENETICS OF DIABETES MELLITUS

Richard A. Guthrie, M.D.

INTRODUCTION

It is becoming increasingly evident through new research data that diabetes mellitus is not a disease but a syndrome. It is a variety of diseases of diverse etiology which happen to affect the same organ, namely the islet cells of the endocrine pancreas. Perhaps this should not be too surprising, since the same is true of many other organs. End-stage kidney, liver, or lung disease looks very much the same whatever the original assaulting force. So may the final common pathway be similar regardless of the original insult to the pancreas.

Thus, we can now separate diabetes mellitus into three broad categories: 1) type I or insulin-dependent diabetes mellitus (IDDM), 2) type II or noninsulin-dependent diabetes mellitus (NIDDM), and 3) other -- a broad category including mechanical problems such as primary pancreatic destruction (pancreatitis, pancreatectomy), hormonal problems (acromegaly, Cushing's disease, etc.), and a variety of unrelated, usually genetic syndromes that may include diabetes mellitus as part of a consequence of the syndrome (acanthosis nigricans, congenital lipodystrophy, Prader-Willi syndrome, progeria, etc.). These individuals may be insulin-dependent or noninsulin-dependent (1).

Although children with type II and other types of diabetes mellitus have been described and may be more common than previously thought, most children with diabetes mellitus are type I IDDM. Consequently, this chapter, and indeed this book will deal predominately with this disease.

PREVALENCE OF DIABETES MELLITUS

Epidemiologic studies indicate that approximately 4-5% of the population of the United States and Canada have some form of diabetes mellitus. The reported prevalence is similar in Northern Europe. The prevalence is somewhat less in Southern Europe and in the less industrialized portions of the world. Eighty-five percent of persons with diabetes mellitus have type II diabetes mellitus. The prevalence of type I diabetes mellitus varies widely in the world, from rare in Asiatic populations to common in certain Northern European areas such as Finland. In the United States and Canada, type I diabetes mellitus constitutes about 15-20% of the population with diabetes. If the prevalence is 5% for diabetes mellitus in the American population of some 230 million people, then there are about 11.5 million people in the United States with diabetes (2). Using a figure of 15% of this population with type I diabetes mellitus, there would be 1,725,000 people with type I diabetes in the United States. This figure agrees reasonably well with drug companies' estimates that about 1.5 million people in the United States currently are taking insulin injections. Assuming some 5% of this population to be children, there would then be about 86,250 children in the United States with diabetes. This figure is in accordance with figures from the National Diabetes Commission of 1976 which estimated that there were about 80,000 children in the United States with diabetes mellitus taking insulin (2).

Surveys of United States schoolchildren indicate a prevalence of 1.6-1.89 per 1000 school-age (6-18 yr) children. The distribution by prevalence by age group is: 1 in 1429 children at age 5 to a peak of 1 in 358 at age 16 (3, 4).

The annual incidence (number of new cases per year) in children under the age of 17 has been estimated to be 0.3 per 1000 or roughly 20,000 new cases per year in the United States. More importantly, the incidence by some estimates may be rising by as much as 6% per year. By these figures, and given the extended life expectancy the numbers of persons with diabetes mellitus in the United States could double every 15 years. Sex prevalence is about equal and white children appear to be affected about two times the prevalence of blacks (2).

Since there is no United States national registry of diabetes, the accuracy of these figures cannot be checked. In a few places (Allegheny Co., Pa. and Alabama) where there are registries, the figures are being checked so that better data may be available in the future. In any event, diabetes mellitus is a common disease (the second most common chronic disease) in children (5) and is the most common of the endocrine-metabolic disorders in children. A national type I diabetes registry, such as that found in several European countries, would be helpful in determining by epidemiologic techniques, incidence, and prevalence of this disease and in studies of etiology, natural history, and outcome.

ETIOLOGY OF TYPE I IDDM

The complete cause of type I diabetes mellitus remains unknown. Modern research, however, is beginning to supply clues that at least allow us to formulate testable hypotheses. Unquestionably, type I diabetes mellitus in children is due to the destruction of B cells of the islets of Langerhans of the endocrine pancreas. Pathologic studies of limited amounts of pancreatic material from diabetic children dying in diabetic ketoacidosis (DKA) or in accidents soon after the onset of diabetes mellitus have indicated that the islets of Langerhans are infiltrated with round cells (6). Newer staining techniques with old and new tissue confirm that these round cells are lymphocytes (7, 8). These observations suggest, then, that there is an inflammatory reaction in the islets and that the inflammation is either secondary to agents which are destroying B cells or is primary, i.e., an autoimmune process in the pancreas. A combination of both factors may be the case. Extensive studies indicate that diabetes mellitus may be caused by direct destruction of B cells by invading agents (most probably viruses, but perhaps also environmental chemicals) (9). Other studies suggest that offending or invading agents may trigger an autoimmune reaction in a genetically susceptible host (10). Whatever the cause, the result is the same — B-cell destruction and ultimate loss of insulin-secreting ability by the endocrine pancreas.

INFECTION AND TYPE I DIABETES MELLITUS

The role of infectious agents in the pathogenesis of diabetes mellitus is not clear and has been the subject of considerable investigation. Many studies suggest a temporal relationship between certain viral infections and the onset of overt diabetes (11-18). Recently, Gamble et al. (19) used serologic techniques to study the interrelationship between newly diagnosed diabetes and a variety of viral infections. Only neutralizing antibody to coxsackie B, especially type 4, appeared more often and in higher titer in diabetic patients than in control subjects.

In 1979 Yoon and his colleagues (20) reported the isolation of coxsackie B_4 virus from the pancreas of a child dying from meningoencephalitis and sudden-onset diabetes. The pancreas of this child exhibited an inflammatory reaction termed insulitis. The coxsackie B_4 virus, which was subsequently isolated, induced insulitis and diabetes in experimentally infected animals.

In infants who were overwhelmingly infected with coxsackie B_4 virus in the neonatal period, insular lesions of the pancreas resembling those shown by Yoon and in experimentally infected animals have been demonstrated. Islets from those infants who died before demonstrating clinical evidence of diabetes showed a mononuclear cell, inflammatory exudate around the islets (21). Similarly, patients with malignant disease who are infected with cytomegalovirus have shown intranuclear inclusions of cytomegalovirus and an inflammatory reaction in the islets of the pancreas (22).

The seasonal incidence of diabetes in children, with a peak in late summer (when school reconvenes) and in midwinter (during the peak of the virus season), suggests a relationship to infectious agents. It is noteworthy that this seasonal variation is seen (with the peak incidence being in winter) in Australia, where the seasons are reversed (23).

The development of diabetes after mumps virus infections is the most obvious viral relationship to diabetes, since mumps virus is known to produce pancreatitis even when it does not produce diabetes. There are numerous anecdotal reports of diabetes after mumps and mumps pancreatitis (12-16). In one family, diabetes developed in two siblings in less than a month after mumps struck the household (24). It is important to point out, however, that the mumps-diabetes relationship is based upon circumstantial-temporal relationships not upon pathologic information. Indeed, the temporal relation to mumps virus or any infecting agent may be that of years, not days, weeks, or months as reported by Sultz (25). In this report, diabetes followed mumps epidemics in New York by several years. Since mumps is known to cause pancreatitis, one would expect insular damage, along with exocrine tissue damage, and diabetes would be the result. The limited autopsy data on the very few children who died early in the course of mumps, however, have *not* documented the insular lesions (26). The evidence for mumps virus as an etiologic agent in diabetes, therefore, remains highly circumstantial.

A number of authors have independently reported the occurrence of diabetes mellitus in infants with congenital rubella (27-31). It is not yet clear if the rubella virus exerts its influence by direct virus and cell interaction, leading to cell death and a mononuclear cell infiltration, or if it causes inhibition of cell replication (32, 33).

Australia and New Zealand sustained rubella epidemics in the early 1960s just before the vaccine became available. This epidemic spread to the United States in 1963. A number of babies with rubella syndrome were born during these years. This author is currently caring for five girls born in 1963-64 with congenital rubella syndrome who also have diabetes mellitus. The diabetes developed when the girls were between 2 and 6 years of age. In Australia, Forrest et al. (30) conducted a systematic follow-up of children with rubella syndrome and found that 20% had abnormal carbohydrate tolerance or frank diabetes. This very high frequency of diabetes was not demonstrated, however, in a study reported from England, although the prevalence of diabetes was increased (34). Persistent rubella virus infection of various tissues, including the pancreas (35, 36), and pancreatitis (31) in infants with congenital rubella have been demonstrated. As in mumps, insular lesions have not been demonstrated in infants dying of congenital rubella syndrome (37). One American study on the follow-up of the 1963-64 epidemic has been recently published (38). In this study, 173 patients with congenital rubella were studied. Twenty-one had diabetes. The HLA (human lymphocyte antigen) were studied. There was an increase in DR3 and a decrease in DR2 in children with rubella syndrome and diabetes but not in children with rubella syndrome without diabetes, indicating that although rubella may have been the trigger for the B-cell destruction, the genes that control susceptibility to diabetes mellitus type I must also be present.

Parenthetically, it must be added that there has been no demonstrated increase in diabetes following the use of either rubella or mumps vaccine, even though this has been studied. There is no reason, therefore, to withhold vaccination to these diseases even in high-risk families.

Results of experiments with animals provide the best evidence for virus-induced diabetes. Burch and others (39) have shown that experimental coxsackie B_4 infection of mice causes damage not only to the exocrine tissue of the pancreas but also to the islet cells. Craighead and coworkers (40-42) noted that a syndrome similar to diabetes resulted in more than 46% of mice that survived induced infection with the M-variant of encephalomyocarditis virus.

In experimental animals, the insular lesions needed to prove a causal relationship of diabetes to the virus can be demonstrated (26). Many viruses have been demonstrated to cause diabetes in various species. It must be pointed out, however, that these viruses are usually species specific. A given virus may cause diabetes in one or several species of animals but not in others. Some are highly specific and some are not. Since many of these viruses are species specific, their studies may not be applicable to man.

Undoubtedly, genetic factors are important in species specificity to viral insulitis, but how the genetic factors control the infection is not known. Yoon and Natkins (43) have suggested that the presence of genetically determined viral receptors on the B-cell surface may determine the susceptibility or resistance of a given species or even a given animal to a certain virus. Craighead (26) believes this explanation to be too simple. He has found a difference in viral inhibitory property of interferon between viral-susceptible and resistant cells (44). In any event, in animals at least, the susceptibility to viruses seems to be mediated by a single recessive gene *not* associated with the major histocompatibility complex (45).

Whatever the mechanism, it is becoming increasingly clear that infectious agents play some role in the cause of diabetes mellitus and as a precipitating factor for symptomatic diabetes and DKA in children. At diagnosis, children with diabetes mellitus almost always have evidence of infection and, indeed in those rare children who die in DKA, infection is still the cause of death in nearly one-third. This infection is, however, a precipitating factor, not an etiologic infection. A source of infection then, must be searched for in all children at the time of diagnosis of the acute diabetic state and treated appropriately.

In the meantime, research continues on the role of viruses in the etiology of diabetes mellitus in children, since this offers us a possible avenue for prevention. If viruses can be proved to be a major etiologic factor, and the viruses identified, vaccines for genetically susceptible individuals may eventually be possible. If immunization is not possible, interferon or antiviral drugs of the future may preserve beta cell function with prompt diagnosis of the disease and intensive therapy.

AUTOIMMUNITY IN DIABETES MELLITUS

Grodsky et al. demonstrated that exogenous bovine insulin could induce an immune response in the normal rabbit (46-49). The bovine insulin produced high titers of anti-insulin antibodies that bound the rabbit's own insulin. Diabetes mellitus, associated with round-cell infiltration of the islets of Langerhans, was produced in the previously normal rabbits. These studies suggest that foreign antigens might induce antibodies that crossreact with a subject's own insulin or islet tissue to produce autoimmune diabetes mellitus. Other studies suggest an association between diabetes mellitus and several autoimmune disorders, including Hashimoto's thyroiditis, hypothyroidism, and idiopathic hypoadrenocorticism.

Newer studies have begun to shed new light on this issue. In 1971, Nerup et al. (50) reported finding antipancreatic activity in 12 of 22 diabetic patients studied. He used a leukocyte migration inhibition system measuring cell-mediated immunity. Subsequent studies showed the presence of this antibody in most young persons with diabetes near onset of the disease, with fading of the antibody with time. This phenomenon has been confirmed by others (51) and probably reflects destruction of the entire B-cell mass.

In 1974, Bottazzo et al. (51) reported finding a circulating antibody to islet cell tissue. This IgG antibody has been identified as a cytoplasmic antibody, is not specific for B cells, and can be identified by immunofluorescence using frozen sections of human pancreas. In a summary of three studies (52-54) by Nerup and Lernmark in 1981 (55), the prevalence of these antibodies was 0.6% in a control population, 4% in first-degree relatives of IDDM patients, 6% in NIDDM patients, 3% in people with autoimmune disease without diabetes, 27% in IDDM without autoimmune disease, and 34% in persons with IDDM and autoimmune disease. The antibodies fade with time to about 5% after 10 to 20 years. They are more likely to remain in persons who are HLA-B8 and DR3 positive.

Islet cell surface antibodies in the circulation may be better markers of autoimmunity than are cytoplasmic antibodies, since they are specific for living cells, while cytoplasmic antibodies may be the result of cell death and necrosis. Cytoplasmic antibodies, then, may reflect a reaction to cellular debris released after cellular destruction and may not be the antibody which destroys the cell. Surface antibodies are more likely to reflect true autoimmunity to the islet cell. Islet cell surface antibodies have been identified in the circulation of persons with IDDM by Lernmark (56). These antibodies were present in 67% of newly diagnosed diabetic children and 3% of controls. The antibodies are organ specific but not B-cell or species specific. Studies of these antibodies are as yet incomplete but may yield very valuable information in the future.

Finally, a clinical observation with practical application has been made. Several investigators, including Nerup (57, 58), Eisenbarth (59), and Fialkow (60) have observed an increased prevalence and incidence of autoimmune disease in organs other than the pancreas in children with diabetes and, conversely, a high prevalence of diabetes in children with other autoimmune diseases, especially diseases of the thyrogastric cluster (thyroid, stomach, adrenal, skin, and hair). Diabetes was present in 15% of children with autoimmune Addison's disease and 7-10% of children with thyroid autoimmune disease. This is a 50% higher than expected association. In children with diabetes, Hashimoto's autoimmune thyroiditis occurs in 15-20% of the cases and thyroid microsomal antibodies may be present in as high as 30-50%. A few children with diabetes may also develop Addison's disease which, if present with thyroiditis, constitutes the Schmidt-Carpenter syndrome (61). Children with diabetes may also have pernicious anemia with antibodies to gastric tissue, and vitiligo and/or alopecia with antibodies to pigment cells in skin and/or to hair follicles. The associations with diabetes and autoimmunity of the thyrogastric cluster of organs are associated with the HLA-B8 and DR3 antigen of the major histocompatibility complex.

The practical implication of these observations (the association of diabetes with autoimmunity in the other organs), of course, is to watch for disease of these other organs (especially thyroid and adrenal) in order to recognize and treat hypothyroidism appropriately and to treat Addison's disease before a life-threatening adrenal crisis develops. Treatment is by means of thyroid and adrenal hormone (including mineralocorticoid in many cases) replacement to prevent delay of growth and development and Addisonian crises.

Goiter is the most common presenting sign of thyroiditis and must be looked for continually in children with diabetes mellitus. It should be borne in mind that while chronic lymphocytic thyroiditis (Hashimoto's thyroiditis) is more common in girls than boys (9:1) in persons without diabetes, this distinction is lost in children with diabetes. Therefore, the disease must be looked for in boys as well as in girls.

Of what importance is the matter of autoimmunity in diabetes? At present autoimmunity is of research interest only since the antibodies so far identified have not been shown to be B-cell specific or even to be cytotoxic. Indeed, most of the antibodies so far demonstrated are probably the *result* of B-cell destruction and not the cause. New techniques for study of autoimmunity are being developed, however, which may demonstrate specific B-cell cytotoxic antibodies. Preliminary studies have been published and more may soon appear. If such antibodies can be discovered and can be shown to cause B-cell destruction, several practical therapeutic avenues may open up as follows: 1) antibodies may become a marker for diabetes mellitus in children long before B cells are destroyed, allowing time to intervene to preserve B-cell function; 2) immunosuppression may be able to preserve B-cell functions even in a newly diagnosed diabetic person by suppression of autoantibodies (studies of immunosuppression with cyclosporin A are now underway, with preliminary data encouraging); and 3) antiantibodies or antireceptor antibodies may be developed to block antibody destruction of B cells.

All of these techniques may be feasible in the next few years if definitive techniques become available that allow early detection of impending overt diabetes mellitus before B-cell destruction. The prevention or reduction of B-cell destruction or at least of complete loss of B-cell function would be highly desirable. Thus, diabetes may be prevented or its severity at least ameliorated by therapeutic intervention stemming from knowledge of autoimmunity.

GENETICS OF IDDM

The relationship of genetic factors to the development of diabetes (or to variations in metabolic processes that may contribute to the development of vascular complications of diabetes) is poorly understood. The interaction between genetic control mechanisms and dietary and other environmental factors needs to be explored in much greater depth.

Diabetes mellitus has been the subject of many genetic studies (62, 63), but the mode of genetic transmission of the disease remains obscure. The carrier state can only be assumed rather than biochemically defined. In most epidemiologic studies in the past, carbohydrate intolerance was considered to be an expression of a single, uniform disease. That is, both the types I and II disease seen in middle-aged or older adults were usually considered to be manifestations of the same genetic abnormality. Since we now know this not to be true, most studies of the past are invalid.

Until recently, an autosomal-recessive pattern has been considered the mode of inheritance for diabetes. The concept was developed from a study of the parents and siblings of patients with type I diabetes (62). Most investigators now favor a multifactorial hypothesis, which states that the diabetic predisposition results from the interaction of a variable number of genetic alleles at different loci (64). As few as two pairs of genes with two abnormal loci could result in as many as nine possible diabetic genotypes with variable clinical expression. It is quite possible that several genetic factors are involved and that the relative importance of any one factor may vary from family to family. One method for obtaining information on possible gene action in multifactorial problems is to compare biochemical or physiologic data on individuals having a close familial relationship with the subject with diabetes (such as identical twins.)

The concept of genetic heterogeneity, i.e., that diabetes is not one but several diseases with many different causes, was first suggested by the following findings: 1) ethnic differences in prevalence and clinical features (type II diabetes is common while type I diabetes is rare in Orientals, for example); 2) the existence of rare genetic syndromes with associated diabetes; and 3) the presence of genetic heterogeneity in animal models.

Twin studies then established a clear difference between types I and II diabetes mellitus. In studies by Tattersall and Pyke (65, 66), identical twins were studied. If one twin developed type II diabetes mellitus, the second twin would also develop the disease 98% of the time and would do so usually within 5 years. This clearly established type II diabetes mellitus as an almost purely genetic disease. Type I diabetes mellitus, on the other hand, was clearly different. In this disease, when one twin developed the disease only 45-55% (mean 50%) of the second twins developed the disease. Furthermore, unless the second twin developed the disease soon after the first twin (within 5 years), there seemed to be no increase in concordance even after 10 years of follow-up.

Such studies would tend to indicate that while type II diabetes mellitus may be a genetic disease, type I diabetes mellitus must have an environmental factor interfacing with a genetic predisposition (50% concordance exceeds that expected in the general population or even in siblings). Current studies implicate viruses and/or the immune system in this interaction, but other factors such as environmental chemicals could still participate in triggering the process which leads to beta-cell destruction.

The fact that diabetes can be caused by a variety of genetic factors is illustrated by the nearly 50 diseases that may have diabetes in association with them. A complete list of these diseases can be found in an excellent article by Rotter and Rimoin (67). Three diseases (Down's syndrome, Klinefelter's syndrome, and Turner's syndrome) are mentioned here because all three of these conditions result from chromosomal abnormalities. The abnormalities in each of the three, however, are different. Children with Down's syndrome have an extra number 21 chromosome, males with Klinefelter's syndrome have an extra X chromosome, and females with Turner's syndrome have a deletion of an X chromosome. Persons with any of these syndromes have a prevalence of concurrent diabetes mellitus significantly higher than the general population even though the genetic abnormality is different. This suggests that there may be several chromosomal relationships to diabetes causing a variety of metabolic derangements and clinical presentations.

There are also familial but nonchromosomal syndromes with concurrent diabetes. Neuromuscular disorders, such as muscular dystrophies and Friedreich's ataxia, and progeroid syndromes, such as Cockayne's or Werner's syndrome, are examples. All these syndromes have different genetics and are thought to be determined by abnormal genes on a variety of chromosomes. The heterogeneity of these diseases associated with diabetes leads to a belief in the heterogeneity of the diabetes syndrome.

New light has recently been shed upon the genetics of the disease with the recent discovery of an association of diabetes mellitus with certain of the HLA tissue types within the major histocompatibility complex.

HLAs are proteins on cell surfaces which are genetically determined by associated genes carried on the short arm of the number 6 chromosome. Four areas or loci have been identified on this chromosome and have been designated A, B, C, and D. Each locus carries a number of genes which have been cataloged and numbered. Since there may be many (65 or more) genes on each locus, the number of possible combinations of any or all genes in each individual is fairly large. Some genes present in one individual may not be present in others. The combination is determined by the parents' HLA types in the usual transmission of genetic material to offspring and is unique for each individual. The complete function of these genes is unknown, but they are thought to contribute to the function of the immune system.

They are at least involved in tissue compatibility and must be matched as closely as possible between individuals for transplant survival.

During the course of tissue typing for organ transplant, it was observed that certain tissue types (HLA types) were highly associated with certain diseases, especially diseases involving the immune system. The first such identification was an association of the HLA-B27 antigen with the disease ankylosing spondylitis. Soon distinct HLA types began to emerge in type I diabetes mellitus.

Two forms of type I diabetes mellitus have now been identified with a third type, also present as a combination or heterozygote of the first two. The first association between diabetes mellitus and HLA type was an association with HLA-B8. This gene now appears to be in disequilibrium linkage with the DW3 (also known as the DR3 or D-related gene depending upon the method of determining its presence). This disease (B8-DR3) is associated with an increased prevalence of pancreatic islet cell antibodies, antipancreatic cell-mediated immunity, and a decreased immune response to exogenous insulin (68). The B8-DR3 positive individuals have a 2.5 times greater prevalence and incidence of diabetes mellitus than the general population and have a high prevalence and incidence of other associated autoimmune diseases (thryoiditis, Addison's disease, etc.).

The second HLA association was described for B15, which is also in disequilibrium linkage to the CW3 and DW4 (DR4) loci. This form of the disease is less well characterized than the B8-DR3 form, but it is not associated with other autoimmune diseases or islet cell antibodies. It is accompanied by an increased antibody response to exogenous insulin. This form of the disease may have an earlier onset than B8-DR3 disease.

There also exists a third form of the disease, i.e., the B8-DR3/B15-DR4 heterozygote. This form of the disease is characterized by a marked increased risk of diabetes mellitus (15-17 times the general population) and an increased prevalence in families (increased prevalence for concordance in twins and an increased risk for developing the disease in siblings). This group may also develop their disease at an earlier age and sustain greater beta-cell damage from the assaulting force (68).

There appears to be no consensus on the mode of inheritance of diabetes mellitus in type I diabetes, and indeed, the inheritance may be different for the different genetic forms of the disease. Some type I diabetes mellitus may be inherited, then, as an autosomal-recessive trait and some by a dominant tract. Indeed, there is a form of type II diabetes mellitus seen occasionally in children (called maturity-onset diabetes of the young or MODY or Mason-type diabetes) that is clearly autosomal dominant in inheritance (66, 69, 70). For most children some form of recessive inheritance associated with environmental factors seems best to describe the inheritance type.

How does heredity play a part? As yet we cannot answer this question completely and intensive investigation continues. Clearly, type I diabetes is a genetic disease or at least some genetic defect is present. The genetic defect is thought to be in the immune system, probably linked to, if not determined by, the presence of the particular B and D locus or other genes. Viruses and perhaps other environmental factors, then, may interact with the defect in immunity triggering the beta-cell destruction. Such destruction may be directly by the virus (or chemical) or through the triggering of an autoimmune process. For the B8-DR3 individuals, autoimmunity seems to play an important role. But how is autoimmunity triggered and sustained? Some investigators have hypothesized that the defect is an inability to kill the virus or eliminate the chemical, allowing it to penetrate the beta cell and alter its proteins, which then triggers an autoimmune reaction to a now-foreign protein (71). Others have shown a defect in the lymphocyte system in which there is an overreaction of killer T cells either because they are overreactive (genetically determined) or because there is a deficiency in number or activity of the T-suppressor cells (55).

In those instances where autoimmunity does not seem to play a part (B15-DR4 individuals), other mechanisms must be in play. Some investigators (43) have suggested that these individuals may have a genetically determined excess of viral receptors on the cell surface. The virus has increased affinity to infect the cell, effecting its destruction. There are perhaps other as yet unsuggested and undiscovered mechanisms for the disease.

SUMMARY

Whatever the external or internal environmental triggers, type I diabetes mellitus is a genetically determined disease. It is probably inherited by autosomal-recessive mechanisms. Either a deficiency or surplus of a number of different genes may cause the disease by a variety of different genetic mechanisms. The majority of the genetic defects probably lead to an over- or underactive immune system interacting with a variety of environmental insults of which viruses may be the most important.

None of this information, of course, alters the management of the disease. However, it may be important in the future prevention or treatment of the disease in its early stages or before it develops.

More importantly, the information is needed for genetic counseling, an important aspect of total diabetes care. What do we tell parents of a diabetic child about the risk in other children? It has been our experience that this is often an urgent and burning question as soon as the shock of the initial diagnosis fades.

To answer this question, it is necessary to clearly establish the type of disease the child has, since types I and II and the rare genetic syndromes have their own inheritance patterns and frequency and must be taken into account during counseling for this disorder.

In general, when a child has type I diabetes mellitus, the increased incidence and prevalence of diabetes mellitus in the family will be for that disease. This is true also for type II disease, although the data are not so solid and some crossover between types I and II diabetes is seen in certain families (67).

For type I disease, the average risk to the siblings is 5-10%. If a parent has type I disease, the risk is 1-2% for the children. For type II disease, the sibling risk is 5-10% for clinical disease and 15-25% for abnormal carbohydrate tolerance (67). For those with abnormal carbohydrate tolerance, the risk of clinical disease is on the order of 5% per year (1). These are relatively low risks (the risk in the general population is 4-5%) so that parental fears can be allayed and parents encouraged to have further children if they so desire.

It might be remembered that our present state of knowledge is very limited and that new tools such as islet cell antibodies, HLA typing, or other as yet undiscovered genetic markers may change our present impressions. Such tools, which are now research tools only, may soon become clinically useful markers of disease and allow us both to study the natural history of the disease more scientifically and to be able to detect the susceptible persons before clinical disease appears. Thus, the future holds the possibility of: 1) better knowledge of the epidemiology and etiology of the disease, 2) better genetic counseling, and 3) the marking of genetically susceptible individuals for interventions aimed at prevention of the disease. The future looks bright for such intervention.

REFERENCES

1. National Diabetes Data Group: Classification and diagnosis of diabetes mellitus and other categories of glucose intolerance. *Diabetes* 28:1039-1057, 1979.

2. Crofford, O., et al.: Report of the National Commission on Diabetes. *U.S. Government DHEW Publication (NIH),* 1976.

3. Gorwitz, K., Thompson, T., and Howen, G. C.: The prevalence of diabetes in school-age children. *Diabetes* 25: 122-127, 1976.

4. Kyllo, C., and Nuttall, F. Q.: Prevalence of diabetes mellitus in school-age children in Minnesota. *Diabetes* 27:57-60, 1978.

5. Dorman, J. S., LaPorte, R. E., et al: The Pittsburg insulin-dependent diabetes mellitus (IDDM) morbidity and mortality study: Mortality results. *Diabetes* 33:271, 1984.

6. VonMeyenburg, H.: Uber insuliti's bei diabetes. *Schweiz. Med. Wochenschr* 21:554-561, 1940.

7. LeCompte, P. M.: "Insulitis" in early juvenile diabetes. *Arch. Pathol.* 66:540-547, 1958.

8. Gepts, W.: Pathological anatomy of the pancreas in juvenile diabetes mellitus. *Diabetes* 14:619-633, 1965.

9. Craighead, V. E.: Viral diabetes. In: Volk, V. W., and Wellman, K. F. (Eds.), *The Diabetic Pancreas,* Plenum Press, New York, 1977, pp. 467-488.

10. MacCuish, A. C., and Irvine, W. J.: Autoimmunological aspects of diabetes mellitus. *Clin. Endocrinol. Metab.* 4:435-71, 1975.

11. Harris, H.: Familial distribution of diabetes mellitus: Study of relatives of 1241 diabetic propositi. *Ann. Eugenics* 15:95, 1950.

12. Harris, H. F.: A case of diabetes mellitus quickly following mumps. *Boston Med. Surg. J.* 140:465, 1899.

13. Patrick, A.: Acute diabetes following mumps. *Br. Med. J.* 2:802, 1924.

14. John, H. J.: The diabetic child: Etiologic factors. *Ann. Intern. Med.* 8:198, 1934.

15. Kremer H. U.: Juvenile diabetes as a sequel to mumps. *Am. J. Med.* 3:257, 1947.

16. Hinden, E.: Mumps followed by diabetes. *Lancet* 1:1381, 1962.

17. McCrae, W. M.: Diabetes mellitus following mumps. *Lancet* 1:1300, 1963.

18. Marble, A.: Infections in diabetes. In: Joslin, E. P., Root, H. F., White, P., Marble, A., and Bailey C. C. (Eds.), *The Treatment of Diabetes Mellitus,* 8th ed. Lea and Febiger, Philadelphia, 1946, p. 523.

19. Gamble, D. R., Kinsley, M. L., FitzGerald, M. G., Bolton, R., and Taylor, K. W.: Viral antibodies in diabetes mellitus. *Br. Med. J.* 3:627, 1969.

20. Yoon, J. W., Austin, M., Onodera, T., and Natkkins, A. L.: Virus induced diabetes mellitus: Isolation of a virus from the pancreas of a child with diabetic ketoacidosis. *N.E.J.M.* 300:1173-1179, 1979.

21. Ursing, B.: Acute pancreatitis in coxsackie B infection. *Br. Med. J.* 3:524-525, 1973.

22. Wyatt, J. P., Saxton, J., Lee, R. S., and Pinkerton, H.: Generalized cytomegalic inclusion disease. *J. Ped.* 36: 271-294, 1950.

23. Fleegler, F. M., Rogers, K. D., Drash, A. et al: Age, sex and seasonal variation of onset of juvenile diabetes in different geographic areas. *Pediatrics* 63:374-379, 1979.

24. Messaritakis, J., and Karabula, C., Kattemics, C., and Matsaniotis, N.: Diabetes following mumps in sibs. *Arch. Dis. Child.* 46:561-562, 1971.

25. Sultz, H. A., Hart, B. A., Zielezny, M. et al: Is mumps virus an etiologic factor in juvenile diabetes mellitus? Preliminary report. *J. Ped.* 86:654-655, 1975.

26. Craighead, J. E.: Viral diabetes mellitus in man and experimental animals. *Am. J. Med.* 70:127-134, 1981.

27. Hay, D. R.: The relation of maternal rubella to congenital deafness and other abnormalities in New Zealand. *N.Z. Med. J.* 48:604, 1949.

28. Forrest, J. M., Menser, M. A., and Harley, J. D.: Diabetes mellitus and congenital rubella. *Pediatrics* 44:445, 1969.

29. Johnson, G. M., and Tudor, R. B.: Diabetes mellitus and congenital rubella infection. *Am. J. Dis. Child.* 120:453, 1970.

30. Forrest, J. M., Menser, M. A., and Burgess, J. A.: High frequency of diabetes mellitus in young with congenital rubella. *Lancet* 2:332, 1971.

31. Bunnel, C. E., and Monif, C. R. G.: Interstitial pancreatitis in the congenital rubella syndrome. *J. Ped.* 80: 465, 1972.

32. Monif, C. R. G., Sever, J. L., Schiff, G. M., and Traub, R. G.: Isolation of rubella virus from products of conception. *Am. J. Obstet. Gynecol.* 91:1143, 1965.

33. Plotkin, S. A., and Vaheri, A.: Human fibroblasts infected with rubella virus produce a growth inhibitor. *Science* 156:659, 1967.

34. Smithsells, R. W., Shepphard, S., Marshall, W. C., and Peckham, C.: Congenital rubella-diabetes mellitus. *Lancet* 1:439, 1978.

35. Monif, G. R. G., Avery, B. G., Karones, S. B., and Sever, J. L.: Isolation of the rubella virus from the organs of three children with rubella syndrome defects. *Lancet* 1: 723-724, 1965.

36. DePrins, F., VanAsshe, F. A., Desmyter, I., DeGroote, G., and Gepts, W.: Congenital rubella and diabetes mellitus. *Lancet* 1:440, 1978.

37. Singer, D. B., Rudolph, A. J., Rosenberg, H. S., Rawls, W. E., and Baniuk, M.: Pathology of the congenital rubella syndrome. *J. Ped.* 71:665-675, 1967.

38. Rubenstein, P., Walker, M. E. et al: The HLA system in congenital rubella patients with and without diabetes. *Diabetes* 31:1088, 1982.

39. Burch, G. E., Tsui, C. Y., Harb, J. M., and Colcolough, H. L.: Pathologic findings in the pancreas of mice infected with coxsackie virus B4. *Arch. Intern. Med.* 128: 40, 1971.

40. Craighead, J. E., and McLane, M. F.: Diabetes mellitus: Induction in mice infected with encephalomyocarditis virus. *Science* 162:913, 1968.

41. Craighead, J. E., McLane, M. F., and Steinke, J.: Virus-induced diabetes in mice. *Metabolism* 17:1154, 1968.

42. Craighead, J. E., and Steinke, J.: Diabetes mellitus-like syndrome in mice infected with encephalomyocarditis virus. *Am. J. Pathol.* 63:119, 1971.

43. Yoon, J. W., and Natkins, A. L.: Virus-induced diabetes mellitus VI. Genetically determined host differences in the replication of encephalomyocarditis virus in pancreatic beta cells. *J. Exp. Med.* 143:1170-1185, 1976.

44. Wilson, G., Craighead, J. E.: Interferon effects of EMC virus in beta cell cultures (In press, 1982).

45. Onadera, T., Yoon, J. W., Brown, K. S., and Natkins, A. L.: Evidence for a single locus controlling susceptibility to virus-induced diabetes mellitus. *Nature* 276:693-696, 1978.

46. Grodsky, G. M.: Production of autoantibodies to insulin in man and rabbits. *Diabetes* 14:396, 1965.

47. Karam, J. H., Grodsky, G. M., and Forsham, P. H.: Coxsackie virus and diabetes. *Lancet* 2:1209, 1971.

48. Grodsky, G. M., Feldman, R., Toreson, W. E., et al: Diabetes mellitus in rabbits immunized with insulin. *Diabetes* 15:579, 1966.

49. Toreson, W. E., Lee, J. C., and Grodsky, G. M.: The histopathology of immune diabetes in the rabbit. *Am. J. Pathol.* 52:1099, 1968.

50. Nerup, J., Andersen, O. O., Bendixen, G., et al: Antipancreatic cellular hypersensitivity in diabetes mellitus. *Diabetes* 20:424-427, 1971.

51. Bottazzo, G. F., Florin-Christensen, A., and Doniach, D.: Islet cell antibodies in diabetes mellitus with autoimmune polyendocrine deficiency. *Lancet* 2:1279-1283, 1974.

52. Lendrum, R., Walker, G., Cudworth, A. G. et al: Islet cell antibodies in diabetes mellitus. *Lancet* 2:1273-1276, 1976.

53. Irvine, W. J., McCollum, C. J., Gray, R. S. et al: Pancreatic islet cell antibodies in diabetes mellitus correlated with the duration and type of diabetes, coexistent autoimmune disease and HLA-type. *Diabetes* 26:138-147, 1977.

54. DelPrete, G. F., Betterle, C., Padovan, D. et al: Incidence and significance of islet cell autoantibodies in different types of diabetes mellitus. *Diabetes* 26:909-915, 1977.

55. Nerup, J., and Lernmark, A.: Autoimmunity in insulin-dependent diabetes mellitus. *Am. J. Med.* 70:135-141, 1981.

56. Lernmark, A., Freedman, Z. R., Hofmann, C. et al: Islet cell surface antibodies in juvenile diabetes mellitus. *N.E.J.M.* 299:375-380, 1978.

57. Nerup, J.: The clinical and immunological association of diabetes mellitus and Addison's disease. In: Bastenie, P.A., and Gepts, W. (Eds.), *Immunity and Autoimmunity in Diabetes Mellitus,* Excerpta Medica, Amsterdam, 1974, pp. 149-152.

58. Nerup, J., and Bender, C.: Thyroid, gastric and adrenal autoimmunity in diabetes mellitus. *Acta Endocrin.* 72: 279-286, 1973.

59. Eisenbarth, G. S., Wilson, P. W., Ward, F., Buckley, C., and Lebovitz, H.: The polyglandular failure syndrome: Disease inheritance, HLA type and immune function. *Ann. Intern. Med.* 91:528-533, 1979.

60. Fialkow, P. J., Zavala, C., and Nielsen, R.: Thyroid autoimmunity: Increased frequency in relation of insulin dependent diabetic patients. *Ann. Intern. Med.* 83: 170-176, 1955.

61. Carpenter, C. C. J., Solomon, N., Silverberg, S. G. et al: Schmidt's syndrome (thyroid and adrenal insufficiency): A review of the literature and a report of 15 new cases including ten instances of coexistent diabetes mellitus. *Medicine* 43:153-180, 1964.

62. Pincus, G., and White, P.: On the inheritance of diabetes mellitus. *Am. J. Med. Sci.* 186:1, 1933.

64. Simpson, N. E.: Multifactorial inheritance: A possible hypothesis on diabetes. *Diabetes* 13:462, 1964.

65. Tattersall, R. B., and Pyke, D. A.: Diabetes in identical twins. *Lancet* 2:1120-1124, 1972.

66. Pyke, D. A.: Diabetes: The genetic connections. *Diabetologia* 17:333-343, 1979.

67. Rotter, J. I., and Rimoin, D. L.: The genetics of the glucose intolerance disorders. *Am. J. Med.* 70:116-126, 1981.

68. Rotter, J. I., and Rimoin, D. K.: Heterogeneity in diabetes mellitus — update 1978. Evidence for further genetic heterogeneity within juvenile onset insulin dependent diabetes mellitus. *Diabetes* 27:599-608, 1978.

69. Tattersall, R. B.: Mild familial diabetes with dominant inheritance. *Q. J. Med.* 43:339-357, 1974.

70. Tattersall, R. B., and Fajans, S. S.: A difference between the inheritance of classical juvenile onset and maturity onset types of diabetes in young people. *Diabetes* 24:44-53, 1975.

71. Nerup, J., Plotz, P., Andersen, O. O. et al: HLA antigens and diabetes mellitus. *Lancet* 2:864-866, 1974.

Chapter 4

PATHOPHYSIOLOGY OF DIABETES MELLITUS TYPE I

Richard A. Guthrie, M.D.

DEFINITION

Diabetes mellitus type I (DMI) is the form of diabetes most commonly encountered in children, adolescents, and young adults. DMI is an endocrinopathy and a disorder of metabolism resulting from a deficiency of insulin. It is the most common endocrine disease in children. Diabetes mellitus, however, should not be considered a single disease but a syndrome, i.e., a group of diseases having common signs and symptoms. Diabetes mellitus is the final common pathway of several disease processes that affect insulin secretion or action resulting in altered metabolism, especially altered carbohydrate metabolism.

Diabetes involves the whole life process. It involves every organ and organ system of the body since it affects such a fundamental process as carbohydrate metabolism. It also affects the total life-style and family relationships. Diabetes is a unique disease in that it requires self-management on the part of the person with the disease and the willingness and ability of the family to support the patient.

Diabetes mellitus type II or noninsulin-dependent (DMII) is a much more common form of the disease but is seen most often in adults -- usually adults over the age of 45 years. DMII is occasionally seen in children and is most often identified when doing oral glucose tolerance testing in children with obesity or in families with a strong family history of DMII. Since many adults with DMII may present with complications, the disease probably begins much earlier, perhaps in childhood, but is so mild as to go unnoticed. One form of DMII seen in childhood is inherited as an autosomal dominant trait and thus manifests a strong family history. This form of the disease is called Mason type DMII.

One important distinction to be made between the various kinds of diabetes mellitus is the form of treatment. All persons with DMI are insulin-dependent; i.e., if their insulin is discontinued after the remission period, they will develop ketoacidosis and cannot survive. Some persons with DMII also may need insulin. These persons are insulin-*requiring,* not insulin-*dependent.* Persons with DMII may need or require insulin to control hyperglycemia intermittently or even permanently, but if the insulin is discontinued they do not develop ketoacidosis and can survive for many years.

PHYSIOLOGY OF CARBOHYDRATE METABOLISM

Insulin is an anabolic hormone which is necessary for the regulation of carbohydrate and lipid metabolism (and, to a lesser extent, protein metabolism). The primary function of insulin in the body is to serve as a storage hormone. Insulin is necessary for the body to store food during times of plenty so that it can be available in times of fasting. Even for animals with a relatively constant source of food such as a fish in the sea or modern man, eating is not constant. The intermittent intake of food requires the storage of the energy in depots to be released as needed between feedings. It is the function of insulin to cause the uptake of energy sources (primarily carbohydrate and fat) into these depots for storage. The depots affected by insulin are the liver and the muscle for the storage of carbohydrate and the adipose tissue for the storage of fat. Carbohydrate is stored as glycogen in the liver and muscle or converted to fatty acids and stored as fat in the adipose tissue.

Insulin works as a storage hormone by interacting with an insulin-specific receptor on the cell membrane. The insuline-receptor interaction causes several reactions to occur. The first effect of the insulin is to alter the permeability of the cell membrane to glucose, to free fatty acids and amino acids, thus facilitating the uptake of these metabolic fuels and building blocks of tissue into the cells. The second effect is that the insulin-receptor interaction causes the formation in the cell membrane of substances which act as second messengers to the organelles of the cell to stimulate whatever function that organelle may have in the metabolic process of that particular cell.

Some of the carbohydrate and fat taken up by the cell will be utilized by the cell for fuel. Insulin interacts here by stimulating the enzymes of the normal glycolytic pathway as glucose is metabolized into the Krebs cycle for energy production. In particular, the enzyme necessary for the first step of the glycolytic pathway, glucokinase IV, which phosphorylates glucose to form glucose-6-phosphate, is insulin-dependent. Insulin also stimulates the enzymes necessary for storage of glucose, such as the glycogen-producing enzymes of the liver and the muscle. Insulin stimulates the lipogenic enzymes of the adipose tissue, which allows fatty acids and glucose to be converted to triglyceride and stored in the adipose tissue. Insulin also suppresses the enzymes that break down energy stores, such as the lipase enzymes of adipose tissue that break down triglyceride to free fatty acid and glycerol and the glycogenolyses enzymes of the liver and muscle which break down glycogen to glucose. Thus, insulin is a key hormone in the entire pathway of all metabolic fuels. An understanding of these functions of insulin and the metabolic pathways leads to a better understanding of the abnormalities of diabetes mellitus, which is a deficiency of this important hormone.

MECHANISM OF INSULIN ACTION

Insulin is secreted from the beta cells of the pancreas under the influence of a glucose stimulus. Other metabolic fuels, hormones, and the central nervous system can contribute to the secretion of insulin, but the primary stimulus is glucose. Insulin is produced as a coiled molecule called proinsulin. Before the molecule is released into the circulation it is split into two molecules — insulin and C peptide. The measurement of C peptide can be used as a measure of endogenous insulin secretion since it is secreted in equimolar amounts with insulin and is present in the circulation (see Chapter 5B).

Insulin which is secreted constantly in small amounts is called basal insulin. Even with prolonged fasting, insulin levels never fall to zero. When food is ingested, insulin levels rise in proportion to the need. This postprandial rise in insulin levels is called the postprandial bolus. It is this basal and bolus effect of physiologic insulin secretion that we attempt to duplicate in the treatment of persons with DMI.

In the complex secretion and action cycle of insulin, many things can go wrong and produce the complex of symptoms and signs we call diabetes mellitus. 1) Insulin secretion can be deficient or abnormal. A defective insulin molecule can be produced and be biologically inactive or the insulin can be bound or destroyed in the circulation. 2) Insulin receptors can be abnormal, deficient, or absent. 3) Finally, the secondary messenger can be absent or defective or the organelles of the cell may not respond to the messenger appropriately. All of these defects have been described (Fig. 4.1). Thus, diabetes is not a single disease but a syndrome, since diabetes due to each of these possible defects has a different etiology and perhaps also different genetics. DMI as it occurs in young people is primarily a defect in insulin secretion caused by damage or destruction of the beta cells thought to be a genetically determined defect in the immune system with subsequent interaction with environmental factors such as viral infections (see Chapter 3).

PATHOPHYSIOLOGY OF DIABETES MELLITUS

When insulin is deficient, there is: 1) decreased glucose uptake by the cells and decreased storage of glycogen and fat; 2) excess breakdown of glycogen to glucose; 3) defective glycolysis; 4) enhanced gluconeogenesis from protein; and 5) excess fat breakdown. There may also be defective protein uptake by the cell or defective protein metabolism. All of these actions result in intracellular starvation and the

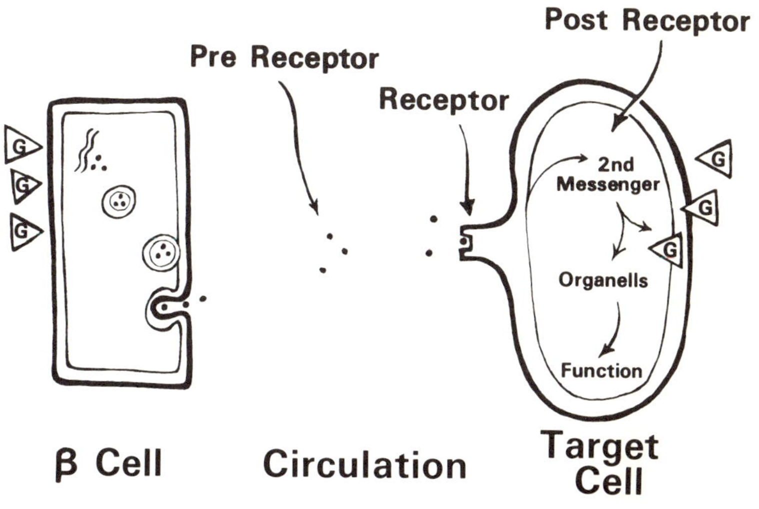

FIGURE 4.1

accumulation of glucose and fat products (free fatty acids and ketones) in the blood. In short, deficient insulin results in deficient anabolism and excessive catabolism.

Excess glucose in the blood (hyperglycemia) results in glucose excretion in the urine. The urinary excretion of glucose carries with it the loss of water resulting in excess urination or polyuria, one of the three cardinal signs of diabetes. Polyuria results in dehydration, which stimulates the thirst mechanism, causing increased fluid intake or polydipsia, the second cardinal sign of diabetes. Cellular starvation results in stimulation of the hunger mechanism, causing excess eating or polyphagia, the third cardinal sign of diabetes. In spite of the polyphagia, there is progressive weight loss, since the food consumed cannot be metabolized due to the insulin deficiency.

Fat breakdown results in increased levels of free fatty acids in the blood. The free fatty acids are quickly converted by the liver to the ketone bodies -- beta-hydroxybutyric acid, acetoacetic acid, and acetone, which are strong organic acids. The accumulation of the acids eventually overwhelms the bodies' buffering capacity and the blood pH is lowered, ultimately resulting in DKA, coma, and death if not corrected (see Chapter 6 D). DKA is, then, the result of fuel deprivation, cellular starvation, and a catabolic state resulting from insulin deficiency, i.e., a reversal of the normal fuel storage effect of insulin. DKA is the extreme of the insulin-deprivation syndrome. Any time insulin is deficient in the tissues, there will be a local catabolic state in which the cells are deprived of the normal metabolic fuels and normal aerobic metabolism. The cellular damage, minute as it may be, is cumulative and, along with the accumulation of glucose in some tissues, results in the long-term damage of diabetes known as the chronic complications of the disease, which are micro- and macroangiopathy and neuropathy (see Chapter 8). The chronic complications of diabetes are devastating problems and can be delayed and possibly prevented by understanding the physiology of insulin secretion and by the replacement of insulin to the deficient individual in a manner that simulates normal physiology as nearly as possible.

COUNTERREGULATORY HORMONES

Glucagon, epinephrine, growth hormone, and adrenocorticosteroids are hormones which counter the actions of insulin. These hormones elevate blood glucose levels and are known as counterregulatory hormones. Glucagon and epinephrine have the duel actions of causing glycogen breakdown by the liver and muscle and also of stimulating ketogenesis by facilitating fat breakdown (Fig. 4.2). Growth hormone exerts its effect primarily on muscle fat and, to a lesser extent, on body fat to also facilitate glucose production and ketogenesis. Adrenocorticosteroids exert their effect on glucose metabolism by promoting gluconeogenesis from protein. This effect is primarily exerted in the liver. Glucagon is the hormone primarily involved in minute-to-minute glucose regulation in a delicate balance with insulin. Epinephrine is involved in crisis glucose regulation as the emergency or fight-flight hormone utilized by the body for sudden, large, and rapid surges of glucose for short-term, intense energy production. Gluconeogenesis from protein is an important standby source of glucose, especially to preserve the energy to the brain during times of fasting when glycogen stores may be depleted.

The secretion of these counterregulatory hormones are controlled by many mechanisms, including the central nervous system (epinephrine), the pituitary (cortisol), the fuel supply, the blood glucose level, and the availability of insulin. Insulin, for example, exerts a suppressive effect on glucagon secretion. Epinephrine, on the other hand, has a suppressive effect on insulin secretion. Thus, intermediary metabolism is a complex interaction between metabolic fuel supplies and needs and several regulatory and counterregulatory hormones. Any imbalance in the system such as insulin deficiency, glucagon excess, or counterregulatory hormonal excess will imbalance the entire system with devastating effects. Insulin

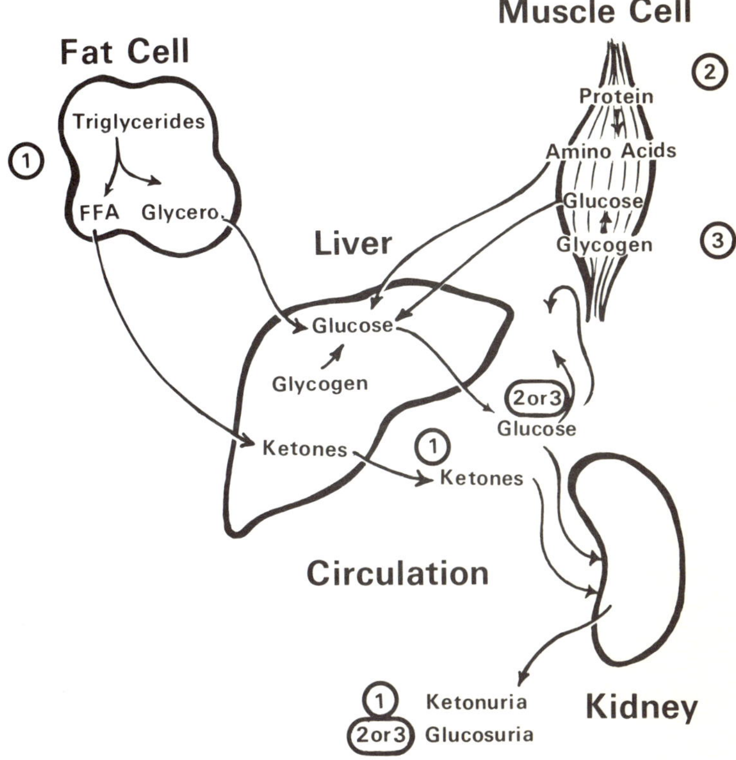

FIGURE 4.2

therefore, should be supplied in as physiologic a manner as possible to restore and maintain the balance.

SUMMARY

DMI is a serious metabolic disease resulting from a deficiency of the hormone insulin. It is a catabolic state which is a reversal of the normal anabolic state promoted by the presence of insulin. An understanding of normal intermediary metabolism is necessary for an understanding of the reversed catabolic state of DMI.

BIBLIOGRAPHY

Brownlee, M.: Etiology/Hormone Physiology, Vol. I. In: *Handbook of Diabetes Mellitus,* Garland STPM Press, New York, 1981.

Brownlee, M.: Biochemical Pathology, Vol. IV. In: *Handbook of Diabetes Mellitus,* Garland STPM Press, New York, 1981.

Rifken, H., and Raskin, P. (Eds.): *Diabetes Mellitus,* Volume V. American Diabetes Association Series. Robert J. Brady Co., Bowie, Maryland, 1981.

Chapter 5

TYPE I DIABETES IN CHILDREN

A. DIAGNOSIS AND DIFFERENTIAL DIAGNOSIS

Robert L. Jackson, M.D.

DIAGNOSIS

When overt diabetes mellitus occurs in childhood, the symptoms and signs of insulin deficiency are usually apparent, as they appear quite abruptly. The child or parents can usually recall the week or even the day when symptoms were first noticed. Symptoms observed are the classic polyuria, polydipsia, polyphagia, and weight loss in spite of polyphagia. The child is often said to have become chronically fatigued and run-down. A younger child may resume bedwetting. The diagnosis of diabetes mellitus is usually made shortly after the appearance of these symptoms, there being greater public awareness recently of the importance of early evaluation of unusual symptoms.

When the onset of overt diabetes occurs during an acute infection, the child often has an accelerated progression of symptoms that leads rapidly to ketoacidosis. For a short period of time after the onset of symptoms, increased intake of food and liquids compensates for the urinary losses. The child may tolerate mild ketosis even though increased catabolism and defective protein synthesis interfere with normal growth. Ketonemia gradually increases and causes anorexia and vomiting, after which ketoacidosis develops rapidly.

The classic history of polyuria, polydipsia, and weight loss in a child with glycosuria, hyperglycemia, and ketoacidosis leaves little room for diagnostic uncertainty. Glucose tolerance testing is not indicated for diagnostic purposes in children with classic symptoms. Glycosuria with a random reliable blood glucose value in excess of 200 mg/dl confirms the diagnosis.

DIFFERENTIAL DIAGNOSIS

During acute infections, children often have decreased food and fluid intake, which leads to depleted glycogen stores and rapid development of ketonemia and ketonuria without glycosuria. Acute infections are the most common cause of ketonuria. When the urine of young children is concentrated, results of the reduction test for glucose may be mildly positive, but testing with glucose oxidase will yield negative results.

The child with salicylate intoxication often has hyperpnea and ketonuria. Glycosuria may appear to be present if a reduction test for urinary glucose is used, but retesting of the urine with glucose oxidase paper strips will indicate either a negative reaction or only a slight trace of glucose. In salicylate poisoning, the ferric chloride reaction for ketones will remain positive after the urine is boiled.

Transient hyperglycemia with or without glycosuria is observed occasionally in infants and children who have other disorders; in these cases, the hyperglycemia may be, but usually is not, complicated by ketoacidosis. 1) Elevated blood glucose often is observed in premature infants receiving parenteral fluids. 2) Hypokalemia and hypernatremia at times may be associated with carbohydrate intolerance and transient hyperglycemia, and in children, severe electrolyte disturbances with hypokalemia and hypernatremia may develop as a result of gastrointestinal and renal disorders. Delayed insulin release, observed during hypokalemia, explains the hyperglycemia. 3) Acute pancreatitis may cause transient hyperglycemia and glycosuria. 4) During the first 24-48 hr of intravenous alimentation, most children have varying degrees of glycosuria. If the hyperglycemia persists for a longer period, it may cause osmotic diuresis and dehydration. 5) Blood glucose levels may be elevated for a short time in children with central nervous system disorders such as encephalitis, head trauma, heat stroke, tumor, or infiltrative process of the hypothalamus. 6) The administration of drugs such as steroids or diuretics also may cause transient hyperglycemia. Steroids cause glucose intolerance by increasing the rate of gluconeogenesis, whereas diuretics may cause hypokalemia, which can then induce hyperglycemia. 7) Severe stress such as extensive burns, trauma, surgical procedures, severe infection, and general anesthesia may produce hyperglycemia and transient glycosuria. Hyperglycemia during severe stress is caused by increased secretion of glucocorticoids, catecholamines, and glucagon (1).

Renal glycosuria may be confused with diabetes in childhood, but it is easily differentiated by a normal response to the glucose tolerance test. Another rare condition in which glycosuria is seen in the absence of hyperglycemia is the Fanconi syndrome with or without cystinosis. Reducing sugars other than glucose, such as galactose, pentose, and fructose, appear in the urine as the result of inborn metabolic errors. Other endocrine disorders may be associated with impaired glucose tolerance and hyperglycemia. These include gigantism or acromegaly, Cushing's syndrome, pheochromocytoma, thyrotoxicosis, and excessive secretion of glucagon (i.e., glucagonoma). These disorders, however, are less likely to produce a diabeticlike syndrome in children than in adults.

Ketoacidosis may also occur with renal insufficiency or as the result of severe gastrointestinal upsets, but in those cases it is not associated with hyperglycemia or glycosuria. The patient with lead encephalopathy may have glycosuria and coma without hyperglycemia. Children with lead encephalopathy also are likely to have increased intracranial pressure and convulsions. The urine of children with alkaptonuria contains homogentisic acid, which yields a positive reaction to the copper reduction test.

EARLY DETECTION OF DIABETES

There is evidence that glucose tolerance in children may be abnormal before the onset of clinical or overt diabetes. The arrows in Figure 5.1 indicate that in the early phase, the glucose intolerance is transient and reverts to normal except during stress, whereas in the late stages the glucose intolerance is progressively more persistent. Because of the shorter time required for development of diabetes in children than in adults, public detection drives (designed for adults) that are based on urine tests for sugar and one or two postprandial blood glucose values will not identify a significant number of children with diabetes. *We therefore recommend that immediate members of a family in whom diabetes is present test their urine for glucose during febrile illnesses and, if transient glycosuria is found, have a standardized oral glucose tolerance test.*

The most opportune time to detect diabetes in prediabetic children is during the stress of an infection. Experience with a number of the siblings of our patients has lead us to develop a simple and relatively effective way to detect children with glucose intolerance. We began with the premise that diabetes is most likely to be found in those children whose parents or siblings are diabetic. When a child of such a family has an infection, the parents are advised to test the child's urine for the presence of glucose after having given the child a simple sugar load: 1) For the child less than 6

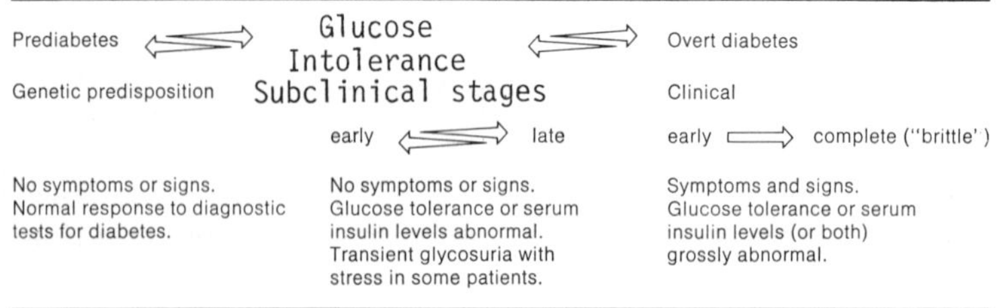

FIGURE 5.1

years old — after emptying his bladder, the child drinks 4 oz of orange juice or 2 oz of grape juice sweetened with 1 tablespoon of sugar. Twenty minutes later, he drinks 3 oz of a sweetened cola (not artificially sweetened or diet cola). 2) For the child 6 years old or more, the quantities are doubled, i.e., 8 oz of orange juice or 4 oz of grape juice sweetened with 2 tablespoons of sugar, followed by 6 oz of sweetened cola.

Two to three hours after having consumed the sugar load, the child is asked to void, and his urine is tested for the presence of glucose. If results of the test are positive (during the stress of infection), the child should have a standardized glucose tolerance test and, if possible, an islet cell antibody determination as soon as it can be conveniently scheduled.

STANDARDIZED ORAL GLUCOSE TOLERANCE TESTS

The oral glucose tolerance test (OGTT) remains the investigation most often used to detect or confirm impairment of carbohydrate metabolism. In pediatric practice, an OGTT is most often done to reassure parents from high-risk families that their children have a normal test. It also identifies the occasional child with a borderline or abnormal test. In these children, the test is repeated periodically, especially during periods of environmental stress, to help elucidate the natural pattern of diabetes in children. It is imperative not only to have standardized methodology but also to have well-defined norms for appropriate age and sex to make possible reliable interpretation of the OGTT.

Previous studies of blood glucose and serum insulin values during the OGTT for normal children from our laboratory and others were published in 1973 (2). Additional observations have been made to permit statistical analysis of differences on the basis of age and sex. We have now analyzed 235 standardized OGTTs of normal children and adolescents to establish normal percentiles for glucose and insulin values in pre- and postpubescent boys and girls. Glucose and insulin percentiles have been determined for both capillary (fingerstick) and venous (venipuncture) sampling techniques.

Capillary Studies

One hundred ninety-six children who had no known family history of diabetes in the preceding two generations were included in the group of normal children having capillary whole blood drawn for glucose determinations. One hundred five also had capillary serum insulin determinations. Only children who were of normal height for age, as compared with Iowa growth charts (3), and whose weights were within 1.5 SD (standard deviation) of the expected weight for their actual height were included in this study. None of the children had any signs or symptoms of infection or were taking any medications for at least 1 month preceding the test.

For 3 days preceding the test the children's meals were planned to ensure the intake of at least 60% of the total daily calories as carbohydrates. A standardized snack was eaten at about 10 p.m. before the start of a 10-hr fasting period. For children 5–8 years, 4 oz of whole milk and 1 graham cracker were eaten; for children 8–12 years, 6 oz of milk and 1 graham cracker; for children over 12 years, 8 oz of milk and 2 graham crackers.

The oral glucose load was given the following morning from 8:00 to 8:30 a.m. as 1.75 g glucose/kg of average weight for actual height using Iowa growth charts as norms. A 30% glucose solution was drunk within 5 min after taking the fasting blood specimen. Capillary blood samples were then obtained by fingersticks by experienced technicians at 30 min and 1, 2, and 3 hr after the glucose was ingested. Urine specimens were collected at the 1-hr time period. A modest amount of physical activity was supervised in the same testing room during the test period.

The quality control of the blood glucose determinations was verified by the Glucose Standardization Laboratory, U.S. Public Health Service, Atlanta, Georgia. The variability in the blood glucose obtained by the fingersticks using the o-toluidine method was within 3 mg/100 ml. Insulin determinations were done in triplicate on the serum by a modification of the double antibody method of Morgan and Lazarow. The sensitivity of our assay allowed for the detection of 5 μU/ml of insulin and a reproducibility within an assay of 3.67% coefficient variation (CV) and between assays of 7.9% CV.

Capillary Glucose Values

Figures 5.2, 5.3, 5.4, and 5.5 demonstrate the normal range of blood glucose levels and serum insulin values for younger and older boys and girls. When the glucose values for the younger girls were compared with those of the older girls, there was no significant difference between the two groups. At 30 min the younger girls tended to have slightly higher values than the older girls but the difference was not highly significant ($0.05 < p < 0.1$). In comparing the younger boys with the older boys there was no significant difference between the two groups. Fasting glucose values of the younger boys tended to be slightly higher than the values of the older boys ($p = 0.01$). Overall, when comparing glucose values of children of the same sex, age does not make a significant difference.

In a similar manner, the glucose values of younger girls were compared with the younger boys and the older girls were compared with the older boys. The glucose values of the younger girls were generally higher than the younger boys, with the 30 min difference being highly significant ($p < 0.002$) and the 1- and 3-hr differences indicating a similar trend ($p < 0.08$ and $p = 0.02$, respectively).

The glucose values of the older girls compared with the older boys also show that the older girls' values are generally higher than the older boys. The differences are highly significant at fasting and 3 hr ($p < 0.01$), and this trend is suggested at the other time intervals as well; 30 min, $0.05 < p < 0.1$; 1 hr, $0.02 < p < 0.05$; and 2 hr, $0.01 < p < 0.02$.

When the glucose values of all girls were compared with glucose values of all boys at the five time periods, *the differences are highly significant at all time periods (each $p < 0.007$), with the girls showing higher values than the boys.*

Capillary Insulin Values

In more recent years capillary serum insulin specimens were obtained at the same time that capillary glucose specimens were collected during the standard 3-hr OGTTs. When the insulin values of younger boys were compared with younger girls, the younger girls' insulin values tended to be higher at 30 min and 2 hr ($0.02 < p < 0.5$). The insulin values of older boys compared with those of older girls also tended to be

ORAL GLUCOSE TOLERANCE NORM FOR GIRLS 5-11 yrs.
CAPILLARY WHOLE BLOOD
GLUCOSE mg/dl
175
150
125
100
75
50
25
91---------169--------136------84%tile-------122-----------------102
79---------146--------114------50%tile-------102------------------86
72---------119----------90----- 16%tile ------- 80------------------68
Fasting 1/2 hr 1 hr 2 hr 3 hr
GLUCOSE
INSULIN
1 Hour Urine
Clinitest:
Acetest
24----------98----------67------84%tile--------66------------------33
15----------72----------37------50%tile--------39------------------22
9----------35----------25------16%tile--------24------------------15
CAPILLARY SERUM
INSULIN uU/ml
125
100
75
50
25
0

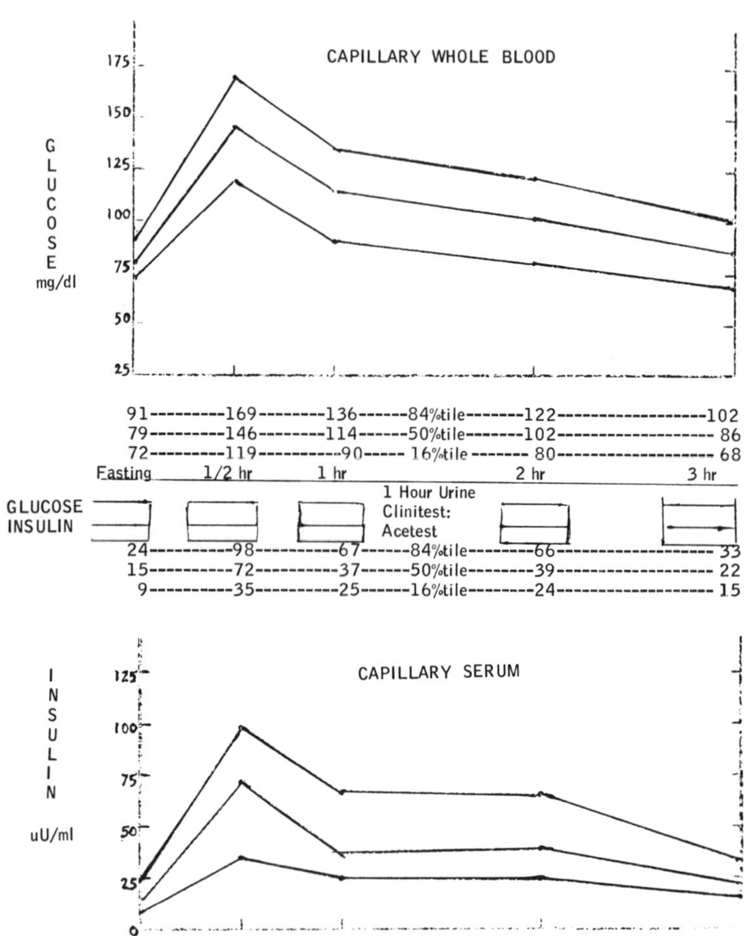

FIGURE 5.2

ORAL GLUCOSE TOLERANCE NORM FOR ADOLESCENT GIRLS
CAPILLARY WHOLE BLOOD
GLUCOSE mg/dl
175
150
125
100
75
50
25
87--------162--------140-------84%tile-------120-----------------106
82--------134--------113-------50%tile-------103-----------------90
75------- 114---------95------ 16%tile--------93-----------------77
Fasting
1/2hr
I hr
2 hr
3 hr
GLUCOSE
INSULIN
1 Hour Urine
Clinitest:
Acetest:
28--------110---------89-------84%tile----------74---------------- 51
21---------73--------50-------50%tile----------52----------------- 32
11--------- 41--------30-------16%tile----------32----------------- 18
CAPILLARY SERUM
INSULIN uU/ml
125
100
75
50
25
0

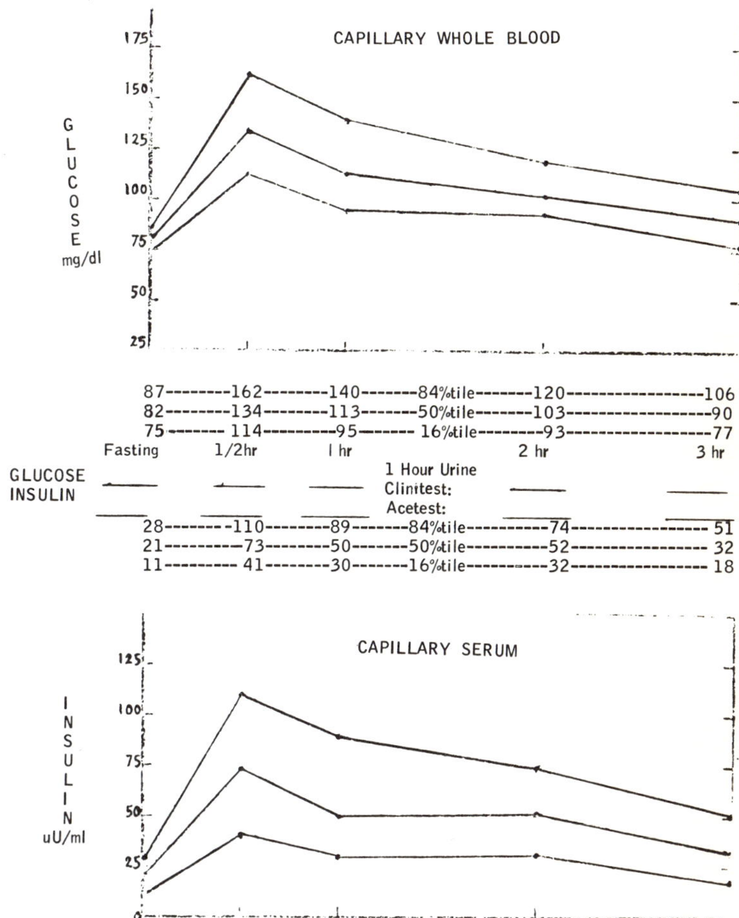

FIGURE 5.3

ORAL GLUCOSE TOLERANCE NORM FOR BOYS 5-13 yrs.
CAPILLARY WHOLE BLOOD
GLUCOSE mg/dl
175
150
125
100
75
50
25
87--------145--------126--------84%tile------113------------------91
80--------124-------- 107------ 50%tile-------97------------------77
71--------107-----------85------ 16%tile-------84------------------ 63
Fasting
1/2hr
1 hr
2 hr
3 hr
GLUCOSE
INSULIN
1 Hour Urine
Clinitest:
Acetest:
23---------73----------56------84%tile--------45------------------24
19---------49----------32------50%tile--------28------------------19
10-------- 21----------22------16%tile--------15------------------12
CAPILLARY SERUM
INSULIN uU/ml
125
100
75
50
25
0

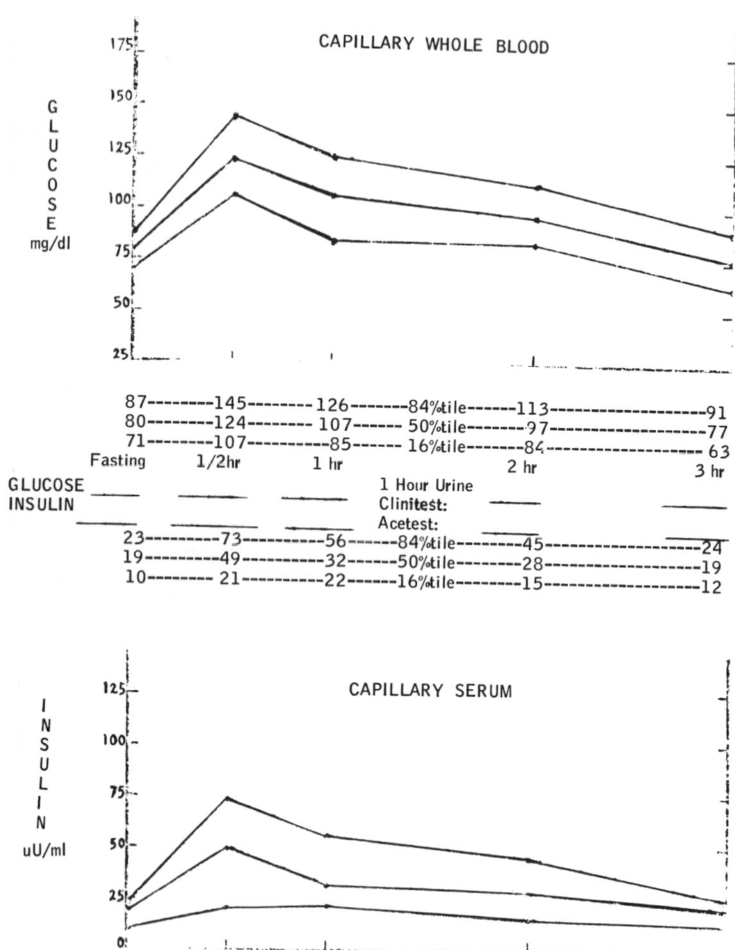

FIGURE 5.4

ORAL GLUCOSE TOLERANCE NORM FOR ADOLESCENT BOYS

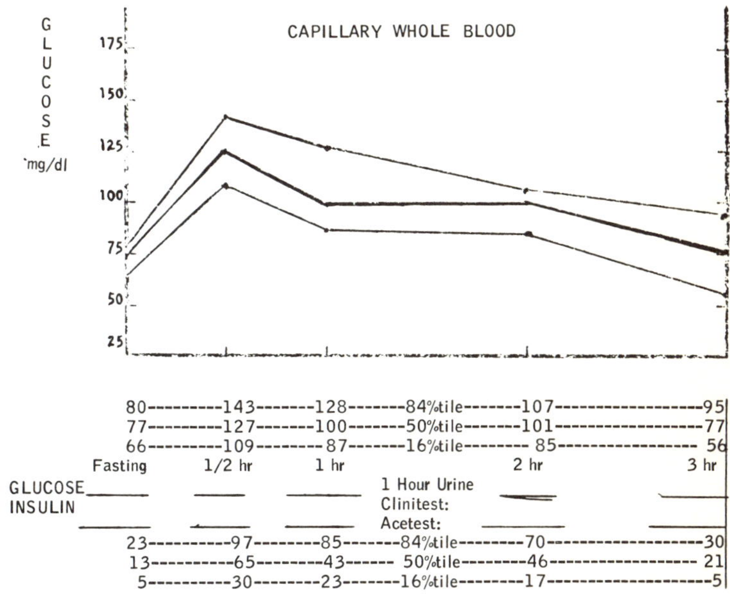

	Fasting	1/2 hr	1 hr		2 hr	3 hr
GLUCOSE	80	143	128	84%tile	107	95
	77	127	100	50%tile	101	77
	66	109	87	16%tile	85	56
INSULIN	23	97	85	84%tile	70	30
	13	65	43	50%tile	46	21
	5	30	23	16%tile	17	5

GLUCOSE______ ______ ______ 1 Hour Urine ______ ______

INSULIN Clinitest:

______ ______ ______ Acetest: ______ ______

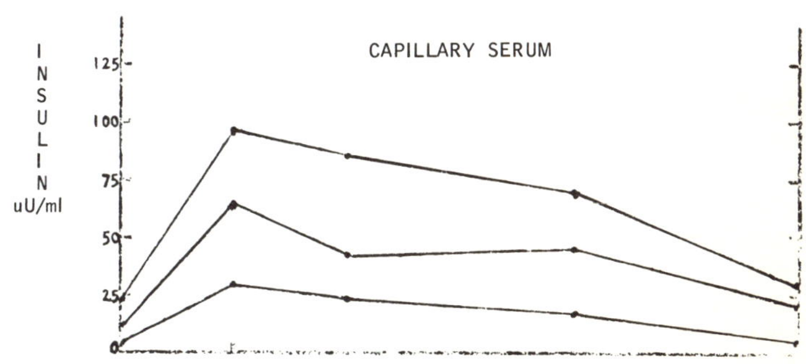

FIGURE 5.5

lower at fasting ($0.01 < p < 0.02$), and at 3 hr ($p < 0.01$). The insulin values of *all girls* compared with the insulin values of *all boys* showed *girls' values to be significantly higher than boys at 30 min, 2 hr, and 3 hr (all ps < 0.01).*

Age differences in insulin response to glucose challenge also were evaluated for both sexes. The insulin values of older and younger girls were significantly different at 3 hr ($p < 0.01$) with the older girls' being higher. The age analysis did not show so strong a trend in boys. At fasting, the older boys' insulin values were somewhat lower than younger boys ($0.05 < p < 0.1$) while at 30 min and 2 hr the older boys' insulin values were somewhat higher ($p = 0.1$ and $0.01 < p < 0.02$ respectively).

Comment

These analyses demonstrate the importance of having a normal range of blood glucose and serum insulin values during OGTTs for children which are sex-specific, if the test is to be used for detecting possible early abnormalities in glucose tolerance.

Venous Studies

Standardized venous studies also were done to provide more reliable OGTT norms for adolescents and young adults. Thirty-nine healthy adolescents and young adults (age range 11-28 years; mean age 15 years, 3 months) were divided by sex (20 male and 19 female). All 39 subjects previously had had one or more capillary OGTTs done in our laboratory with blood glucose and serum insulin values within the 84th and 16th percentile range. All tests were done using the same standard procedures and laboratory methods as previously defined.

All subjects also had normal height for age (as compared with the Iowa growth charts or the Metropolitan Life charts) and normal weight for height (within 1.5 SD of expected weight for actual height). All subjects were free of symptoms and signs of infection for more than 1 month prior to testing and had received no medications (including oral contraceptives) for more than 2 months prior to test. All subjects had stable weights for more than 6 months and during this period had not engaged in weight modification programs.

No significant differences ($p < 0.10$) were found for glucose or insulin values between male or female groups. The 84th, 50th, and 16th percentile venous whole blood glucose and serum insulin values for these 39 older children and young adults are depicted in Figure 5.6.

Figure 5.7 compares mean capillary whole blood glucose values (mg/dl) during OGTTs in normal children receiving 1.75 g of glucose/kg of body weight by our laboratory with values reported by five other laboratories using comparable methods (4-8). Note how similar all of the blood glucose values are, especially at fasting and at 2 hr.

Serum or plasma glucose values are about 12-15% (not mg%) higher than whole blood values because concentration of glucose is about 30% greater in plasma than in red cells. This relationship is not entirely constant because it varies according to the hematocrit level (e.g., if the hematocrit is low, the difference is diminished). Conversion of whole blood glucose values into estimates for the plasma levels are needed for comparison of data between different reported studies. Figure 5.8A depicts the calculated 50th percentile (median) curve for plasma glucose by our laboratory. Figure 5.8B compares the calculated 50th percentile curve for adolescents and young adults (16-30 years of age) with the 50th percentile curves by other research groups using comparable methods for normal subjects within the same age range. Fajan's data also are confined to the same age range. Note how close the median values are at each time period (9-13).

DISCUSSION

Many oral glucose tolerance studies of normal children and adults have been published. However, the results of many of the studies are not comparable because of different glucose loads and lack of standardization of other procedural practices and laboratory methods. *Of major importance is standardization of the glucose load in order to avoid giving an excessive amount of glucose to overweight subjects or an insufficient amount to those who are underweight.*

In 1976, the International Study Group on Diabetes in Children and Adolescents directed its attention to the need for standardization of OGTTs for children. In 1978 (10), B. Weber of the International Study Group reviewed the world

ORAL GLUCOSE TOLERANCE TEST
VENOUS CONTROLS
ADOLESCENTS AND YOUNG ADULTS
Sugar (mg%)
VENOUS WHOLE BLOOD
200
175
150
125
100
75
50
25
0
F
1/2
1
2
3
82----------123---------112-------84%tile--------91---------------------78
74----------112----------88-------50%tile--------76---------------------66
71-----------94----------69-------16%tile--------69---------------------49
Fasting
½ hr
1 hr
1 Hour Urine
Clintest:
Acetest:
2 hr
3 hr
SUGAR
INSULIN
17----------121---------100-------84%tile--------75---------------------46
10-----------89----------64-------50%tile--------55---------------------26
7-----------55----------47-------16%tile--------29----------------------9
Insulin (uU/ml)
VENOUS SERUM
175
150
125
100
75
50
25
0
F
1/2
1
2
3

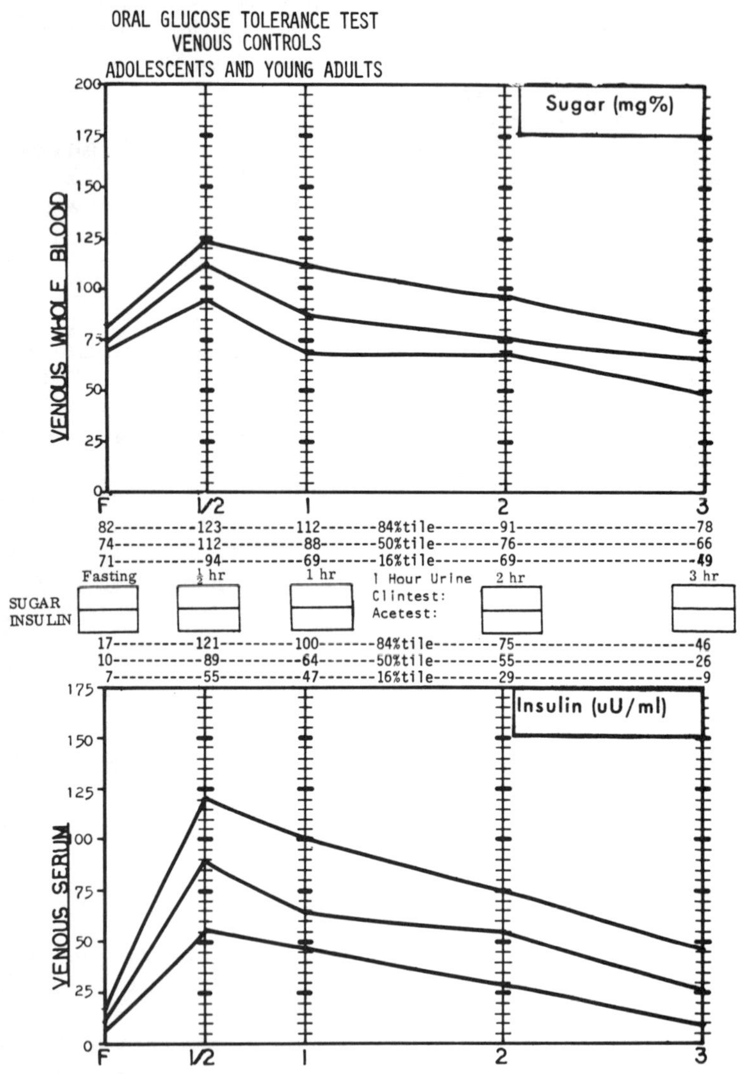

FIGURE 5.6

MEAN CAPILLARY WHOLE BLOOD GLUCOSE VALUES (mg/dl) DURING O.G.T.T.'s
IN NORMAL CHILDREN RECEIVING 1.75 g/kg BY SIX RESEARCH GROUPS
+ 2 S.D.
- 2 S.D.
G L U C O S E mg/dl
150
125
100
75
50
0
1/2
1
2
3
time (hrs.)

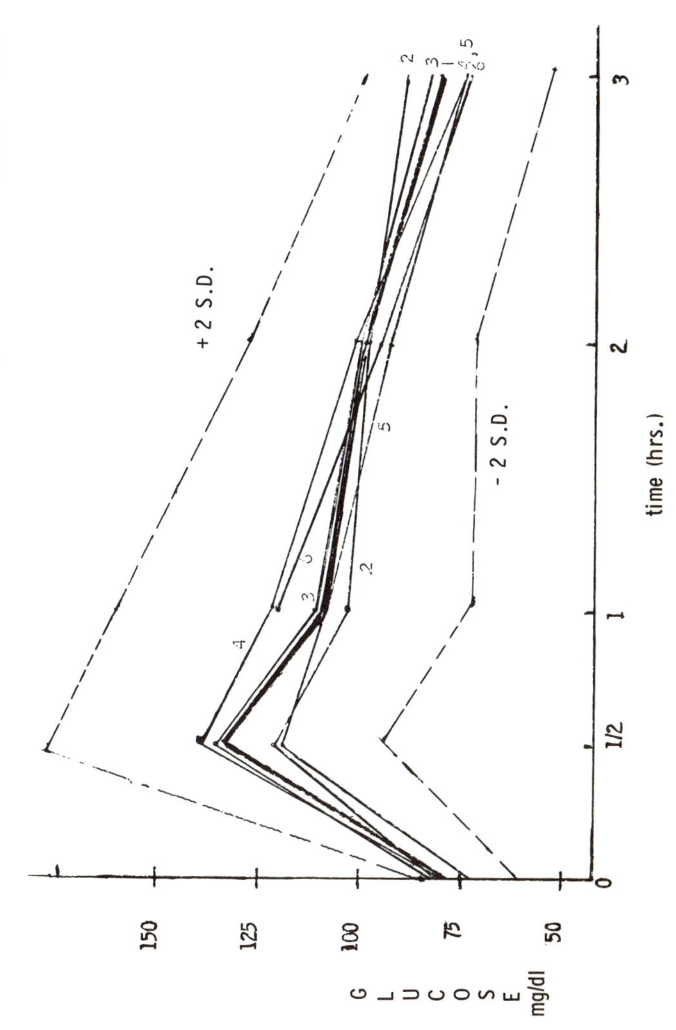

FIGURE 5.7

ORAL GLUCOSE TOLERANCE TEST

The broken line represents the calculated 50th percentile for plasma glucose in adolescents and young adults in our laboratory.

ADOLESCENTS AND YOUNG ADULTS--OUR LAB

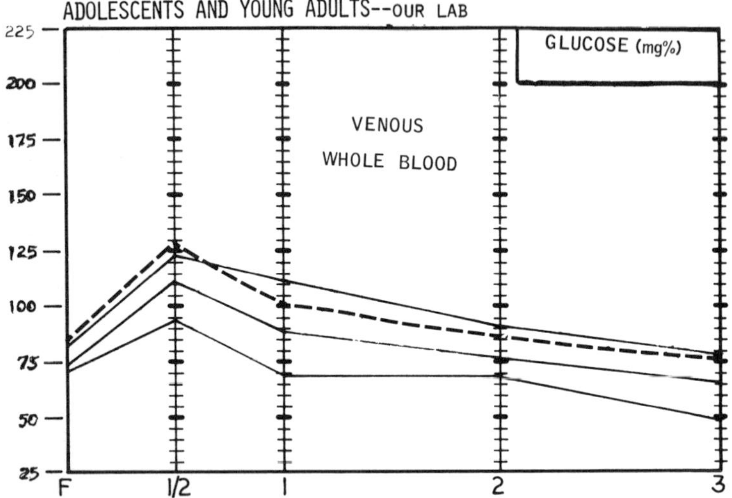

COMPARISON OF OUR PLASMA GLUCOSE VALUES IN ADOLESCENTS AND YOUNG ADULTS WITH THREE OTHER RESEARCH GROUPS

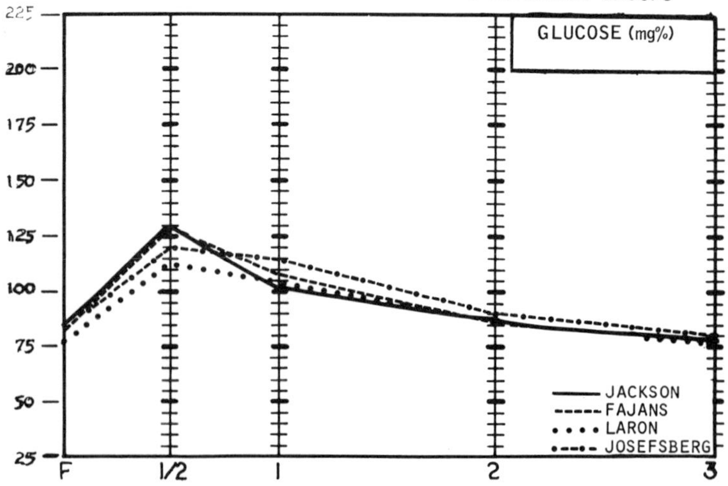

FIGURE 5.8

literature and recommended detailed guidelines for the performance of OGTTs in children. In 1979, Weber and Burger (14) as well as L. Matajc, L. Brus et al. (15) found that either 1.75 g/kg of ideal body weight or 45 g/m^2 are equally well suited as a glucose load in normal children. Comparable mean values for both serum glucose and insulin levels were found using both doses in the same individuals given two OGTTs within 1 to 3 weeks of each other. The heights and weights of all the healthy children studied by both Weber and Matajc were within the normal range for age and sex using Tanner and Iowa growth charts. *On the basis of endogenous insulin response, lower glucose loads have been found insufficient for older children.* (10).

On the basis of the studies selected from the literature and from the extension of our data using comparable procedures, we believe that we now have well-defined guidelines for performing OGTTs and reliable norms for both capillary and venous blood glucose and serum insulin values for children and young adults.

In 1979 the following questions were directed by the National Diabetes Data Group of the U.S.A. National Institute of Health to the Lawson Wilkins (American) Pediatric Endocrine Society (16):

1. What age and sex adjustment, if any, needs to be made for children?
2. What criteria are necessary to make a diagnosis of insulin-dependent diabetes in children and to establish an impaired glucose tolerance in children?

After considerable discussion, the following consensus of opinion was reached by the Lawson Wilkins Pediatric Endocrine Society at their May, 1979 meeting: The greatest divergence of opinion was with the definition and significance of an impaired glucose tolerance:

1. That glucose tolerance testing is not indicated for diagnostic purposes in children with classical symptoms of diabetes and a random reliable and confirmed true whole blood glucose value in excess of 200 mg/dl is diagnostic.

2. That in the child who is asymptomatic a diagnosis of diabetes be restricted to those with a fasting blood glucose ≤ 120 mg/dl for whole blood or ≤ 140 mg/dl for venous plasma and a 2-hour postglucose tolerance test value of ≤ 180 for whole blood or ≤ 200 mg/dl for venous plasma and with an intervening value at or about the 2-hour value on more than one occasion under standard conditions for glucose tolerance testing, i.e., absence of infection, stress such as trauma, drugs known to adversely affect OGTTs and with appropriate dietary preparation including three days of adequate carbohydrate intake. That the dose of glucose given be 1.75 g/kg *ideal* body weight with a maximum of 75 g. *Available evidence indicates no need for age adjustment of glucose responses to OGTT under the conditions outlined above,* despite abundant evidence that the insulin responses do increase with age so that the interpretation of insulin response during OGTTs requires age-adjusted criteria. *That the term impaired glucose tolerance (I.G.T.) be used to replace chemical diabetes.*

3. That, for the present, *I.G.T.* be confined to children with fasting capillary or venous whole blood glucose values < 120 mg/dl or < 140 mg/dl for venous plasma and *in addition* with a 2-hour capillary or whole blood glucose values < 120 mg/dl or < 140 mg/dl for venous plasma.

The criteria finally adopted by the National Diabetes Data Group for the *diagnosis* of overt insulin-dependent diabetes in children will protect children with only questionably abnormal OGTTs from having an unwarranted diagnosis of diabetes. We believe it is inadvisable to classify any child to have an IGT (previously designated as chemical diabetes) on the basis of only one abnormal test regardless of the degree of deviation from the standard curve. We require serial tests to classify a child to have either probable or possible IGT.

Since 1958, whenever possible, we have done OGTTs on the siblings of the children in our clinic with overt insulin-dependent diabetes (17). We have found that about 13% of the post-pubescent siblings have some glucose and/or insulin values outside the normal range. Only occasional prepubescent children have been found to have an IGT during intercurrent infections (18). A few younger and older siblings with high-glucose and low-insulin values have developed overt diabetes in a relatively short period of time. Many of the adolescent siblings have had less deviant tests after their period of rapid growth. To our knowledge, none of the siblings with only elevated insulin levels has developed overt insulin-dependent diabetes in early adult life. We believe additional longitudinal research studies of siblings of patients with type I diabetes are needed to reexamine the criteria and indications for doing OGTTs and islet cell antibody determinations. These studies are needed to help elucidate the natural pattern of development and the clinical course of type I diabetes and to determine if insulin replacement during periods of stress might be indicated before the onset of overt diabetes. The ability of children who receive prompt insulin replacement soon after the onset of symptoms to restore and preserve beta cell function (19), and the declining rate of insulin release after a glucose load in siblings with impaired glucose tolerance suggests that transient insulin replacement may be indicated.

REFERENCES

1. Bilginturan, H. N., and Jackson, R. L.: Transient hyperglycemia in infancy and childhood. *Clin. Ped.* 17:338-342, 1978.

2. Guthrie, R. A., Murthy, D. Y. N., Jackson, R. L., and Lang, L.: Standardization of the oral glucose tolerance test and the criteria for diagnosis of chemical diabetes in children. *Metabolism* 22:275-282, 1973.

3. Jackson, R. L., and Kelly, H. G.: Growth chart for use in pediatric practice. *J. Ped.* 27:215-229, 1945.

4. Pickens, J. M., Burkeholder, J. N., and Womack, W. N.: Oral glucose tolerance tests in normal children. *Diabetes* 16:11-14, 1967.

5. Sachsse, R.: Standardization of the oral glucose tolerance test. International Study Group on Diabetes in Children and Adolescents, *Bulletin* 2:24, 1978.

6. Drash, A. L.: Diabetes mellitus. In Nelson: *Textbook of Pediatrics,* 10th ed., W.B. Saunders Co., Philadelphia, 1975, pp. 1259-1271.

7. Knopf, C. F., Cresto, J. H., Dujovne, I. L., Ramos, O., and De Majo, S. F.: Oral glucose tolerance test in 100 normal children. *ACTA Diabetol.* Lat. 14:95, 1977.

8. Cole, H. S., and Bilder, J. G.: Capillary blood sugar values in infants and children during oral glucose tolerance tests. *Diabetes* 19:176-181, 1970.

9. Josefberg, A., Vilunski, E., Hanukuglu, A., Bialik, O., Borwn, M., Karp, M., and Laron, Z.: Glucose and insulin responses to an oral glucose load in normal children and adolescents in Israel. *Isr J Med Sci* 12:189-194, 1976.

10. Weber, B.: Standardization of the oral glucose tolerance test. International Study Group on Diabetes in Children and Adolescents, *Bulletin* 2:23, 1978.

11. Balsam, M. J., Kaye, R., and Baker, L.: Chemical diabetes in children: Glucose tolerance tests. *Metabolism* 22:283-287, 1973.

12. Theodoridis, C. G., Brown, G. A., Chance, G. W., and Tayner, P. H. W.: Growth-hormone response to oral glucose in children with simple obesity. *Lancet* 1:1068-1069, 1969.

13. Fajans, S., Personal communication, 1978.

14. Weber, B., and Burger, W.: Standardization of the oral glucose tolerance test. International Study Group on Diabetes in Children and Adolescents, *Bulletin* 3:7, 1979.

15. Matajc, L., Brus, L., Krzisnik, C., and Zemva, Z.: Glycaemia and insulinaemia during oral glucose tolerance test using various glucose loads. International Study Group on Diabetes in Children and Adolescents, *Bulletin* 3:7, 1979.

16. National Diabetes Data Group. Classification and diagnosis of diabetes mellitus and other categories of glucose intolerance. *Diabetes* 28:1039-1057, 1979.

17. Burkeholder, J. N., Pickens, J. M., and Womack, W. N.: Oral glucose tolerance test in siblings of children with diabetes mellitus. *Diabetes* 16:156-160, 1967.

18. Jackson, R. L., and Waiches, H.: *Do infectious agents cause diabetes mellitus:* International Beilinson Juvenile Diabetes Symposium. S. Karger, New York, 394-398, 1977.

19. Jackson, R. L., Bilgenturin, N. A., Terry, C. W., and Hewitt, J. E.: Beta cell function. *J. Kansas Med. Soc.* 84:321-330, Nov. 1, 1983.

B. PARTIAL REMISSION PERIOD*

Robert L. Jackson, M.D.

The exogenous insulin requirement of most children with recent onset of diabetes decreased rapidly and predictably to a relatively low level (0.15-0.40 U/kg/day) when prompt physiologic insulin treatment is given (1-3). This state of partial remission (honeymoon period) occurs but once, except in rare cases, and persists for a variable period of time. In 1971, we reviewed the records of 63 children with recent onset of diabetes to compare responses of children with early diagnosis and prompt insulin replacement with the responses of children

---

*This subchapter is a modification of a previous publication, "Beta Cell Function", by R.L. Jackson, Nihat A. Bilginturan, M.D., Carolyn W. Terry, M.D., and John E. Hewett, Ph.D., published in the *Journal of the Kansas Medical Society,* June 1983. Reproduced with permission from the *Journal of the Kansas Medical Society.*

with delayed diagnosis and treatment (4). We found that the earlier the diagnosis was made and insulin was given, the lower the maintenance insulin requirement and the easier it was to attain and maintain a high degree of metabolic control with minimal risk of hypoglycemia. When parents continued the treatment plan at home, partial remission persisted for as long as 4–5 years. In 1978, we reviewed the records of an additional 90 children under continuous care in our clinic since onset of diabetes who had remained in a high degree of control. After stabilization, the insulin requirement of these children, 7–12 years of age, was 0.16–0.42 (mean 0.32) U/kg/day. Forty-four remained in partial remission (i.e.. required less than 0.60 U/kg/day to maintain aglycosuria and to permit normal growth) for 4–60 (mean 26) months; 40 at the time of their last observations were still in partial remission for 8–42 months; and the other six were older children in their growth spurt who required from 0.64 to 0.68 U/kg/day after stabilization. We also have observed that the maintenance insulin requirements for adolescents who have completed their growth spurt before the onset of diabetes is lower and extends for longer periods of time than for younger children, as reported by Madsbad et al. (5).

Until the recent development of the C-peptide assay, there was no precise method available to determine endogenous insulin secretion. Previous studies were based on histologic examination of the pancreases obtained from patients, most of whom died in the initial coma or after more than 10 years after onset of their disease. These studies proved that the total islet cell mass is invariably reduced (6). Wrenshall (7) correlated the extractable insulin of the pancreas with pathologic and clinical findings in diabetic and nondiabetic subjects. He found that the insulin-dependent diabetics had very low values as compared with the nondiabetic control subjects, but that a few long-standing diabetics continued to have some extractable insulin.

When the insulin radioimmunoassay became available, studies of patients with insulin-dependent diabetes in remission demonstrated the presence of endogenous insulin secretion, but at a low level (8). Highly developed immunocytochemical staining methods also revealed the presence of beta cells in most patients with insulin-dependent diabetes at the time of onset of their disease (9).

The recent development of a more sensitive laboratory method to measure C-peptide levels (as low as 0.10 ng/ml) made it possible to observe the beta cell secretory capacity of the pancreas during the course of insulin-dependent diabetes. C peptide is cleaved from proinsulin during its conversion to insulin and is secreted by the beta cell in equimolar amounts with insulin. C peptide provides an accurate index of endogenous insulin. Rubenstein and Gonen (10) and Gonen et al. (11) reviewed the literature and published C-peptide studies of children and young adults with insulin-dependent diabetes. Assessment of pancreatic insulin reserve was done by measuring C-peptide levels after stimulation by either the ingestion of a meal or intravenous injection of 1 mg of glucagon. Hendrickson, Faber, Dryer, and Binder (12) found an increase above fasting C-peptide levels at 1 and 2 hr in response to both of these challenges in 64 insulin-dependent diabetic subjects and a significant correlation between the magnitude of the response and the fasting C-peptide level. Faber and Binder (13) also found that the diabetic subjects with the highest fasting C-peptide concentrations had the lowest exogenous insulin requirements and a more stable metabolic status. Ludvigsson and Heding (14) did serial fasting C-peptide determinations on 12 diabetic children for almost 1 year after the time of diagnosis. At the time of diagnosis all subjects had very low but measurable fasting C-peptide values. At about 1 month after insulin replacement therapy, all of them had higher fasting C-peptide values. During the subsequent 9 months with semiconventional management there was a steady decrease in C-peptide levels with values below the normal range except in one of the children. An index of metabolic control was calculated from home records of fractional urinary glucose analysis. A significant correlation was found between C-peptide levels and the diabetic control index in the children who received more intense treatment. These findings indicate that more intense therapy may prolong pancreatic islet cell function. Gonen et al. (11), using HbA_{1c} levels, have confirmed these observations. They found that nonobese insulin-dependent diabetic subjects with fasting C-peptide concentrations above 0.1 pmol/ml (0.29 ng/ml) had significantly better metabolic control than did those with lower values. They also found that patients with onset after 20 years of age had higher fasting C-peptide values and higher values after stimulation. They postulated that good metabolic control may contribute to the preservation of insulin secretory capacity and concluded that additional studies are needed to resolve this important question. Mirouze et al. (15), by means of an external artificial pancreas, also have recently demonstrated that the institution of control shortly after the diagnosis of diabetes is associated with enhanced preservation of beta cell function. During the period of partial remission we have not found it necessary to use insulin infusion pumps to attain and maintain essentially physiologic control.

For children with insulin-dependent diabetes, we define insulin requirements to be that amount of exogenous insulin per unit of normal body weight required daily to maintain aglycosuria and approximate normal blood glucose levels when the child is ingesting adequate calories and essential nutrients to permit normal growth and avoid excessive weight gain.

By extensive clinical experience we have found that if the diabetic child receives early and adequate insulin replacement therapy, the exogenous insulin requirement after nutritional repletion usually will remain relatively constant from day to day. We also have found that the rate of increasing insulin requirement is usually predictable and intimately interrelated with the normal increase in body weight for height and the normal growth and maturation pattern of children, as well as the effectiveness of the plan of treatment in maintaining a high degree of metabolic control (16). *By years of trial and error, we have observed that as long as the insulin requirement remains less than about 0.70 U/kg/day, it is not only possible but also practicable to maintain an essentially euglycemic state with freedom from glycosuria and hypoglycemic episodes.*

However, when the exogenous insulin requirement begins to exceed about 0.70–0.80 U/kg/day, we have found it necessary to modify our objective of management to a slightly lower degree of control. At this time we reinstruct the parents and children to accept minimal transient glycosuria to widen the threshold of safety for preventing hypoglycemia. The recent studies of Liljenquist et al. (17) have confirmed our assumption that a slight overdosage of exogenous insulin, during the period of partial remission, would be compensated for by suppression of endogenous insulin. These authors demonstrated inhibition of endogenous insulin in normal men by use of the C-peptide assay.

We recently assessed pancreatic beta-cell function in 60 children with diabetes maintained in a high degree of metabolic control documented by HbA_{1c} determinations (18). Fasting and 1- and 2-hr postprandial serum glucose and C-peptide levels were determined after a 10-hr overnight fast and after the ingestion of a standard liquid breakfast. Ten normal nonobese children and adolescents (five girls and five boys) had a standardized Sustacal tolerance test as a control group. All of these control subjects previously had had normal serum glucose and insulin concentrations during oral glucose tolerance tests with values between the 84th and 16th percentiles. The mean C-peptide, insulin, and glucose values of these ten healthy control subjects are depicted in Figure 5.9 and the mean $\pm$ 1 SD values also are recorded in the caption. The closely similar curves for C peptide and insulin with a very narrow excursion of blood sugar values are demonstrated.

Figure 5.10 depicts the mean fasting, 1- and 2-hr postprandial C-peptide values of 11 children after regulation of diabetes for less than 1 month and after 1 to 6 months when they had attained nutritional repletion and a stable insulin requirement.

A Sustacal tolerance test was also done in an 8-year-old diabetic girl before she received insulin replacement therapy. Three weeks before admission to our clinic this child, during an upper respiratory infection, was seen by her family physician. At this time she was found to have glycosuria with a fasting blood glucose values of 134 mg/100 ml and a 2-hr postprandial value of 245 mg/100 ml. Although her symptoms diminished and her urine became sugar free within a few days, she was referred to our clinic for evaluation and management. At the time of admission to the medical center she had glucosuria of 1% during a standard oral glucose tolerance test with a high normal fasting blood glucose level but the 30 min, 1-, and 2-hr glucose values all were more than 2 SD above mean values for normal girls. Her serum insulin levels also were more than 1 SD below mean values for normal girls. A Sustacal tolerance test was done the day after the oral glucose tolerance test and just prior to the initiation of insulin replacement therapy. The test was repeated 3 months later after she had remained in physiologic control with an insulin requirement of less than 0.3 U/kg/day. Results of the tests done before and after treatment are

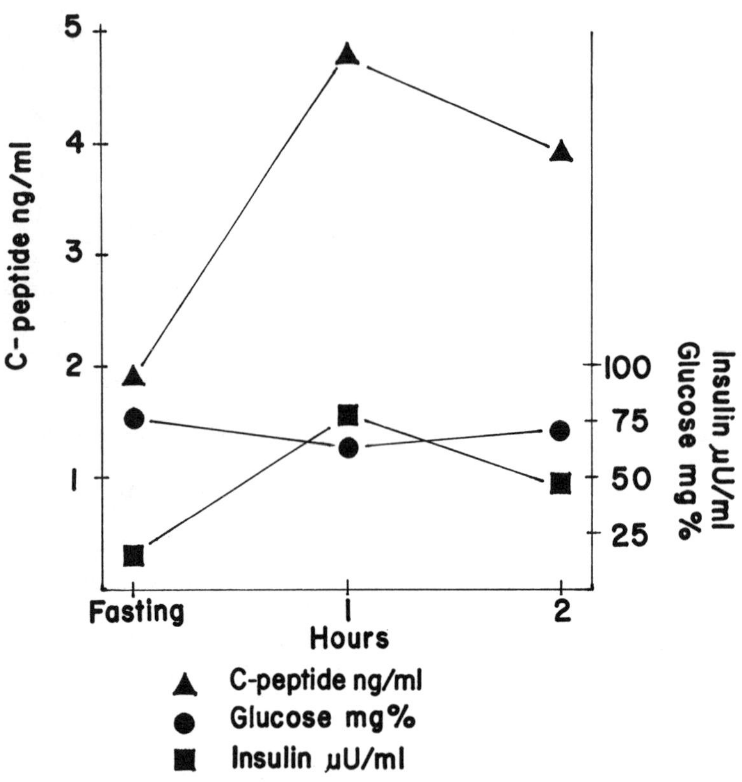

FIGURE 5.9 Mean fasting, 1- and 2-hr C-peptide, insulin, and glucose values of ten healthy control subjects with no family history of diabetes and with normal oral glucose tolerance tests. The mean ± SD fasting, 1- and 2-hr C-peptide values (ng/ml) were: 1.95 ± 0.8, 4.8 ± 1.6, and 3.0 ± 1.6.

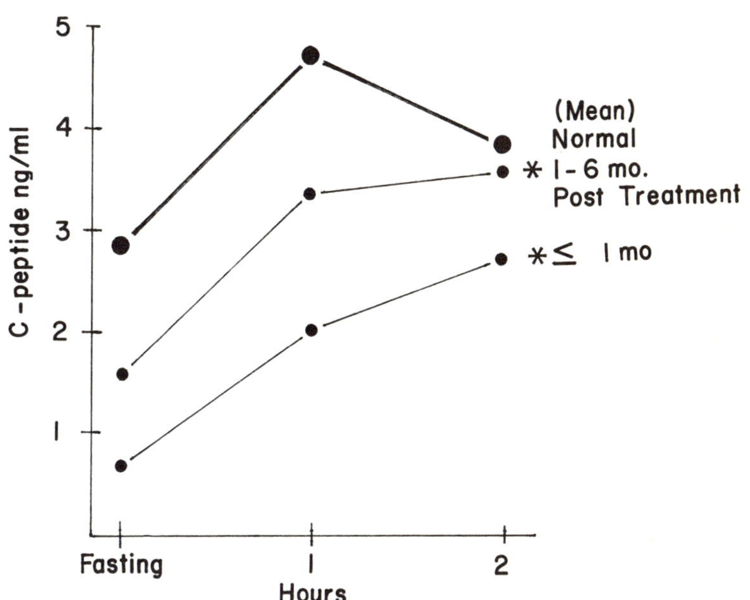

FIGURE 5.10 Mean fasting, 1- and 2-hr postprandial C-peptide values of children with recent onset after regulation of diabetes for less than 1 month and after 1 to 6 months.

depicted in Figure 5.11. This confirms that the pancreas may recuperate some secretory abilities under good metabolic control.

Table 5.1 summarizes the clinical and laboratory data of the diabetic subjects. The subjects are subdivided on the basis of their daily insulin requirement expressed as U/kg/day. Figure 5.12 demonstrates the consistent progressive decrease in C-peptide levels as the exogenous insulin requirement increases.

The availability of a reliable and sensitive C-peptide assay offers the opportunity of undertaking additional systematic animal and human studies to extend our knowledge of how to prevent destruction, to promote regeneration, and to preserve function of beta cells in insulin-dependent diabetic subjects.

REFERENCES

1. Jackson, R. L., and Boyd, J. D.: 1940 stabilization of the diabetic child. *Am. J. Dis. Child.* 59:332-341.

2. Jackson, R. L., Guthrie, R. A., and Murthy, D.: 1977 clinical course of diabetes in children. In: *Diabetes in Children,* S. Karger (Ed.), New York, pp. 22-23.

3. Ludvigsson, H., and Heding, L. G.: 1978 Beta cell function in children with diabetes. *Diabetes* 27 (Suppl. 1): 230–244, 1978.

4. Jackson, R. L., Onofrio, J., Waiches, H., and Guthrie, R. A.: The honeymoon period: Partial remission of juvenile diabetes mellitus. *Diabetes* 20 (Suppl. 2):361, 1971.

5. Madsbad, F., Faber, O. K., Biner, C., McNair, P., Christiansen, D., and Transbol, I.: Prevalance of residual beta cell function in insulin-dependent diabetes in relation to age at onset and duration of diabetes. *Diabetes* 27 (Suppl. 1):260–262, 1978.

6. Gepts, W.: Pathologic anatomy of the pancreas in juvenile diabetes mellitus. *Diabetes* 14:619–632, 1965.

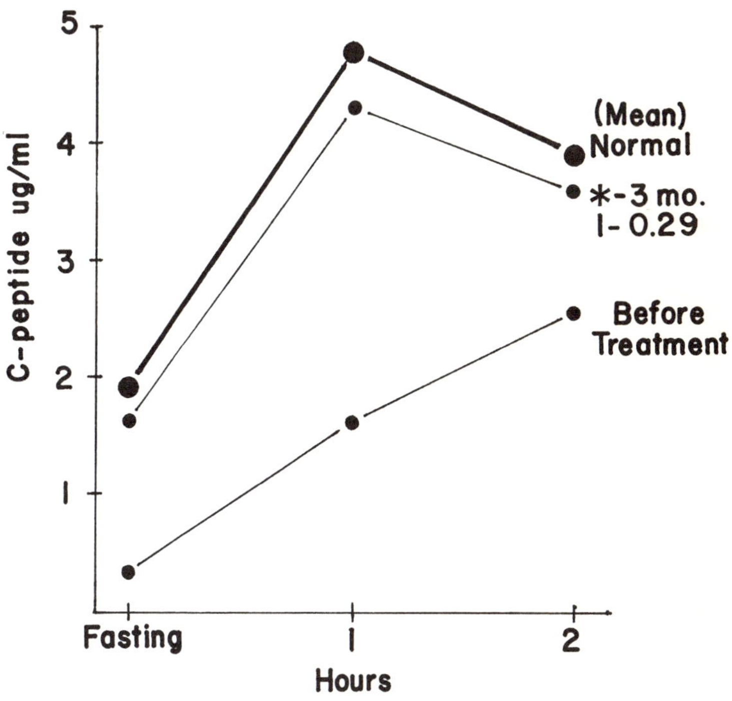

FIGURE 5.11 Note the low fasting C-peptide value and delayed response to the ingestion of food at the time of diagnosis and the approximately normal response after maintaining metabolic control for 3 months, reflecting restoration of B-cell function.

TABLE 5.1 Clinical and Laboratory Data of Diabetic Children Maintained in High Degree of Metabolic Control Subdivided on Basis of Exogenous Insulin Requirement

Insulin requirement U/kg/day	< 0.30	0.30–0.40	0.40–0.50	0.50–0.60	0.60–0.70	0.70–0.80	> 0.80
No. of subjects	18	17	11	10	10	11	12
	* +						
Age at onset years	10.7 7/16	11.0 9/16	11.0 9/12	10.0 5/15	9.0 7/15	9.9 4/15	10.8 7/14
Duration years	0.9 0.1/2.1	0.7 0.1/4.3	1.0 0.1/2.3	1.6 0.9/3.8	2.4 1.0/4.3	2.4 0.9/4.6	3.8 0.5/4.6
Insulin/kg/day	0.21 0.10/0.29	0.34 0.34/0.39	0.44 0.40/0.47	0.57 0.50/0.59	0.65 0.62/0.68	0.75 0.70/0.79	0.94 0.84/1.14
% HbA_1C	5.6 4.2/7.1	6.7 4.6/8.6	6.9 4.5/8.5	6.4 5.2/7.3	5.8 4.8/7.2	6.7 5.2/8.6	7.4 6.4/8.6
Fasting C peptide	1.70±0.78	1.54±0.64	1.39±0.53	1.33±0.40	1.08±0.23	0.80±0.41	0.65±0.33
1-hr C peptide	3.63±1.15	3.16±1.16	2.50±0.90	1.89±0.71	1.91±0.86	1.23±0.62	0.96±0.42
2-hr C peptide	3.43±1.09	3.35±1.06	2.57±1.04	2.37±0.79	1.82±0.60	1.32±0.68	0.83±0.45

*Mean
+Range
±1 SD

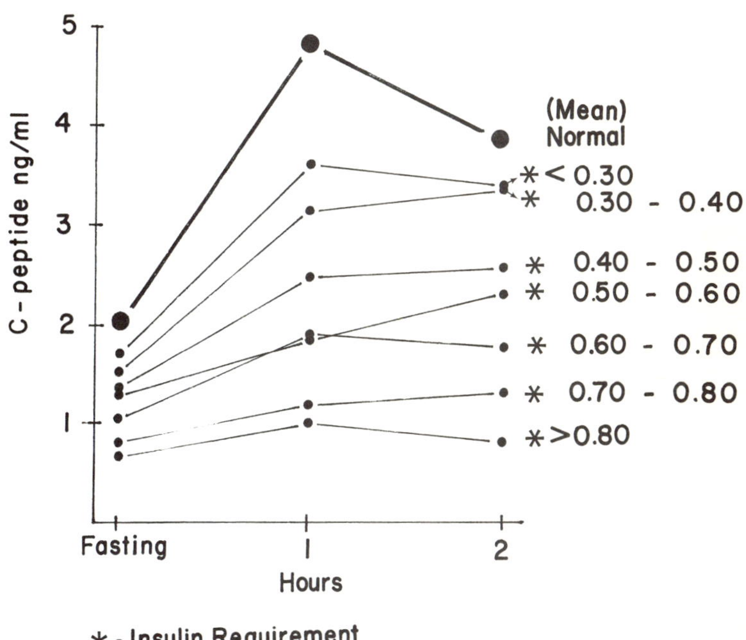

FIGURE 5.12 Consistent, progressive decrease in fasting and postprandial C-peptide levels with increasing exogenous insulin requirement in groups of well-controlled diabetic children. The rate of C-peptide release is also decreased as the insulin requirement increased.

7. Wrenshall, G. A., Bogoch, A., and Ritchie, R. C.: Extractable insulin of pancreas: Correlation with pathological and clinical findings in diabetic and nondiabetic cases. *Diabetes* 1:87-107, 1952.

8. Johansen, K., and Orskov, J.: Plasma insulin during remission in juvenile diabetes mellitus. *Br. Med. J.* 1:676-682, 1969.

9. Gepts, W., and De Mey, J.: Islet cell survival determined by morphology: An immuno-cytochemical study of the islets of Langerhans in juvenile diabetes mellitus. *Diabetes* 27 (Suppl. 1):251-261, 1978.

10. Rubenstein, A. H., and Gonen, B.: Clinical significance of C-peptide. *Ad. Exp. Med. Biol.* 124:15-19, 1979.

11. Gonen, B., Boldman, J., Baldwin, D., Goldberg, R., Tyan, W., Blix, P., Schanzlin, D., Fritz, L., and Rubenstein, H.; Metabolic control in diabetes patients: Effects of insulin secretory reserve (measured by plasma C-peptide levels) and circulating insulin antibodies. *Diabetes* 28:749-754, 1979.

12. Hendrickson, C., Faber, O. K., Dryer, T., and Binder, C. L.: Prevalence of residual beta cell function in insulin treated diabetes evaluated by the C-peptide response to intravenous glucagen. *Diabetologia* 13:280-288, 1977.

13. Faber, O. K., and Binder, C.: Beta cell function and blood glucose control in insulin-dependent diabetic within the first month of insulin treatment. *Diabetoligia* 13:263-271, 1977.

14. Ludvigsson, H., and Heding, L. G.: Beta cell function in children with diabetes. *Diabetes* 27 (Suppl. 1):230-244, 1978.

15. Mirouze, J., Salem, J. L., Pham, T. C.. Mendoza, E., and Orsetti, A.: Insulin-induced remission of juvenile diabetes by means of an external artificial pancreas. *Diabetologia* 14:223-227, 1978.

16. Jackson, R. L., Holland, E., Chatman, I. D., Guthrie, D., and Hewett, J. E.: Growth and maturation of a child with insulin-dependent diabetes mellitus. *Diabetes Care,* 1(2):96-107, 1978.

17. Liljenquist, M. D., Horowitz, D. L., Jennings, A. S.; Chiasson, J., Kellery, U., and Rubenstein, A. H.: Inhibition of insulin secretion by exogenous insulin in normal man as demonstrated by C-peptide assay. *Diabetes* 27:563-569, 1978.

18. Jackson, R. L., Bilginturan, N. A., Terry, C. W., and Hewat, J. E.: Beta cell function. *J. Kansas Med. Soc.* 84:321-353, 1983.

19. Guthrie, R. A., Murthy, D. Y. N., Jackson, R. L., and Lang, L.: Standardization of the oral glucose tolerance test and criteria for diagnosis of chemical diabetes in children. *Metabolism* 22:275-283, 1973.

Chapter 6

TREATMENT AND MANAGEMENT

A. INTRODUCTION

Robert L. Jackson, M.D.

The child with overt diabetes has hypoinsulinism so severe that he cannot survive without exogenous insulin. As stated before, we believe that every child with overt diabetes should receive insulin therapy as soon as the diagnosis is confirmed. Emergency treatment for ketoacidosis preferably may be done in a local hospital by an experienced family physician or pediatrician before referring the child to a diabetic treatment and education center.

The exogenous insulin requirement will vary depending upon how early the diagnosis is made and how soon insulin is given. The earlier the diagnosis is made, the lower the insulin requirement and the easier it will be to attain and maintain a high degree of control with little risk of hypoglycemia.

Replacement therapy should be designed to maintain a state as physiologic as possible, both to permit normal growth and development and to delay or prevent the insidious development of fascular complications. To attain that objective, the parents and, ultimately, the child must learn how to adjust insulin dosage and food intake to control the child's glycosuria, yet allow him to participate fully in all activities of his peer group without fear of an insulin reaction. The task is not easy. It requires understanding, judgment, self-discipline, and acceptance of the concept of maintaining optimum health so as to avoid the need for intensive treatment or periodic episodes of ketosis. The parents have to teach these basic principles to their child by example.

Continuity of care by the health team is necessary for the parents to learn those principles. The plan of treatment must be clear-cut and flexible and must provide a threshold of safety as wide as is practical. Members of the health team must be in agreement about treatment to avoid giving conflicting advice to the parents or child.

As stated in the introduction, children with overt diabetes should be admitted to a hospital, preferably a pediatric unit, not only for the treatment of acute complications such as ketoacidosis but also to establish nutritional status, to determine the maintenance insulin requirement, to explore and identify difficult psychosocial areas, and to educate both the parents and the child. To attain these goals, the undernourished diabetic child with recent onset of diabetes requires hospital care for about 3 weeks. The pediatric unit should have a school and recreational facilities so the child can continue his education and have structured physical activity.

In contrast to the child with recent onset of diabetes, the child with total diabetes, admitted to the hospital to attain a higher degree of control of his diabetes, will not have a period of partial remission; consequently, a shorter period of hospital care is required. If such a child is undernourished, he will need a somewhat higher caloric intake and insulin dosage until his nutritional stores are repleted and a normal growth rate is reestablished. The daily insulin requirement for children with total diabetes is about 0.7-1.5 U/kg/day. Children with total diabetes should be admitted to the hospital for 1-2 weeks to determine insulin and caloric requirements and to educate the parents and child how to continue the program at home. It is generally fruitless to attempt either that education or modification of a treatment program outside the hospital.

Time spent in the hospital for regulation of a child with recent onset of diabetes can be divided into three periods. The first period, usually only a few days in length, is characterized by rapid clinical improvement. During this time, complications such as acidosis are treated and a regimen is established to control ketonuria and gross glycosuria. Within a few days the well-contrilled patient will be ambulatory, free from symptoms, cating well, and gaining weight. The urine will have become free from acetone and essentially glucose free, and a close approximation of the insulin dosage will have been established. The second period, of about 2 weeks, can be described as one of metabolic recovery. During this time, the patient's insulin requirement in relation to food intake gradually decreases from day to day. and the child's nutritional status improves markedly. Careful supervision of physical activity food intake, and insulin dosage is needed to control glycosuria and avoid insulin reactions. The insulin and caloric requirements become relatively constant as the nutritional status approaches normal, provided the pattern of physical activity is relatively constant each day. The third and final period is one in which the patient's insulin and food requirements becomc stable.

The frequent occurrence of insulin reactions and recurrence of glycosuria from overtreatment of hypoglycemia have discouraged many doctors from attempting to attain physiologic control during the recovery period. Consequently, many children return home after only a week or 10 days of hospital care to receive a once-daily injection of insulin and a diabetic meal plan.

Figure 6.1 illustrates the typical response to treatment in our clinic of a child with diabetes of recent onset. Degree of glycosuria represents the average qualitative values of the four daily fractional urine specimens. Blood glucose values are those of the mean, maximum, and minimum of eight blood samples obtained at specific times during a 24-hr period. These diurnal observations demonstrate to medical students and house officers that physiologic (excellent) control of blood glucose throughout the entire 24 hr is attainable. A few days before the child goes home from the hospital, the parents and child should assume primary responsibility for meal plans, insulin administration, urine and blood glucose tests, and keeping a daily home record (Figure 6.2).

When the diagnosis of diabetes is made or confirmed, the parents and child need emotional support from the family doctor. Parents need assurance that their child's condition can be treated effectively and that they can look forward to having a healthy child again in a few weeks — a child who

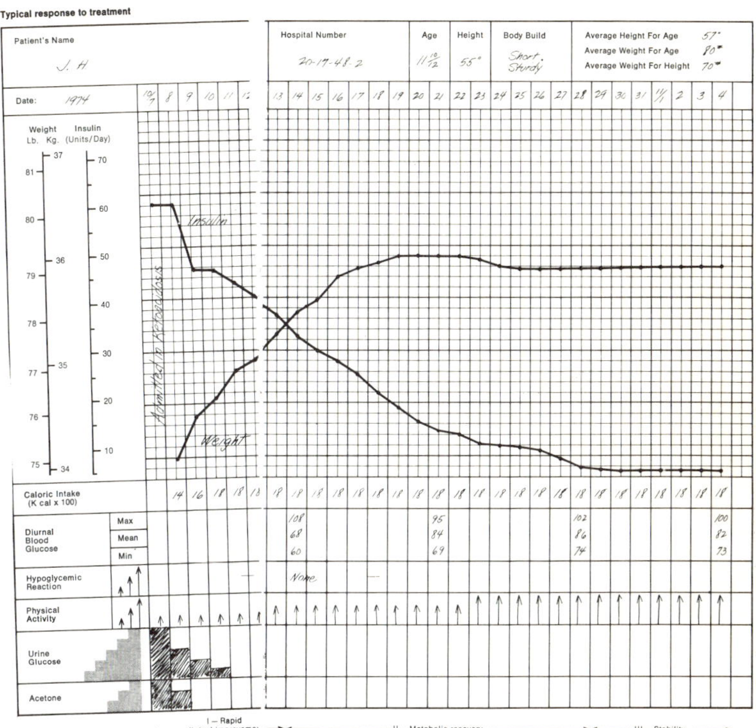

FIGURE 6.1 Typical responses to treatment.

can grow and develop normally. This is a very important role for the family physician. As soon as the child is admitted to the hospital, the pediatrician, as director of the team, should have an educational conference with the parents to confirm the assurance given to them by the family physician. Parents also need to be told that it will take a few days for them to become adjusted to the reality of the situation, as it has been for other parents when they were faced with the same situation. At this time the roles of the various members of the health team are explained. The team should consist of a pediatrician, a nurse specialist, a dietitian,

HOME RECORD

Date	Day	Insulin:		Urine Tests:				Exercise:			Food:			Comments:
		AM	PM	AM	N	PM	EV	AM	PM	EV	AM	PM	EV	
	S													
	M													
	T													
	W													
	T													
	F													
	S													

Past week evaluation and Questions. Next week's plan.

Date	Day	Insulin:		Urine Tests:				Exercise:			Food:			Comments:
		AM	PM	AM	N	PM	EV	AM	PM	EV	AM	PM	EV	
	S													
	M													
	T													
	W													
	T													
	F													
	S													

Past week evaluation and Questions. Next week's plan.

FIGURE 6.2 Home record.

and a medical social worker. At this conference we also explain why the child needs to remain in the hospital for a few weeks. The parents must understand that with daily improvement in the child's nutritional status, the insulin requirement will decrease until the condition becomes stable enough for them to feel confident to continue the management at home. We also explain that by the time the child is ready to go home, only two small daily doses of insulin will be needed and that by dividing the daily dose the child will be protected from the likelihood of insulin reactions. An introductory section of an instruction manual including only limited, basic, reassuring information is given to the parents. The parents then are asked to read the manual independently and discuss the contents with each other. After a few days, most parents are ready for an intensive educational program under the direction of a physician with the help of the nurse specialist and the dietitian. During the first few days, the medical social worker provides additional emotional support and helps the parents make arrangements for meeting the child's and their needs. We prefer to have one of the parents remain with the child during the first days of rapid clinical improvement to provide emotional support. Arrangements need to be made for both parents to be available for instruction as outlined in Chapter 7.

B. PATHOPHYSIOLOGY OF DIABETIC KETOACIDOSIS

Wayne V. Moore, M.D. and
Teresa M. Clabots, M.D.

Insulin and glucagon serve as a bihormonal control system in the development of ketoacidosis. Recent evidence suggests that a simple deficiency of insulin is not sufficient to explain the metabolic derangements that take place in diabetic ketoacidosis (DKA) (1). It is now obvious that the ketogenesis and hyperglycemia classically associated with insulin deficiency are due not only to an absolute or relative decrease in the amount of insulin but also to an absolute or relative increase in an important counterregulatory hormone, glucagon (2). The insulin/glucagon ratio may actually be more important than the absolute levels of each hormone (2). The other counterregulatory hormones, cortisol, growth hormone, and catecholamines, also play a facilitatory role. Insulin's major action is to transport glucose into the cell, especially fat and liver cells, for the synthesis of fatty acids from glucose. In the liver, insulin stimulates glycogen synthesis and inhibits gluconeogenesis and glycogenolysis. In adipose tissue, insulin inhibits lipolysis. In muscle, insulin enhances glucose uptake and utilization and protein synthesis while inhibiting proteolysis. Overall, the absence of insulin results in decreased glucose utilization, lipolysis (with increased circulating free fatty acids), proteolysis, and gluconeogenesis. In contrast to the actions of insulin, glucagon exerts its major effect in the liver, where it stimulates gluconeogenesis and ketogenesis and inhibits glycolysis. In the normal individual the interaction between these metabolic pathways forms a system by which the blood glucose is maintained within the normal range. However, in the pathologic state of relative or absolute insulin deficiency with glucagon excess, the metabolic pathways are interrupted, resulting in decreased glucose utilization, gluconeogenesis, glycogenolysis, and ketogenesis. These processes, if not reversed, result in the syndrome of diabetic ketoacidosis.

The insulin deficiency results in an *intra*cellular hypoglycemia due to decreased intracellular transport of glucose. This causes the alpha cells of the pancreatic islets to increase glucagon secretion. Glucagon-enhanced gluconeogenesis in the liver exacerbates the elevation of the blood sugar due to decreased utilization and the characteristic hyperglycemia of DKA.

The hyperosmotic state leads to additional important changes. The hyperglycemia results in glycosuria when the renal threshold for glucose is exceeded and an osmotic diuresis with the attendant loss of fluid and electrolytes (Na, K) in the urine and volume depletion, thus causing thirst and dehydration. Over time, calories lost in glycosuria cause starvation and weight loss in the face of increased food intake. If the dehydration is acute, the hyperosmotic state also results in fluid shifts from tissues such as the brain, resulting in varying degrees of central nervous system depression.

The ketogenesis occurring in the ketoacidosis results primarily from increased oxidation of the free fatty acids. These are delivered to the liver after fat tissue is broken down into triglycerides because of the lack of insulin. In the nonstarving state, ketone body formation is suppressed by inhibition of carnitine acyltransferase I by malonyl-CoA, where malonyl-CoA is the first committed intermediate leading from glucose through glycolysis to fatty acid synthesis (2). Carnitine acyltransferase I converts fatty acyl-CoA to fatty acylcarnitine, which is transported across the mitochondrial membrane as a substrate for oxidation (Figure 6.3).

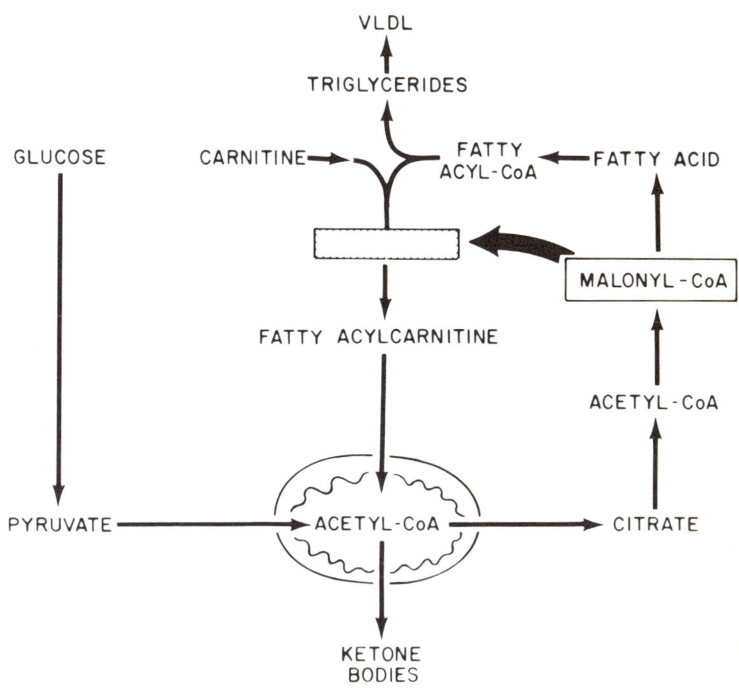

FIGURE 6.3 Interrelations between the pathways of fatty acid synthesis and oxidation in liver. (Reproduced from Ref. 2 by copyright permission of the author.)

In a state of intracellular starvation such as diabetes, the glucose concentrations in the cell are decreased, leading to decreased glycolysis and subsequent decreased formation of malonyl-CoA. Glucagon also inhibits glycolysis in the liver and may cause further suppression of malonyl-CoA levels in diabetes. Without the inhibitory effect of malonyl-CoA, the carnitine acyltransferase I activity is increased and the transport of fatty acids into the mitochondria is enhanced (Figure 6.4). The primary oxidation of the fatty acids in the mitochondria leads to the profound ketogenesis that occurs in diabetic ketoacidosis. Interestingly, ketosis suppresses mobilization of gluconeogenic amino acids from the muscle and may lead to sparing of muscle protein. The ketones and ketoacids (acetoacetate, betahydroxybutyrate, and acetone) are formed at a rate faster than they can be metabolized in the

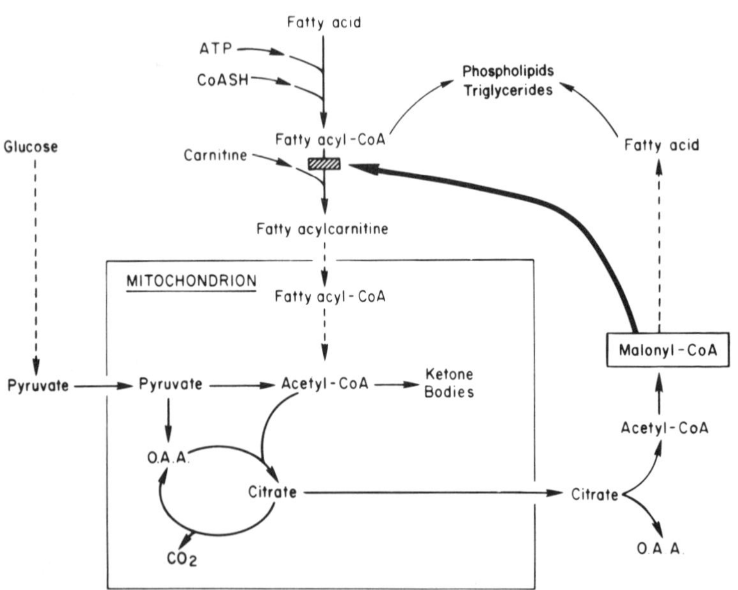

FIGURE 6.4 Interrelations between fatty acid biosynthesis, fatty acid oxidation, and ketogenesis in liver. (Reproduced from Ref. 21 by copyright permission of the author.)

body by the TCA cycle and accumulate in the blood, resulting in ketonemia, and are excreted in the urine, resulting in ketonuria.

The production of the ketones acetoacetate and betahydroxybutyrate also results in the production of hydrogen ions and causes a metabolic acidosis that requires buffering in the extracellular fluids and urine (except for acetone, which does not require buffering). The hydrogen ions from the ketoacids are buffered primarily by the serum bicarbonate. The metabolic acidosis leads to tachypnea in an attempt at compensation by respiratory alkalosis. Kussmaul's respiration is noted (i.e., breathing that is deep and rapid) and the fruity odor in the patient's breath is obvious. The serum acidosis is reflected in a cerebrospinal fluid acidosis and eventually results in further depression of the central nervous system and possible coma if no intervention is made. In an effort to further reduce the amount of H^+ present, hydrogen ion exchanges with intracellular potassium, which is subsequently lost in the urine with the osmotic diuresis or by accompanying the ketoacids and other anions in the urine. The cumulative effects of these metabolic derangements are hyperglycemia, glycosuria, hyperlipidemia, ketonuria, severe dehydration, and electrolyte imbalance with possible *hyper*kalemia, (even though there may be a significant total body depletion of potassium), acidosis, and hyponatremia. The serum sodium, although low at the time of presentation of DKA, may be artificially depressed because of the osmotic effect of glucose (3). These metabolic abnormalities define the derangements that must be corrected in the treatment of DKA. The rational treatment protocol for DKA must include attention to the following: 1) volume expansion, 2) insulin, 3) glucose or calories, 4) electrolytes (sodium and potassium), 5) alkali and acid-base abnormalities, 6) phosphate, 7) calcium, 8) magnesium, and 9) paradoxical states.

TREATMENT OF DKA

Each of the metabolic derangements in DKA may require attention in the therapy regimen. The rationale for the treatment is discussed briefly in this section, followed by an abbreviated treatment protocol for easy reference (4-6).

Volume Expansion: The Most Important Aspect of Early Treatment of DKA

If weights are not available, it is reasonable to assume a 5-10% or greater dehydration in moderate to severe ketoacidosis. Weight loss in a newly diagnosed diabetic is divided into long-term weight loss, which occurs secondary to the loss of calories plus fat and protein catabolism, versus short-term weight loss due to dehydration. This is an important factor to remember when calculating percentage dehydration based upon weight. If hypotensive, generally a volume expansion is accomplished with an isotonic solution (0.9% NaC1, lactated Ringers, 5% albumin, or plasmanate). This is supplied as 300 ml/m^2 over 30 min and may be repeated if hypotension or oliguria persist. Use of this fluid also avoids rapid infusion of free water which will induce complications as discussed later.

If blood pressure is essentially normal or after the successful volume expansion, the patient should receive a solution of less osmolality, such as half-normal sodium chloride solution (0.45%). We generally assume 5% dehydration in a child with mild to moderate DKA. One-half of the total deficit is given in the first 8 hr of rehydration in addition to maintenance fluids (1500 ml/m^2/day). The hyperosmolality of hyperglycemia will artificially lower the serum Na so that administration of solutions containing more than half-normal saline is not necessary (unless the patient is hypertensive). For each 100 mg/dl increase in blood glucose, the serum sodium will be lowered by 1.6 mEq/L.

$$\frac{140\ \text{mEq}}{\text{L}} - 1.6 \times \underline{\text{observed glucose} - \text{normal glucose}} =$$

$$\text{patient's Na}\ \frac{\text{mEq}}{\text{L}}$$

Hyperlipidemia will also cause an apparent depression in serum sodium because the lipid fraction of the serum does not contain electrolytes. This makes the use of serum sodium an inaccurate determinant for degree of dehydration. If $NaHCO_3$ is to be used to correct the base deficit, the final concentration of Na should still be approximately half-normal saline. Monitor closely and be sure that the fluids in are greater than fluids out. Diuresis occurs during early treatment due to increased kidney perfusion (resulting from volume expansion) and the osmotic diuresis (due to hyperglycemia with glycosuria). On the other hand, be aware that overcorrection with hypotonic fluids may lead to cerebral edema.

Insulin

Only *rapid-acting* (regular) insulin should be given. Patients with ketoacidosis are refractory to the action of insulin, so they require relatively large doses of the hormone. *Insulin dosage should always be calculated on the basis of body weight.* The initial dose and route of administration should be determined by the clinical condition of the child as well as by the degree of the ketosis and acidosis. There are four methods available for the initial insulin therapy: 1) continuous intravenous infusion; 2) hourly intramuscular administration; 3) intermittent subcutaneous, intramuscular, and intravenous administration; and 4) intermittent subcutaneous administration (6-11). We generally prefer continuous intravenous infusion in the treatment of moderate to severe DKA ($HCO_3 < 15$); however, the hourly intramuscular regimen appears equally effective, and the intermittent subcutaneous, intramuscular, and intravenous regimen has been the standard therapy for years. The intermittent subcutaneous regimen is reserved for cases of mild to moderate ketoacidosis, the most common form in our experience due to the early recognition and detection of new diabetics.

Glucose or Calories

In the patient with ketoacidosis, it is desirable to control acidosis and ketonuria before controlling glycosuria so as to ensure adequate caloric replacement and end the intracellular starvation. Dextrose should always be given in quantities sufficient to accommodate the relatively large amount of insulin being administered. Dextrose should be added to the parenteral therapy after partial correction of dehydration and acidosis has been accomplished. *Because the undernourished ketoacidotic child has a poor glycogen reserve and will have been given a relatively large dose of insulin, the administered fluids should contain 5% dextrose within 1-2 hr after starting intravenous (IV) therapy or certainly when the blood sugar reaches 250 mg/dl.* Most multielectrolyte solutions contain 5% dextrose. The total amount of dextrose administered intravenously and by mouth in the first 24 hr should be 5-8 g/kg of body weight. *Intravenous administration of dextrose should be continued until oral intake is assured.* It is dangerous to rely upon the patient's level of consciousness as a measure of response to treatment. The patient may remain unconscious after acidosis is corrected or may become severely hypoglycemic without ever gaining consciousness. *Overdosage of insulin may cause irreparable damage to the central nervous system or even death of the patient.* As long as ketonuria persists, blood glucose levels should be above 150 mg/dl and mild glycosuria is desirable as evidence of freedom from hypoglycemia.

The use of continuous IV insulin should be continued until the acidosis is largely corrected rather than until blood glucose concentrations have fallen to arbitrarily selected levels. Since the time to achieve the former may follow the latter by several hours, glucose should be added to the IV fluids to maintain blood glucose concentrations between 150 and 300 mg/dl until subcutaneous insulin therapy is begun. Generally we observe that infusion of 5% dextrose in the proper electrolyte solution at maintenance fluid replacement levels is sufficient to accomplish this goal. IV insulin may be discontinued when venous pH is greater than 7.3 or when the bicarbonate is greater than 15 mEq/L. This allows for continuation of IV insulin and correction of the acidosis without causing hypoglycemia.

Electrolytes

After the initial volume expansion, the sodium concentration of the IV fluid should be approximately half-normal saline. This has proved sufficient to compensate for fluid deficits and continued fluid and electrolyte losses secondary to the osmotic diuresis when given at a rate to provide fluid maintenance plus deficits. The need for supplying intracellular electrolytes, especially potassium, has been well established (1, 6). The total body depletion of potassium is usually accompanied by a normal or even elevated serum potassium before insulin therapy due to the acidosis. Both correction of the acidosis and insulin treatment cause a transfer of K^+ intracellularly, and hypokalemia will develop if K^+ is not given during therapy (since it was previously lost from the cells into the serum and cleared by the kidneys causing a total body K^+ depletion).

Replacement with K^+ should begin as soon as renal flow is restored. The potassium deficit usually ranges from 3 to 10 mEq/kg. It is advisable to add at least 40 mEq of potassium/L of administered fluids. On accasion, concentrations of 60 mEq/L of potassium have been necessary to prevent hypokalemia.

Unless prevented by administration of potassium salts, hypokalemia will develop with muscle paralysis or weakness, cardiac arrhythmia, gastric atony, or intestinal ileus and is potentially fatal. Therefore, one frequently should monitor and adjust, if necessary, the concentration of potassium in the plasma. Hypokalemia can also be detected by changes in electrocardiographic tracings since hypokalemia causes a prolonged Q-T interval with wide low-amplitude T waves and U waves. This makes continuous cardiac monitoring desirable during the treatment of DKA.

Alkali

We recommend the administration of intravenous alkali only when the critically ill patient has a plasma-bicarbonate concentration of less than 10 mEq/L or the arterial pH is 7.2 or less and in the occasional older patient with cardiovascular and renal impairment. It may be advisable then to administer bicarbonate but only in a quantity sufficient to raise the plasma-bicarbonate level to about 12-15 mEq/L or to replace one-half of the base deficit. Direct, rapid administration of the molar solution (containing 892 mEq/L) may raise the effective osmotic pressure of extracellular fluid enough to cause dehydration of body cells, especially those of the central nervous system (12, 13). In addition, administration of hyperosmolar bicarbonate or attempts at rapid correction of the acidosis with bicarbonate may result in a paradoxical intracellular and CSF (cerebrospinal fluid) acidosis that can depress further the level of consciousness (14, 15). *The acidosis will not correct until sufficient fluids are given to correct the dehydration and sufficient insulin is administered to reverse the production of the ketoacids. Several controlled studies have demonstrated that the rapidity of the correction of the acidosis is not altered by the administration of bicarbonate in addition to insulin.* The acidosis itself may be important in several theoretically protective mechanisms. These are: 1) hyperventilation and compensation of the metabolic acidosis by respiratory alkalosis; 2) increased oxygen dissociation to compensate for low 2,3-DPG levels; and 3) increased cardiac contractibility at pH between normal and 7.2. The decreased cardiac contractibility at pH < 7.2 (corresponding $HCO_3 = 15$) is the basis for considering inclusion of bicarbonate in the electrolyte therapy of selected patients with severe ketoacidosis.

Dilution Acidosis or Paradoxical Acidosis

As volume expansion occurs with reperfusion of previously hypoxic areas, the metabolic products of anaerobic glycolysis (i.e., lactic acid) are circulated and there will be a paradoxical lowering of pH and serum bicarbonate (as the patient improves clinically, his laboratory values may worsen). This may even occur after normalization of the blood sugar and aglycosuria and appears as prolonged acidosis, hypocarbia, and ketonuria (6).

Phosphate

A general depletion of high-energy phosphates is observed in DKA since acidosis causes increased renal excretion of phosphate. Decreased ATP and 2,3-DPG has been observed in adult patients with diabetic ketoacidosis. Some investigators suggest that the decrease in 2,3-DPG levels is not sufficient to significantly alter tissue oxygenation in children. Furthermore, in diabetic adults with ketoacidosis 2,3-DPG values remained strikingly low for up to 5 days after the start of treatment. In ketoacidotic children, however, the mean 2,3-DPG value reverted to normal within 24 hr after the onset of treatment (16).

Phosphate therapy may accelerate regeneration of erythrocyte 2,3-DPG (17) but there may be an exaggeration of hypocalcemia in phosphate-treated patients (18). Phosphate therapy may be indicated, especially in patients with other reasons for hypoxia which would be further compromised by hypophosphatemia and low erythrocyte 2,3-DPG. These include patients more susceptible to hypoxia, such as those with anemia, congestive heart failure, and pneumonia. It should be given with caution and monitored closely. Once oral intake is tolerated, phosphate may be provided through milk and milk products.

Calcium

Hydrogen ions compete with calcium for albumin-binding sites, and as calcium is displaced it is excreted by the kidneys (3). Acute hypocalcemia may cause convulsions, nuchal rigidity, irritability, disorientation, laryngeal spasm (stridor), choked disk, prolonged Q-T interval, hyperreflexia, Trousseau's sign and Chvostek's sign, abdominal cramps, and/or intestinal ileus. This is usually seen in 24 hr and especially during overvigorous bicarbonate or phosphorus therapy. Plasma calcium concentration normally falls during the initial 48 hr of DKA therapy but usually can be replaced by food intake.

Magnesium

Magnesium also is lost in DKA due to renal wasting (3). Even though Mg levels may be normal or elevated at the onset, there is a marked fall during treatment. Resumption of normal food intake is usually sufficient to replace magnesium. Only rarely will the hypomagnesemia need correction. In our experience this has occurred when the hypomagnesemia has caused persistent hypocalcemia due to the role of magnesium in parathormone secretion and calcium homeostasis.

Hyperglycemic, Nonketotic Coma and Ketoacidosis with Low Blood Sugars

These two paradoxical states are frequently observed in a large population of children and adolescents with diabetes. The hyperglycemic (blood sugars of 800-1000), nonketotic state occurs primarily in newly diagnosed or mildly insulin-deficient individuals following a large intake of simple sugars. In contrast, severe ketoacidosis with low blood sugars (< 300) occurs in poorly controlled diabetics during periods of decreased food intake, such as episodes of vomiting due to gastroenteritis or gastroparesis. Each of these conditions requires special attention since the blood sugars will correct quickly or precipitously following the institution of insulin therapy. The hyperglycemia in the nonketotic patient will correct rapidly due to renal clearance of the blood glucose and the presence of insulin sensitivity. The hyperglycemia in the starving ketoacidotic patient will correct quickly in the presence of insulin resistance due to intracellular transfer and metabolism of glucose in a state of glycogen depletion. In contrast, the ketoacidosis may be refractory to the usual treatment and require prolonged IV glucose administration and insulin supplementation until the body stores of glycogen are replenished.

For classification of diabetic ketoacidosis, protocol for management of moderate diabetic ketoacidosis, and protocol for management of severe diabetic ketoacidosis by constant IV insulin infusion, see Appendixes A-C at the end of this chapter.

REFERENCES

1. Ellenberg, M., and Rifkin, H.: *Diabetes Mellitus: Theory and Practice,* 3rd Ed. Medical Examination Publishing Co. Inc., New Hyde Park, NY, 1983.

2. McGarry, J. D.: Lilly lecture 1978: New perspectives in the regulation of ketogenesis. *Diabetes* 28:517-523, 1979.

3. Hung, W., Gilbert, P. A., and Glasgow, A. W.: *Pediatric Endocrinology: Medical Outline Series.* Medical Examination Publishing Co. Inc., New Hyde Park, NY, 1978.

4. Williams, R. H.: *Textbook of Endocrinology,* W.B. Saunders Co., Philadelphia, 1981.

5. Szabo, A. J.: Diabetic ketoacidosis: Practical guide to emergency treatment. *Pract. Diabetol.* 2:1-20, 1983.

6. Jackson, R. L., and Guthrie, R. A.: *The Child with Diabetes Mellitus, Current Concepts,* Upjohn & Co., Kalamazoo, MI., 1975.

7. Alberti, K. G. M. M., Hockaday, T. D. R., and Turner, R. C.: Small doses of intramuscular insulin in the treatment of diabetic "coma." *Lancet* 2:515-522, 1973.

8. Smith, L., and Martin, H. E.: Responses of diabetic coma to various insulin dosages. *Diabetes* 3:287-295, 1954.

9. Sonksen, P. H., Srivastava, M. C., Tompkins, C. V., and Nabarro, J. D. N.: Growth hormone and cortisol responses to insulin infusion in patients with diabetes mellitus. *Lancet* 2:155-160, 1972.

10. Lightner, E. S., Kappy, M. S., and Revsin, R.: Low dose intravenous insulin infusion in patients with diabetic ketoacidosis: Biochemical effects in children. *Pediatrics* 60(5):681-688, 1977.

11. Martin, M. M., and Martin, A. L. A.: Continuous low-dose infusion of insulin in the treatment of diabetic ketoacidosis in children. *J. Ped.* 89:560, 1976.

12. Clements, R. S., Prockop, L. D., and Winegrad, A. I.: Acute cerebral edema during treatment of hyperglycemia. *Lancet* 2:384-386, 1968.

13. Young, E., and Bradley, R. F.: Cerebral edema with irreversible coma in severe diabetic ketoacidosis. *N.E.J.M.* 276(12):665-669, 1967.

14. Bureau, M. A., Begin, R., et al: Cerebral hypoxia from bicarbonate infusion in diabetic acidosis. *J. Ped.* 96: 968-973, 1980.

15. Kaye, R.: Editor's column: Diabetic ketoacidosis — The bicarbonate controversy. *J. Ped.* 87:156-159, 1975.

16. Kanter, Y., Gerson, J. R., and Berman, A. N.: 2,3-Diphosphoglycerate, nucleotide phosphate, and organic and inorganic phosphate levels during the early phases of diabetic ketoacidosis. *Diabetes* 26(5):429-433, May, 1977.

17. Keller, U., and Berger, W.: Prevention of hypophosphatemia by phosphate infusion during treatment of diabetic ketoacidosis and hyperosmolar coma. *Diabetes* 29:87-95, 1980.

18. Fisher, J. N., and Kitrabchi, A. E.: A randomized study of phosphate therapy in the treatment of diabetic ketoacidosis. *J. Clin. Endocrinol. and Metabolism* 57:177-180, 1983.

19. Clements, R. S., Jr., and Vourgant, B.: Fatal diabetic ketoacidosis: Major causes and approaches to their prevention. *Diabetes Care* 1:314-325, 1978.

20. TsliKian, E., et al: Electroencephalographic changes in diabetic ketosis in children with newly and previously diagnosed insulin dependent diabetes mellitus. *J. Ped.* 98:355-359, 1981.

21. McGarry, J. D., Mannaertz, G. P., and Foster, D. W.: *J. Clin. Invest.* 60:265-270, 1977.

C. ESTABLISHING GLYCEMIC EQUILIBRIUM

Robert L. Jackson, M.D.

THE POSTACIDOTIC STAGE

As soon as vomiting is controlled and the child requests something to drink, small amounts (1-2 oz) of sweetened, carbonated fluids such as ginger ale should be offered at 15-30-min intervals by a parent or close member of the family. Fruit juice (diluted with an equal amount of water and 2 teaspoons of table sugar for each 8 oz) alternated with skimmed or low fat (2%) milk then should be offered in gradually increasing amounts. Fruit juices and milk are good sources of water, sugar, protein, and electrolytes, including potassium and magnesium. Usually, parenteral fluid infusion, if needed, can be discontinued after 12 to 36 hr.

The child will continue to require special attention for a few days and having a parent or close member of the family provides emotional support for both. Regular insulin should now be given at 4- or 6-hr intervals. The total daily insulin requirement for the postacidotic period will approximate 2.0 U/kg of body weight. The first dose of insulin, therefore, should be about 0.5 U/kg. A simple meal consisting of fruit or fruit juices, skimmed milk, meat broth, custard, gelatin dessert, and toast or crackers is offered about 30 min after the insulin is administered. During the first 24 hr, the patient should be offered only about 30-40 Kcal/kg divided into four or six small feedings. Caloric intake can be increased rapidly as the child's tolerance for food improves.

For the first few days, four or six daily doses of regular insulin are continued with four or six small meals at about 6- or 4-hr intervals. (Infants and preschool children require more frequent and smaller meals and insulin injections.) The daily insulin dosage for each child given prescribed meals is determined by the trial and error method, and each dose will depend upon the child's response and the results of repeated tests for urinary glucose and acetone. Repeated tests for blood glucose levels usually are not necessary if the child is urinating. Repeated fingersticks are not well tolerated by young children. As stated before, the initial 24-hr dose of insulin will usually approximate 2 U/kg of body weight and the child usually will ingest and tolerate about 30-40 Kcal/kg. Thus, if a child weighs about 30 kg, the insulin requirement will be about 60 U and the food intake should be about 900-1200 Kcal in the first 24 hr. The total insulin dose should be divided into four doses and given 30 min before each small meal. For example, the first insulin dose would be 15 U of regular *purified pork* or *human* insulin. The first feeding, supplying about 250 Kcal, should be given as fluids in small amounts (4 oz) at about 30-min intervals. If the urine collected during the next 6 hr continues to have over 3% glucose concentration and is free from acetone, the next insulin dose should be increased to 17-18 U of regular insulin and the next meal should supply 250-300 Kcal. If the urine becomes essentially glucose-free, the insulin dose should be reduced to 12-13 U. If food has been tolerated well, the caloric content of the next meal should be increased by an additional 50-100 Kcal. If the urine continues to have only small amounts of glucose during the next 6 hr and if the child's hunger is not satisfied, the food intake should be increased another 50-100 Kcal and the regular insulin dose should be reduced to 10-12 U.

For the first four or eight feedings, it is most practical to use simple foods that are readily available and do not require special preparation by the dietary department. These feedings need not coincide with usual mealtimes. For gross calculation, it is helpful and advisable for the physician to write orders for specific foods. Each of these food servings provides about 100 Kcal: 8 oz fruit juice, 6 oz 2% butterfat milk, four 2 in x 2 in graham crackers, eight 2 in x 2 in soda crackers.

The sum of the four doses of insulin given in the previous 24-hr period will give an approximation of the total insulin dosage needed for the next day (e.g., 15 + 17 + 12 + 10 + = 54). The child's response to food intake during that period also will serve as a good guide to the adjustment of the caloric intake for the next day. Simply stated, close observation of the child, repeated tests for glycosuria, and adjusted orders every 4-6 hr for insulin doses and food intake provide a sound basis for therapy.

MODIFYING INSULIN AND DIET

Once treatment of the disease is initiated, most diabetic children have a rather uniform pattern of recovery. Before treatment with insulin, the child with diabetes has depleted nutritional stores. In the initial phase of management, the child is rebuilding body tissue and nutritional stores back to normal. During this time, the requirements for insulin, calories, and other nutrients are much higher than maintenance requirements. To calculate a meal plan suitable for the child, one can estimate protein and caloric needs on the basis of his age and body weight (Table 6.1). During early childhood and the prepubescent growth spurt, a minimum daily intake of 1 g of high-quality protein/kg of body weight is recommended. The meals at varying caloric levels are designed to furnish 1 g or more of protein/kg of body weight and all other essential nutrients (Tables 6.2, 6.3, 6.4).

A daily regimen of four injections of insulin and four small meals with increasing caloric content is continued only during the first few days of rapid clinical improvement. As soon as the patient's response becomes relatively predictable, a mixture of two parts of purified pork or human NPH insulin to one part regular insulin is given 30 min before breakfast and 30 min before the evening meal. The insulins are mixed by injecting them proportionately into a sterile bottle; this method is more efficient and convenient and provides greater accuracy than does measuring and mixing the insulins in a syringe. Two-thirds of the total daily dose is given as a 2:1

TABLE 6.1 Average Caloric Intake of Children with Diabetes in Good Control and Growing at a Normal Rate

Age (Years)	Boys: Average* total Kcal/day	Boys: Average* Kcal kg/day	Boys: Average* Kcal lb/day	Girls: Average* total Kcal/day	Girls: Average* Kcal kg/day	Girls: Average* Kcal lb/day
2	1250	95.0	40.0	1150	95.0	40.0
3	1350	75.0	35.0	1250	75.0	35.0
4	1500	75.0	35.0	1350	75.0	35.0
5	1650	75.0	35.0	1450	70.0	32.5
6	1800	70.0	32.5	1600	70.0	32.5
7	1850	70.0	32.5	1800	70.0	32.5
8	2050	70.0	32.5	1900	70.0	32.5
9	2100	65.0	30.0	2000	65.0	30.0
10	2300	65.0	30.0	2050	65.0	30.0
11	2400	60.0	27.5	2150	60.0	27.5
12	2450	60.0	27.5	2250	55.0	25.0
13	2600	55.0	25.0	2250	50.0	22.5
14	2750	55.0	25.0	2200	45.0	20.0
15	2950	50.0	22.5	2000	40.0	17.0
16	3050	50.0	22.5	1800	35.0	15.0
17	3000	45.0	20.0	1600	30.0	14.0
18	3000	45.0	20.0	1500	27.5	13.0

*Values are only approximate. Kcal/day and Kcal/U of body weight have been rounded off to multiples of 50 and 2.5, respectively.

TABLE 6.2 Meal Planning and Food Groups*

List 1:	Milk (A good source of protein, calcium, phosphorus, and riboflavin. Fortified milk is a good source of vitamins A and D.) 240 ml whole milk = 8 g protein, 10 g fat, 12 g carbohydrate; about 170 Kcal. 240 ml 2% butterfat milk = 9 g protein, 5 g fat, 13 g carbohydrate; about 135 Kcal. 240 ml skimmed milk = 9 g protein, 11 g carbohydrate; about 80 Kcal.
List 2:	Bread (fortified grain products provide iron, thiamine, riboflavin and niacin.) One slice = about 2 g protein, 15 g carbohydrate; about 70 Kcal.
List 3:	Vegetables (provide essential nutrients: vitamins A and C.) One-half cup = about 2 g protein, 5 g carbohydrate; about 25 Kcal.
List 4:	Fruits (provide vitamins C and A.) One serving = 10 g carbohydrate; 40 Kcal.
List 5:	Eggs-Meat-Meat Substitute (a good source of protein, iron, thiamine, niacin.) One ounce = about 7 g protein, 5 g fat; 75 Kcal.
List 6:	Fats (a good source of vitamin A.) A high-quality margarine is also a good source of <u>un</u>saturated fatty acids. One serving = about 5 g fat; 45 Kcal.

(Each listed serving portion should be measured or weighed. Refer to complete ADA lists for serving portions.)

It is wise to plan meals and snacks that contain a wide variety of foods to ensure an adequate intake of all essential nutrients and to provide maximum benefits for growth and health. Protein foods should be included with each meal and snack.

*Adapted from *Meal Planning with Exchange Lists,* American Diabetes Association, 18 East 48th Street, New York, NY 10017.

TABLE 6.3 Examples of Meal Patterns for Children with Diabetes Mellitus*

Kilocalories**	1000±50	1600±50	2000±50	2400±50	3000±50
Breakfast Kcal	220	350	450	530	665
Food Group			Serving Portion		
Milk 2%	½	½	1	1	1 whole milk
Bread	1	2	2	3	3
Fruit	1	1	1	1	2
Meat	1	1	1	1	1
Fat	0	1	1½	2	3
Midmorning Kcal	110	175	220	265	330
Milk 2%	½	½	1	1	1 whole milk
Bread	½	1	3/4	1	1
Meat	0	½	0	1	1
Fat	0	0	0	0	½
Noon Kcal	300	465	580	690	855
Milk 2%	½	½	1	1	1 whole milk
Bread	1	2	2	3	4

TABLE 6.3 Examples of Mejal Patterns for Children with Diabetes Mellitus* (Cont'd)

Kilocalories**	1000±50	1600±50	2000±50	2400±50	3000±50
Noon Kcal (Cont'd)					
Fruit	½	1	1	1	2
Meat	1	2	2	2½	3
Vegetable	1	1	1	1	1
Fat	1	1	2	2	2
Midafternoon Kcal	55	90	110	135	170
Milk 2%	½	½	½	0	½ whole milk
Bread	0	½	3/4	1	1
Meat	0	0	0	1	½
Evening Kcal	300	465	580	680	855
Milk 2%	½	½	½	1	1 whole milk
Bread	1½	2	2½	3	4
Fruit	½	1	1	1	1
Meat	1½	2	3	3	4
Vegetable	1	1	1	1	1
Fat	0	1	1½	2	2

Bedtime Kcal	55	90	110	135	190
Milk 2%	½	½	0	0	½ whole milk
Bread	0	½	1	1	1
Meat	0	0	½	1	½

*Using food lists prepared by the American Dietetic Association and American Diabetic Association.

**Kilocalories divided 4/18, 2/18, 5/18, 1/18, 5/18, and 1/18.

TABLE 6.4A Meal Plan for One Day*

Breakfast: 400 Kcal	
Food Group and Serving	
1 Milk	240 ml (8 oz) 2% milk
2 Bread	2 slices toast
1 Fruit	100 ml orange juice
1 Meat	50 g poached egg
1 Fat	5 g (1 tsp) margarine
Midmorning snack: 200 Kcal	
1 Bread	20 g (6–8) crackers (round)
1 Fruit	15 g (1 tbsp) raisins
1 Meat	15 g (1 tbsp) peanut butter
Lunch: 525 Kcal	
1 Milk	240 ml (8 oz) whole milk
2 Bread	70 g hamburger bun
1 Vegetable	lettuce/tomato salad
2 Meat	60 g (2 oz) hamburger
1 Fat	15 g (1 tbsp) French dressing
Midafternoon snack: 100 Kcal	
½ Bread	10 g (2–3) saltine crackers
1 Meat	30 g cheese
Evening Meal: 525 Kcal	
½ Milk	120 ml (4 oz) 2% milk
2 Bread	100 g baked potato
	25 g dinner roll
1 Vegetable	100 g carrots
1 Fruit	100 g fruit cocktail (unsweet)
3 Meat	90 g (3 oz) baked chicken
1 Fat	5 g (1 tsp) margarine
Bedtime snack: 100 Kcal	
½ Milk	120 ml (4 oz) 2% milk
½ Bread	10 g cornflakes

*An example (1800 Kcal): (Three meals and three between-meal snacks: 1800 Kcal divided 4/18, 2/18, 5/18, 1/18, 5/18, 1/18. About 20% protein, 35% fat, 45% carbohydrate.)

TABLE 6.4B Meal Plan for a Diabetic Child with an Intercurrent Illness*

Breakfast: 320 Kcal	
Food Group and Serving	
1 Milk	240 ml (8 oz) skim milk
2 Bread	2 slices toast
1½ Fruit	120 ml (4 oz) apple juice
1 Fat	1 tsp margarine
Midmorning snack: 160 Kcal	
1 Bread	1 slice toast
½ Fruit	50 ml orange juice
1 Meat	1 poached egg
Lunch: 400 Kcal	
1 Milk	240 ml (8 oz) skim milk
2 Bread	2 slices bread
1½ Fruit	150 ml orange juice
1 Meat	30 g sliced turkey
1 Fat	1 tsp margarine
Midafternoon snack: 80 Kcal	
½ Bread	10 g (about 3) saltine crackers
½ Fruit	50 ml orange juice
½ Meat	15 g cheese
Evening meal: 400 Kcal	
2½ Bread	½ cup chicken soup
	2 slices bread
1 Fruit	100 g applesauce (unsweetened)
2 Meat	60 g cheese
1 Fat	1 tsp margarine
Bedtime snack: 80 Kcal	
½ Milk	120 ml (4 oz) skim milk
½ Bread	10 g (1) graham cracker

*An example (1450 kilocalories): When a diabetic child has an intercurrent illness, the three-meal, three-snack meal pattern is continued (with the usual caloric distribution of 4/18, 2/18, 5/18, 1/18, 5/18, 1/18), but his usual daily caloric allowance is reduced by 20%. An 1800 Kcal meal plan, for example, would be reduced to provide 1450 Kcal daily. In addition, the proportion of fat is reduced and the proportion of carbohydrate is increased, thus allowing more juices and simple carbohydrates, which are better tolerated and preferred by the child who is ill. Nutritional composition of the plan is then approximately 20% protein, 20% to 25% fat, and 50% to 55% carbohydrate.

mixture of NPH: regular 30 min before breakfast. The remaining one-third of the same mixture is given 30 min before the evening meal (Figure 6.5). The regular insulin in the mixture acts quickly and makes it feasible and physiologically appropriate for the child to eat breakfast about 30 min after the morning injection; the intermediate insulin in the mixture will be about at peak activity during midday. The usual dietary distribution used with this insulin regimen and with the standardized physical activity prescribed in our hospital is one in which four-eighteenths of the daily caloric intake is given at breakfast, followed by a midmorning snack supplying two-eighteenths of the day's calories. The noon meal provides five-eighteenths of the caloric intake; a midafternoon snack, one-eighteenth, and the evening meal, five-eighteenths. The remaining one-eighteenth of the daily intake is given as a bedtime snack. The snacks are taken about 2-3 hr after the preceding meal. Timing of insulin injections in relation to food intake also is shown in Figure 6.5.

For purposes of testing urine, the day is divided into four collection periods, which end at 6:00 a.m., 11:00 a.m., 4:00 a.m. and 11:00 p.m. All urine collected during each of these periods is pooled, measured, and tested as a fractional specimen. (The collection of a double-voided urine specimen at the end of each period would be helpful but is generally an impractical technique when dealing with small children.) The quantity of glucose in each urine specimen can be estimated from the volume and qualitative test, using the two-drop Clinitest method. The enzymatic paper strip methods are not quite as accurate for estimating the degree of glucose concentration. The presence of acetone in the urine is checked by the Acetest method. After ketonuria is controlled, it is *not* necessary to test for acetone unless glucose content of the urine exceeds 3%. Depending on the total amount of glucose in the four fractional urine specimens, the total *daily*

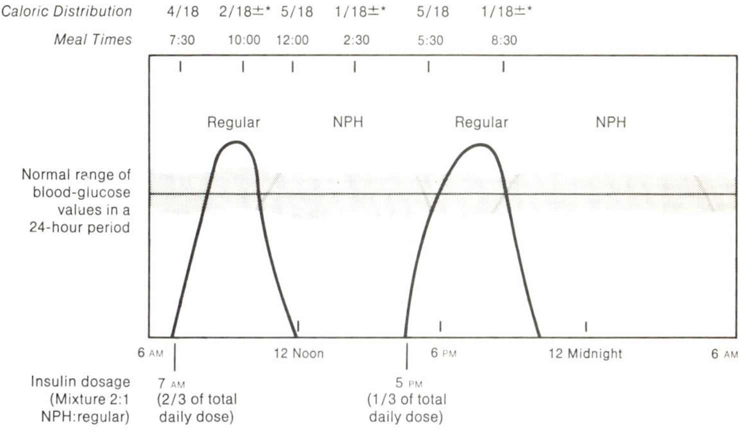

FIGURE 6.5 A schematic illustration of the relationship of food and insulin. The patient's daily food is given as three meals and three between-meal snacks (which is the most common and desirable pattern of food intake for nondiabetic American children). Insulin is given as two doses daily of a 2:1 mixture of NPH:regular. Two-thirds of the total daily dose is given in the morning and the remaining one-third is given in late afternoon. Regular insulin takes effect quickly and lasts for only 4 to 6 hr. NPH insulin, on the other hand, acts for a longer period and lasts for about 12-14 hr. Thus, the regimen provides for maintenance of blood-glucose levels as normal as possible for the diabetic child throughout a 24-hr period, and it helps prevent both urinary "spilling" of glucose and hypoglycemia.

*The quantity of food consumed as between-meal snacks (and thus the proportion of the daily caloric allotment) is varied with decreased or increased physical activity.

dose of insulin is increased or decreased, with maintenance of about the same percentage distribution. As soon as the child becomes aglycosuric, the insulin dose is reduced proportionally, *by percentage,* from the previous day (Table 6.5). As soon as the urine is glucose-free, it becomes necessary for parents, nurses, teachers, and physicians to observe the child closely for early symptoms or signs of an insulin reaction. If the child's urine is glucose-free and he has symptoms of hypoglycemia, the insulin dosage should be decreased at a slightly faster rate or the patient's caloric intake should be increased.

For example, a patient receiving 57 U of insulin in 24 hr (38 U of NPH:regular mixture before the morning meal and 19 U of the mixture before the evening meal) would receive 54 U the following day (36 and 18 U, respectively). The next day, the patient would receive 51 U in the same percentage and time distribution. This daily diminution of dosage continues until transient glycosuria recurs or until insulin requirements have been reduced to about 0.3 U/kg/day. Preferably, the insulin orders should be written each day by the same house officer in charge of the patient with the guidance of the attending physician.

As noted earlier, many children with insulin-dependent diabetes receive delayed and inadequate treatment for months or even for years after onset of the disease. Only when they begin having major clinical problems, especially recurrent episodes of ketoacidosis and hypoglycemia, are they referred for specialized care. In these suboptimally treated children (who usually have been given once-daily doses of insulin), insulin deficiency has gradually progressed until it has become total. Unlike those with recent onset of the disease, these children with total diabetes (which is the advanced stage of the disease) do not have a comparable recovery period, and their maintenance daily insulin requirement will be much higher (0.7-1.5 U/kg/day). To maintain a good to fair degree of control in children with total diabetes, they must receive at least two doses of insulin daily and close dietary supervision. Although most of these children will have a good response to a structured meal plan and twice-a-day insulin dose program as outlined, some will have a better response to more frequent injections of insulin as outlined in Chapter 12.

TABLE 6.5 Insulin Requirements During the Period of Metabolic Recovery in the Hospital

In the hospital, during the period of metabolic recovery, insulin requirements decrease about 7% daily as calibrated. Insulin is given as a mixture of two parts NPH to one part regular. The insulin should be mixed in a bottle, not in a syringe. Varying strengths of insulin are used, depending on the patient's total daily insulin requirement. Diluting fluid for preparation of strengths less than U100 is available. One part U100 insulin to one part diluting fluid = U50 insulin. One part of U100 insulin to three parts diluting fluid = U25 insulin. One part U100 insulin to nine parts diluting fluid = U10 insulin. When the child is in the hospital, a fixed daily caloric intake is prescribed. Every attempt must be made, therefore, to keep the daily physical activity pattern constant. When the child returns home, the caloric intake and distribution of calories will need to be modified, according to the physical activity pattern.

Distribution of daily calories:

Breakfast	4/18
Midmorning snack*	2/18
Lunch	5/18
Midafternoon snack*	1/18
Evening meal	5/18
Bedtime snack*	1/18

*2-3 hr after meals

TABLE 6.5 Insulin Requirements During the Period of Metabolic Recovery in the Hospital (Cont'd)

U100: used when the child's total daily dose is more than 50 U (each 0.01 ml = 1 U)

T	120	114	108	103	98	93	88	84	80
B	0.80	0.76	0.72	0.69	0.66	0.62	0.59	0.56	0.54
E	0.40	0.38	0.36	0.34	0.32	0.31	0.29	0.28	0.26

U50: used when the child's total daily dose is less than 50U but more than 20 U (each 0.02 ml = 1 U)

T	48	46	44	42	40	38	36	34	32
B	0.64	0.61	0.59	0.56	0.54	0.51	0.48	0.46	0.43
E	0.32	0.31	0.29	0.28	0.26	0.25	0.24	0.22	0.21

U25: used when the child's total daily dose is less than 20 U but more than 7.5 U (each 0.04 ml = 1 U)

T	19.0	18.0	17.0	16.0	15.0	14.0	13.0	12.0	11.5
B	0.51	0.48	0.46	0.43	0.40	0.37	0.35	0.32	0.31
E	0.25	0.24	0.23	0.21	0.20	0.19	0.17	0.16	0.15

U10: used when the child's total daily dose is less than 7.5 U (each 0.10 ML = 1U)

T	7.2	6.8	6.5	6.2	6.0	5.7	5.5	5.2	5.0
B	0.48	0.46	0.44	0.42	0.40	0.38	0.37	0.35	0.33
E	0.24	0.22	0.21	0.20	0.20	0.19	0.18	0.17	0.16

T = total daily dose of insulin

B = dose of insulin (in ml at strength indicated) to be given 30 min before breakfast

E = dose of insulin (in ml at strength indicated to be given 30 min before evening meal

U100: used when the child's total daily dose is more than 50 U (each 0.01 ml = 1 U)

76	72	68	65	62	59	56	53	50
0.51	0.48	0.46	0.44	0.42	0.40	0.38	0.36	0.34
0.25	0.24	0.22	0.21	0.20	0.19	0.18	0.17	0.16

U50: used when the child's total daily dose is less than 50 U but more than 20 U (each 0.02 ml = 1 U)

30	28.5	27	25.5	24	23	22	21	20
0.40	0.38	0.36	0.34	0.32	0.31	0.29	0.28	0.27
0.20	0.19	0.18	0.17	0.16	0.15	0.15	0.14	0.13

U25: used when the child's total daily dose is less than 20 U but more than 7.5 U (each 0.04 ml = 1 U)

11.0	10.5	10.0	9.5	9.0	8.5	8.0	7.5
0.29	0.28	0.27	0.25	0.24	0.23	0.21	0.20
0.15	0.14	0.13	0.13	0.12	0.11	0.11	0.10

U10: used when the child's total daily dose is less than 7.5 U (each 0.10 ml = 1 U)

4.7	4.5	4.2	4.0	3.7	3.5	3.2	3.0
0.31	0.30	0.28	0.27	0.25	0.23	0.21	0.20
0.16	0.15	0.14	0.13	0.12	0.12	0.11	0.10

A period of hospital care for the child with total diabetes also is necessary to attain a higher degree of control and to determine the child's insulin requirement. For a short period of time the insulin and food requirements may be relatively higher as a result of an accelerated growth spurt. Hospital care also will free the parents for a period of intensive education. The patient receives the same basic plan of treatment as outlined for the newly diagnosed child. *To avoid hypoglycemia, however, it may be desirable to permit transient glycosuria with a somewhat wider range of diurnal blood sugar levels.* For the child with total diabetes to metabolize food intake appropriate for age and body build, the total daily insulin requirement will be greater than 0.8 U/kg/day. *The relatively high insulin requirement makes it desirable to err on the side of giving too little rather than too much insulin at first.* The daily dose can then be increased gradually on the basis of clinical response.

After a period of management in which the children with total diabetes have received only once-daily doses of insulin and relatively lax supervision of their meal plan, it becomes difficult for them to accept a plan of treatment that requires more self-discipline. For acceptance, both the child and the parents need to understand the basic principles of treatment and the reason for them. Because these children have a much lower threshold of safety than do recently diagnosed children, special attention must be given to teaching them and their parents how to adjust food intake with varying degrees of physical activity to prevent insulin reaction (see section on physical activity).

BLOOD GLUCOSE DETERMINATIONS

Repeated blood glucose determinations are not necessary in regulating most diabetic children except during ketoacidosis when the child may be anuric. Accurate collecting and testing of the four daily fractional urine specimens provides a reliable estimate of the timing and extent of blood glucose fluctuations than can be obtained by sporadic blood glucose measurements. A few fasting and postprandial blood glucose measurements are useful as stabilization nears and the need for reduction of insulin dosage ends. Serial blood glucose determinations are especially useful if properly interpreted by the doctor or nursing specialist to modify a basic regimen to meet the varying needs of individual children. Blood glucose testing at home is described in detail (see Chapter 12).

PREVENTING INSULIN REACTIONS

A severe, prolonged hypoglycemic reaction can have a catastrophic effect not only on the central nervous system of the child with diabetes but also on the morale of the parents and the child. There are two types of insulin reactions. The more common type is caused by a rapid shift in the blood glucose level accompanied by a stimulation of the sympathetic nervous system through increased epinephrine secretion. Early symptoms and signs are irritability, restlessness, hunger, weakness, pallor, sweating, and dilated pupils. The other type of hypoglycemic reaction is more profound and serious. It results from an excessive and continuous overdosage of insulin, which results in a gradual, marked lowering of blood glucose which may deplete the glycogen reserves. The onset is insidious, and frequently the patient will complain only of headache or weakness. The patient's condition rapidly deteriorates, with signs of central nervous system involvement, including unconsciousness and convulsions. Severe insulin reactions are preventable. They should be avoided because severe, prolonged hypoglycemia may result in irreparable damage to the central nervous system, especially in infants and preschool children who have developing central nervous systems.

The mild type of insulin reaction responds readily to orally administered glucose. Depending upon the age and weight of the child, 1-2 teaspoonfuls or packets of sugar dissolved in 2-4 oz of water usually suffices. If symptoms persist, the patient should be given another 2-4 oz of sugar water in 5-10 min. Time must be allowed for absorption of the glucose. Too often, excessive amounts of glucose are given without considering that fact. Mild insulin reactions may occur shortly before a meal. In that case, one can give some part of the meal (a small amount of fruit or half a glass of milk, for example) early and have the child rest for a few minutes before he slowly eats the remainder of the meal. Even mild insulin reactions usually can be avoided during the period of hospitalization if the insulin dosage is reduced gradually as previously outlined and if the pattern of physical activity is kept relatively constant each day. Overtreatment of insulin reactions leads to recurrence of glycosuria. If the cause of this glycosuria is not recognized, the next insulin dose may be increased unnecessarily. The patient so treated will fluctuate between glycosuria and insulin reactions. This problem is frequently observed and explains why many physicians have become convinced that one must permit varying degrees of glycosuria to avoid insulin reactions.

With more severe insulin reactions, gastric stasis is usually present, and time is frequently lost trying to give sugar orally. Intravenously administered dextrose or intramuscularly administered glucagon should be given at once to a child with a more severe insulin reaction. Usually it is preferable to give 5% or 10% dextrose in water, 100-120 ml over a 10- to 30-min period, rather than to give a more concentrated solution by more rapid injection. Intravenous administration of dextrose will usually restore the patient to consciousness within a matter of minutes. The dose of glucagon is 0.5 mg for a child 3 years of age or less and 1 mg for a child older than 3 years. Clinical improvement is usually seen within 10 to 15 min with an increase in level of consciousness and return of the swallowing reflex. Two teaspoonfuls of sugar in 2-3 oz of water should be given by mouth as soon as the child responds to the glucagon. After a *severe* reaction, the child should be kept in bed, and when nausea subsides, small amounts of fluids (2-4 oz of fruit juice or skimmed milk) should be given orally at about 30-min intervals for the next 2-3 hr. If nausea persists, small amounts of a sweetened, carbonated beverage such as ginger ale should be given in 15- to 30-min intervals for a few hours.

The basic meal pattern used for diabetic children in our clinic evolved from observing the eating habits of normal, active children and from the accumulated experience of treating many children with diabetes. The two-dose insulin regimen not only makes it possible for the child to eat meals and snacks at the usual times during the day, but it also lessens the probability of insulin reactions provided physical activity is structured to be relatively the same each day the child is in the hospital. The therapeutic objective is to have the child free from any symptoms of hypoglycemia, free from glycosuria, and for the blood glucose values to be essentially within the normal range during the entire 24-hr period.

There are major differences in the management of children with diabetes in our center as compared with that in many other centers. At the time of onset of the disease, we provide intensive hospital care for the child long enough (about 3 weeks) to attain maximum recovery of endogenous insulin production. We can thereby determine the exogenous insulin required to metabolize an adequate caloric intake with little likelihood of inducing even mild insulin reactions. The longer period of hospital care also provides time for the family and child to learn about the disease and feel secure in how to continue treatment at home. Another difference is that we use at least two doses of insulin daily from the beginning of therapy to provide the additional exogenous insulin at times needed throughout the day (i.e., 24 hr). Thus, there is sufficient insulin available so that the child can eat meals and snacks in quantities and at times customary of well-fed American children. Our experience indicates that maintaining this high degree of control extends the period of partial remission. It demonstrates to the parents and children that insulin-dependent diabetes can be controlled.

As previously discussed, the exogenous insulin requirement of most children with recent onset of diabetes mellitus decreases rapidly to a relatively low level for a variable period. This state of temporary, partial remission is known as the "honeymoon period." During the period of partial remission, glucosuria can be controlled completely without symptoms or signs of an insulin reaction.

The amount of insulin required and the duration of the metabolic recovery period is related to how long the state of hypoinsulinism and catabolism was present before institution of insulin therapy. After the recovery period of a few weeks, the insulin requirement becomes fairly constant. Table 6.6 consists of four subtables indicating when to use varying strengths of insulin. The legend provides instructions as to when to adjust the insulin dosage on the basis of daily urine tests. During the period of hospitalization, the weight of the child increases rapidly and the height remains almost stationary. However, within a short period the child's growth rate begins to accelerate, and concurrent with the increase in growth rate, the caloric and insulin requirements invariably increase somewhat.

There is a close interrelationship between the changing insulin requirement and physical growth. It is therefore important to know and be able to predict the insulin requirement of a given child. The insulin requirement gradually rises in the prepubertal child as a result of increase in body weight, but the ratio of insulin dosage to ideal body weight increases only slightly. During the prepubertal growth spurt, there is a sharper rise in insulin requirement and control is more difficult to maintain. After puberty, the insulin requirement will decrease and remain relatively constant during adulthood. We have not found that age at onset of the disease significantly influences the insulin requirement per unit of *ideal* body weight. As adulthood is reached, it is important that insulin dosage and caloric intake be reduced gradually to the person's adult requirement. The adolescent girl is especially prone to become obese if her insulin dosage and caloric intake are not adjusted to a lower requirement in keeping with her age. It is much easier to prevent than to treat obesity.

A knowledge of insulin requirements and growth rates at varying age periods of well-controlled diabetic patients helps in the prediction of insulin and nutritional requirements for maintaining good control of the disease and a normal growth pattern as discussed in Chapter 8.

D. INSULIN PREPARATION

Richard A. Guthrie, M.D.

The original insulin preparations were relatively impure and of low concentration. Only short-acting regular insulin was available. Thus, frequent injections were needed. Impurities often caused allergy and skin reactions. Insulin has been purified and modified in many ways over the years. In the 1930s, insulin was purified and concentrated to U80. U40 and U80 were the standard commercial concentrations used until the 1970s.

Early in the course of insulin therapy. it became evident that modification was needed to extend the duration of action. An early modification was in 1931 with the introduction of protamine zinc insulin (PZI). This insulin had several drawbacks, including very low absorption, a peak action time of about 18 hr, and a duration of action of over 24 hr. PZI therefore had only limited use and could control blood glucose levels only when combined with multiple injections of regular insulin.

TABLE 6.6 Alteration of Insulin Dosage After Stabilization — Home Care

---

Daily insulin dosage should be kept as constant as possible when the child returns home after the period of metabolic recovery in the hospital. If there is persistent or intermittent glycosuria, however, insulin dosage should be increased the next day by one or two steps as calibrated. If the child is aglycosuric and has even mild symptoms suggesting hypoglycemia, the food intake should be increased or the insulin dosage decreased by one or two steps. Average caloric intake during the day is recorded, but this average distribution is modified, as necessary, according to the physical activity of the child; it may need to be readjusted daily. Insulin is given as a 2:1 mixture of NPH: regular. The preparation should be premixed in a bottle rather than a syringe. Varying strengths of insulin are used, based on the child's total daily insulin requirement. Diluting fluid for preparation of strengths less than U100 is available from various manufacturers of commercial insulin. One part of U100 insulin to one part of diluting fluid = U50 insulin. One part U100 insulin to three parts diluting fluid = U25 insulin. One part U100 insulin to nine parts diluting fluid = U10 insulin.

Distribution of daily calories:

Breakfast	4/18
Midmorning snack*	2/18
Lunch	5/18
Midafternoon snack*	1/18
Evening meal	5/18
Bedtime snack*	1/18

*2–3 hr after meals

TABLE 6.6 Alteration of Insulin Dosage After Stabilization — Home Care (Cont'd)

U100: used when the younger child's total daily dose is more than 30 U and, for older children, when the total daily dose is over 20 U (each 0.01 ml = 1 u)

T	120	117	114	111	108	105	102	99	96
B	0.80	0.78	0.76	0.74	0.72	0.70	0.68	0.66	0.64
E	0.40	0.39	0.38	0.37	0.36	0.35	0.34	0.33	0.32

T	69	66	63	60	57	54	51	48	45
B	0.46	0.44	0.42	0.40	0.38	0.36	0.34	0.32	0.30
E	0.23	0.22	0.21	0.20	0.19	0.18	0.17	0.16	0.15

U50: used when the child's total daily dose is less than 30 U but more than 20 U (each 0.02 ml = 1 U)

T	28.5	27	25.5	24	22.5	21
B	0.38	0.36	0.34	0.32	0.30	0.28
E	0.19	0.18	0.17	0.16	0.15	0.14

U25: used when the child's total daily dose is less than 20 U but more than 7.5 U (each 0.04 ml = 1 U)

T	20.25	19.5	18.75	18	17.25	16.5	15.75	15	14.25
B	0.54	0.52	0.50	0.48	0.46	0.44	0.42	0.40	0.38
E	0.27	0.26	0.25	0.24	0.23	0.22	0.21	0.20	0.19

U10: used when the child's total daily dose is less than 7.5 U (each 0.10 ml = 1 U)

T	7.2	6.9	6.6	6.3	6	5.7	5.4	5.1	4.8
B	0.48	0.46	0.44	0.42	0.40	0.38	0.36	0.34	0.32
E	0.24	0.23	0.22	0.21	0.20	0.19	0.18	0.17	0.16

T = total daily dose of insulin

B = dose of insulin (in ml at strength indicated) to be given 30 min before breakfast

E = dose of insulin (in ml at strength indicated) to be given 30 min before evening meal

U100: used when the younger child's total daily dose is more than 30 U and for older children, when the total daily dose is over 20 U (each 0.01 ml = 1 U)

93	90	87	84	81	78	75	72
0.62	0.60	0.58	0.56	0.54	0.52	0.50	0.48
0.31	0.30	0.29	0.28	0.27	0.26	0.25	0.24

42	39	36	33	30	27	24	21
0.28	0.26	0.24	0.22	0.20	0.18	0.16	0.14
0.14	0.13	0.12	0.11	0.10	0.09	0.08	0.07

U25: used when the child's total daily dose is less than 20 U but more than 7.5 U (each 0.04 ml = 1 U)

13.5	12.75	12	11.25	10.5	9.75	9	8.25	7.5
0.36	0.34	0.32	0.30	0.28	0.26	0.24	0.22	0.20
0.18	0.17	0.16	0.15	0.14	0.13	0.12	0.11	0.10

U10: used when the child's total daily dose is less than 7.5 U (each 0.10 ml = 1 U)

4.5	4.2	3.9	3.6	3.3	3
0.30	0.28	0.26	0.24	0.22	0.20
0.15	0.14	0.13	0.12	0.11	0.10

Globin insulin was the first intermediate-acting insulin; that is, intermediate in action between short-acting regular insulin and long-acting PZI. Globin insulin was introduced in 1937 and came into general use in the early 1940s. Globin insulin was made by attaching the globin molecule to regular insulin. The larger molecule slowed absorption, giving the insulin a longer action than regular insulin. Globin insulin was very useful and was widely used until the 1950s when NPH and the Lente series became available. Globin insulin was usually used in combination with regular insulin, with which it was compatible and could be premixed, both being acid pH. Globin was made by Burroughs-Welcome in England and by Squibb in the United States. Burroughs-Welcome discontinued both European and American production of globin insulin in the late 1960s and Squibb discontinued manufacture in 1981.

In 1953, Dr. Hagedorn working in Denmark developed neutral pH protamine intermediate-acting insulin. This insulin became known in the United States as NPH insulin for Neutral Protamine Hagedorn, denoting that the insulin is of neutral pH (previous insulins were acid), that protamine is the attached molecule giving an action longer than regular, and honoring Dr. Hagedorn as the developer. NPH insulin proved very useful with a duration of action comparable to globin insulin. NPH insulin or a combination of NPH and regular insulin before breakfast rapidly became the preferred method of insulin replacement in the 1950s.

It had long been evident with globin insulin, and now with NPH insulin, that insulins containing foreign proteins could cause a variety of allergic problems. It has become evident recently that foreign proteins in the insulin (now removed) may have contributed to some of the allergies, but at the time they were ascribed to the globin or protamine. The allergy problems led to a search for protein-free insulins. This search led eventually to the development of the Lente series of insulins.

There are two basic insulins in the Lente series: Semilente and Ultralente. Semilente is a short-acting, amorphous insulin similar in action to regular insulin except slightly longer acting. Ultralente is a crystalline insulin. The crystals are large, thus reducing the surface area for absorption and slowing the entry into the circulation. Lente insulin, the most commonly used insulin in the series, is a mixture of 30% Semilente and 70% Ultralente. Lente has an action intermediate to Semilente and Ultralente and is roughly equivalent to NPH in its time-action curve.

No further changes have been made in the time action of insulin. The more recent changes have been in insulin purity and the development of monospecies insulin. We are then left with three basic insulins: 1) short-acting, 2) intermediate-acting, and 3) long-acting insulins. There are two insulins available today in each group: 1) short-acting -- regular and Semilente, 2) intermediate-acting -- NPH and Lente, and 3) long-acting -- PZI and Ultralente. Other insulins such as protamine sodium insulin have been tested, but none as yet have been marketed.

INSULIN PURITY

The early insulins contained glucagon, proinsulin, desamido-insulin (insulin damaged during processing), and other proteins. The primary contaminant was proinsulin. Proinsulin is a precursor of insulin in the beta cell, and a considerable amount of proinsulin is extracted from the pancreas along with the insulin. Proinsulin was not identified until the 1970s, so the primary contaminant of insulin was unknown until that time.

With the identification of proinsulin and other contaminants, a purification process of insulin began. In 1972, Eli Lilly released new insulins in the U100 concentration purified and neutralized. These insulins went from about 87% purity to over 98% purity. The proinsulin content was reduced to about 20-50,000 parts per million (ppm). Soon thereafter, the Danish insulin companies, Nordisk and Novo, began to release insulins into the American and, more recently, the Canadian market. The Danish insulins are highly purified to less than 1 ppm of proinsulin. Eli Lilly further purified their insulins in 1980 to < 50 ppm proinsulin for their standard insulins and < 10 ppm for their monospecies purified Iletin II insulins. The Danish insulins are slightly more purified than the Lilly insulins (Table 6.7). The value of this difference (< 10 ppm for Lilly Iletin II and < 1 ppm for Danish insulins) remains to be determined. All of these more purified insulins accomplish two things: 1) they reduce insulin allergy and 2) reduce lipoatrophy (see Chapter 11).

TABLE 6.7 Purity of Insulin Preparations

Name or Type	Purity-ProInsulin Content (Parts per Million)
USP Insulin	20-50,000 ppm
Lily Standard	< 50 ppm
Lily Iletin II	
Pork	< 10 ppm
Lily Human	0
Nordisk Pork	< 1 ppm
Nordisk Human	0
Novo Pork	< 1 ppm
Novo Human	0
Squibb Standard	< 50 ppm

U40 (40 U/cc) was the initial concentration of insulin. This was soon diluted to U20 and to U10. These concentrations of insulin were not enough (especially after the development of longer acting insulins and few injections per day) so the concentration was doubled to U80 insulin. In 1972, U100 insulin was introduced in the United States. The purpose of U100 insulin was to put insulin concentration into the metric system (a U100 insulin syringe is essentially a 1 cc tuberculin syringe) and to eliminate confusion with multiple concentrations (i.e., U40 and U80). U80 insulin has now been discontinued in the United States, but U40 is still available, although little used. U40 insulin will be doscontinued in the future, leaving only U100 insulin available for standard use. U500 insulin also is available from Eli Lilly Company for special purposes. *U100 insulin can be diluted with special diluting fluid (the buffer base for the insulin) which can be obtained at no cost from the pharmaceutical companies.* For small children, especially during the recovery and remissions periods, such dilution to U50, U25, or even U10 may be needed. *Without dilution, it is impossible to make changes of less than 1 U at a time. For a very small child in partial remission, a 1 U change could be a 20-30% change in dose, which might be equivalent to a 15-25 U change in an adult on the usual insulin dosage. Dilution of insulin is easy to accomplish and to teach to parents and is mandatory for small children on small dosages of insulin.*

The pH of insulin was also adjusted in 1972 when purified U100 insulin was introduced. Prior to 1972, NPH and regular insulin could not be premixed and stored because of the pH difference (regular was acid). Jackson et al. (1) found that neutral regular insulin (unbuffered regular insulin with pH adjusted to neutrality), retained almost full potency when stored at room temperature for 12 months; the potency of acid regular insulin had meanwhile dropped 20%. The increased stability of neutral regular over that of acid regular insulin may be related to a slower rate of deamination of the insulin protein at the neutral pH. Neutral insulins, therefore, do not need refrigeration during usage and can be stored at room temperature. When neutral regular and acid regular insulins were administered in combination with NPH or Ultralente, comparable time-activity responses were elicited. Animal studies in our laboratory in 1973 showed that neutral regular and NPH insulin premixed in a 2:1 ratio remain stable at least 4 weeks. Recent studies by Jawadi (2) using Nordisk insulins confirmed the stability of premixed insulins up to 3 months. The insulins retained their biphasic regular and NPH activity when premixed and stored for up to 3 months at room temperature.

Human insulin is now commercially available. Until recently, standard insulin preparations were beef-pork insulin mixtures. Beef insulin differs from human insulin by three amino acids in the A chain. Pork insulin differs from human insulin by only one amino acid, the terminal amino acid of the B chain (theonine in human insulin and alanine in pork). The difference in amino acid sequences confers some immunogenicity to the insulins of animal origin. Beef insulin is more antigenic than is pork. Beef insulin or beef-pork mixtures have been the standard insulin for many years because of availability and lower cost.

The immunogenicity of insulin of beef or pork origin is low and usually is of little consequence. All persons with diabetes are known to produce insulin-binding antibodies after a few months of insulin therapy. These antibodies usually peak by 6 months of therapy and remain relatively stable thereafter in most individuals. Dosage can be easily adjusted to compensate for the insulin binding.

Occasional individuals may have severe insulin binding, which can be persistent or may occur in crises. Dosage can become quite high in some cases requiring U500 insulin and even multiple doses or continuous IV insulin to compensate. In such cases a change to pure pork insulin should be tried (3). If unsuccessful, then a trial of human insulin is indicated. Insulin resistance in such cases is defined as an insulin requirement in excess of 200U/day in adults or 4 U/kg in children. Doses between 100 and 200 U/day in adults and between 2 and 4 U/kg/day in children is considered insulin insensitivity, probably a mild or early stage of insulin resistance (4).

It is hoped that the use of human insulin might eliminate the problem of insulin-binding antibodies. Although antibodies are rarely a clinical problem (true insulin resistance is rare), still the presence of antibodies and insulin-antibody complexes may conceivably cause some damage of which we are today unaware. It has been speculated, for example, that insulin-antibody complexes may contribute to vascular damage in a similar way as antigen-antibody complexes contribute to autoimmune renal disease. Such speculations have not been proved. Nonetheless, if we could eliminate antibodies, it might have some benefit. This speculation contributed part of the rationale for the development of human insulin.

Another rationale for the development of human insulin is an economic one. The supply of animal pancreases for insulin extraction is diminishing while the need for insulin is increasing. The supply and demand lines may someday cross, causing a deficiency of insulin and a marked increase in cost. An inexhaustible supply of insulin is needed.

There are two approaches to making human insulin. The Danish companies (Novo and Nordisk) have taken the approach of making human insulin from the porcine insulin molecule. In this approach, pork insulin is dealinated at the terminal amino acid of the B chain, then theonine is placed at that position. This approach presupposes an adequate supply of pork pancreas. Semi-synthetic human insulin (SSHI) made by Novo is available in the United States and is marketed as regular and Lente insulins.

The Eli Lilly Company has taken a different approach -- the recombinant DNA approach. In this method of making human insulin, no pancreas source is needed. Utilizing now standard recombinant DNA techniques in *E. coli* bacteria, the insulin gene can be inserted into the plasmid of the bacterium. When the bacteria reproduce, they pass the genetically engineered plasmid to the daughter cells. The daughter cells now can produce insulin in essentially unlimited quantities. The techniques of recombinant DNA technology developed by Genentech in San Francisco have now been applied to production of the Eli Lilly Co. This insulin is known as biosynthetic human insulin (BHI). BHI has been under test in the United States for 3 years and was released by the Food and Drug Administration (FDA) for sale in July, 1983 as Humulin. Humulin is available as regular and NPH. Lente is under test.

The original promise of no antibody formation of human insulin has not proved to be the case. During the first 6 months of therapy with BHI or SSHI, antibodies rise essentially identical to those of pure pork insulin. If beef insulin is used, levels of antibodies are higher and continue to rise. With purified pork insulin, antibodies level off or rise only slightly after 6 months. With BHI or SSHI, antibodies peak at 6 months, then begin to fall or level off and are somewhat lower at 1 year than with pork insulin. Lower antibody levels may give an advantage to human insulin, but this has not as yet been proved.

The time-action curve of human insulin is very similar to that of pork insulin but has a slightly shorter duration of action. The shortened duration of action could be advantageous in the split-mix or multiple-dose insulin regimens as it may produce less nocturnal hypoglycemia and overlap between doses. The shorter duration of action could be a disadvantage in single-dose therapy, which is not recommended.

CURRENT RECOMMENDATIONS

Although absolute advantages to pure pork and human insulins have not as yet been proved, there are indications for their use.

1. Absolute indications:
    a) In the presence of proved allergy to beef insulin, pork or human insulin must be used. If pork insulin allergy is proved, then human insulin is indicated.
    b) Insulin resistance to beef or pork insulin.

There are no other absolute indications for these insulins.

2. Relative indications:
   a) Intermittent therapy -- if for some reason insulin therapy is to be interrupted (rare in children), then the least immunogenic insulin available should be used to prevent the immunization effect of intermittent therapy.
   b) Newly diagnosed patients -- until the data are absolute that antibodies or insulin-antibody complexes are not harmful, we feel that all newly diagnosed patients who have no antibodies at the beginning should be given the benefit of the least immunogenic insulin available. Human insulin where available or pure pork insulin should be used in every newly diagnosed patient, particularly in children.
   c) Insulin insensitivity and diabetic instability. Sometimes insulin antibodies can contribute to high dosage and diabetic instability. In such cases a trial of pure pork or human insulin should be carried out. A reduction in antibodies may improve stability in some cases.

Some investigators believe all patients should be changed to pure pork or human insulin. When patients are doing well with beef-pork mixtures (standard insulin), we are not at present proposing a change since standard insulins are more economical than the new insulins. As data accumulate on complications, it may be necessary to change this policy.

The junior author has been involved in testing human insulin and pure pork (Nordisk) insulin for the past 3 years. We are convinced of the safety and efficacy of these insulins and their usefulness in many cases of instability. The majority of our patients are currently receiving either human or pure pork insulin. These insulins are, however, more expensive than standard insulins and will probably not replace standard insulins until cost decreases or standard insulins are discontinued. We would recommend that all newly diagnosed patients or anyone in whom therapy will be interrupted and restarted be given one of the new pure pork or human insulin preparations.

TIME ACTIONS OF INSULINS (TABLE 6.8)

Knowledge of the time-action curve for an insulin is a vital piece of knowledge in diabetes therapy. Many factors affect the kinetics of insulin absorption (where injected, dosage, exercise, a hot bath, etc.) so that definitive time action curves cannot be precisely defined. Pharmaceutical companies must provide definitive data to the FDA for approval of their product. They, therefore, determine pharmacologic time-action curves for insulin by testing under carefully controlled conditions, often in nondiabetic volunteers or in animals. Such data become part of the package insert and is translated into textbooks and into therapeutics. Such pharmacologic time-action curves may not be applicable, however, to therapy in many diabetic patients in whom we must use therapeutic time action curves. Pharmacologic time-action curves for publication may be defined as time-action curves based upon the presence of some insulin in the bloodstream following the subcutaneous injection of the insulin. The therapeutic time-action curves may be defined as the period of time that there is a sufficient amount of the injected insulin in the bloodstream to control the blood glucose level. It is the therapeutic time-action curve in which we are interested in the treatment of persons with diabetes mellitus. Table 6.8 contains therapeutic time-action curves for the various insulins available in the United States. The range of values for each insulin indicates individual variation, as well as other variables such as injection site, injection depth, etc.

An important principle of diabetes therapy is the need to duplicate what nature normally does, i.e., to provide physiologic insulin replacement. In the person with diabetes, a small amount of insulin is secreted continually. Twenty-four hours a day, every day, some insulin is present in the bloodstream and in the tissue. This is called basal insulin. When food is consumed, there is a rise in blood insulin levels called a bolus of insulin. It is this basal and bolus effect that must be duplicated to provide normal metabolism and physiology for persons with diabetes mellitus. By reference to Table 6.8 it should be evident that it is possible to provide 24-hr basal insulin and a bolus with each meal with presently available insulins used in various combinations. It should be equally evident, however, that with presently available insulins, it is not possible to provide physiologic insulin replacement of

TABLE 6.8 Insulin Preparations — Therapeutic Time Actions

Type	Action	Appearance	Onset of Action	Maximum Action (Hrs)	Total Action (Hrs)
Regular	Rapid	Clear		2–4	6–8
Semilente		Turbid	1/2–1		8–10
NPH	Intermediate	Turbid	1–2		
30% amorphous				4–8	12–14
70% crystalline				6–10	14–16
PZI	Long	Turbid	3–4	12–18	24–36
Ultralente			2–4	8–12	24–36

the insulin with less than two injections per day with a combination of short-acting (regular or Semilente) insulin and an intermediate-acting (NPH or Lente) insulins. Physiologic control can be provided with various three-dose or four-dose per day (or even more injections per day) programs but cannot be provided with less than two doses per day of combination therapy. This two-dose per day regimen of short- and intermediate-acting insulins is known as split-mix insulin therapy and today (1984) is considered conventional insulin therapy In our program we begin with this program and move to three- or four-dose insulin regimens when we can no longer maintain adequate metabolic control with conventional therapy. We never hesitate to move to a three- or four-dose per day program (intensive insulin therapy) when glucose control by conventional split-mix regimen is no longer adequate.

REFERENCES

1. Jackson, R. L., Stervick, W. O., Hollinden, C. S., Stroeh, L., and Shultz, J. G.: Neutral regular insulin. *Diabetes* 21:235, 1972.

2. Jawadi, H., Ho, L., Childs, B., and Guthrie, R. A.: Stability of premixed Nordisk insulins when used in vivo. Submitted for publication, 1984.

3. Guthrie, R. A., Murthy, D. Y. N., and Womack, W.: Insulin resistance in diabetes in juveniles. *Pediatrics* 40:642, 1967.

4. Murthy, D. Y. N., Guthrie, R. A., Womack, W. N., and Jackson, R. L.: Insulin binding in children with diabetes mellitus. *Pediatrics* 43:558, 1969.

E. NUTRITIONAL MANAGEMENT

Robert L. Jackson, M.D.

As previously stated, the basic meal plan which we advocate evolved over many years from observing the eating habits of healthy, nondiabetic children and adolescents and from treating many children with diabetes. We prefer to use the term meal plan rather than diet because diet has the connotation of fasting and denial.

The child with diabetes needs the same kinds and amounts of food that every other well-fed child of similar age, height, and weight should eat, but the amounts and distribution of the foods must be carefully planned to match the action of the insulin administered. Insulin injections are necessary to allow the child to utilize his food properly. *Since the insulin injections have to be given at a certain time, meals and snacks also need to be eaten in keeping with the kind and amount of insulin injected.*

For a sound beginning the dietitian should have a preliminary conference with each family to establish rapport and to obtain detailed information about their present eating habits, schedule, and preferences. Only then can a meal plan be devised most suitable for the child and family. *At first it is important to teach the mother and child how to use high-quality common foods to prepare simple menus.* Then, as the mother and child gradually become more familiar with planning meals and snacks, they can be taught how to use combinations of food and recipes most enjoyed by their family. The education is best done by short, repeated teaching sessions with time in between for study and learning how to apply the information.

Meal planning is taught via food groups advocated by the American Dietetic Association and American Diabetic Association (see Table 6.2 for explanation). Emphasis is placed on the use of a wide variety of foods to ensure an adequate intake of all essential nutrients. Families are encouraged to include plenty of fruits, vegetables, whole-grain products, and legumes to increase daily consumption of dietary fiber. Use of foods containing large amounts of simple sugar is discouraged. No emphasis is placed on maintaining the same carbohydrate distribution at each meal. Thus, foods from the various food groups may be interchanged as long as the calories are subdivided into the meals and snacks and high-quality foods are included in each meal and most of the snacks. When the caloric content of the meals and snacks are the major consideration, a wide variety of food combinations for meals and snacks is attainable and recipes combining several different food groups are easier to calculate. Calorie counting is simplified by the use of the point system originally developed by Virginia Stuckey (75 calories ± = 1 point). Table 6.9 contains the distribution of calories in points.

After the child has regained normal weight for height and age, it is relatively easy to predict the gradual increase in calories for normal growth. We use the child's appetite as our major guide, but we also accurately assess and plot height and weight measurements at each office visit to evaluate growth and to avoid excessive weight gain.

As previously mentioned, meal Kcal/kg of body weight for a group of diabetic boys and girls, recorded in Table 6.1, may be used as a rough guide for the caloric maintenance requirement for children and adolescents. However, a wide range of caloric intake may be expected at each age. The needs of each child are variable and depend not only upon the patient's age and sex, but also upon body build, rate of growth, type and amount of activity, amount of rest, and emotional stress.

The education in sound nutrition for the family continues at each office visit after the relatively simple but basic instructions are completed and the mother and child have gained experience and confidence. The food intake needs to be adjusted as the child grows and develops. The parents and child also are taught the basic principles of how to adjust calorie intake to compensate for wide variation in daily physical activity and for illness (see Table 6.4B).

In our opinion, it is not desirable to permit children, diabetic or not, to eat without some supervision and direction. Many American children have poor dietary habits characterized by erratic food intake and excessive intake of unessential foods. Improved eating patterns should be encouraged for all children. The family of the child with diabetes needs to understand that the child's meal plan is reasonable and desirable for all members of the family. *One of the most effective ways for the family to help is to establish regularity in meal patterns, avoid the use of poor quality foods, and adopt the same basic food plan advocated for the child with diabetes.* The use of low-calorie "dietetic" sweets should be

TABLE 6.9 Calorie Points Division*

Calories	Breakfast 4/18	Snack 2/18	Lunch 5/18	Snack 1/18	Dinner 5/18	Snack 1/18	Total Calorie Points
800	2½	1	3	1	3	½	11
900	2½	1½	3	1	3	1	12
1000	3	1½	3½	1	3½	1	13½
1100	3	1½	4	1	4	1	14½
1200	3½	1½	4½	1	4½	1	16
1300	4	2	5	1	4½	1	17½
1400	4	2	5	1	5½	1	18½
1500	4½	2	5½	1½	5½	1	20
1600	5	2	6	1½	6	1	21½
1700	5	2½	6½	1½	6½	1	23
1800	5½	2½	6½	1½	6½	1½	24
1900	5½	3	7	1½	7	1½	25½
2000	6	3	7	1½	7½	1½	16½
2100	6	3	7½	1½	8	1½	28
2200	6½	3½	8	1½	8	1½	29
2300	7	3½	8½	2	8½	1½	31
2400	7	3½	9	2	9	1½	32
2500	7½	3½	9	2	9½	2	33½
2600	8	4	9½	2	9½	2	35
2700	8	4	10	2	10	2	36

2800	8½	4	10½	2	10½	2	37½
2900	8½	4½	11	2	11	2	39
3000	9	4½	11	2	11½	2	40
3100	9	4½	11½	2½	11½	2½	41
3200	10	5	11½	2½	12	2½	42
3300	10	5	12	2½	12	2½	44
3400	10	5	12½	2½	12½	2½	45
3500	10½	5	13	2½	13½	2½	47
3600	10½	5½	13½	2½	13½	2½	48
3700	11	5½	13½	3	13½	3	49½
3800	11½	5½	14	3	14	3	51
3900	11½	6	14½	3	14	3	52
4000	12	6	15	3	14½	3	53½

*One (1) calorie point equals approximately 75 (±15) calories.

discouraged except for special occasions. (Cultivating and perpetuating a "sweet tooth" and substituting empty calories for sound nutrition is a habit all of us, not just the child with diabetes, would do well to avoid.) Adherence to proper nutritional principles can benefit all members of the family and will diminish the child's feeling of being different.

GOALS FOR MANAGEMENT

To summarize, these are goals of management related to food intake:

1. Establish regular times for eating meals and snacks each day.
2. Have about the same amounts of high-quality foods in each of three regular meals.
3. Avoid foods and drinks containing large amounts of simple sugar (i.e., candy, frostings or other foods such as sherbet or carbonated drinks which contain primarily simple sugar).
4. Adjust both the kind and the amount of food in meals and snacks for variability in physical activities.
5. Adjust food intake during illness (see Table 6.4B).
6. Adjust the amounts of food in the meals and snacks to satisfy the appetite of the child and to sustain proper weight for his body build with growth.

F. DIABETES AND EXERCISE

Robert L. Jackson, M.D. and Libbie Russo, M.D.

Normal physical activity is as necessary for the child with diabetes as it is for children in general. As previously stated, the physical activity of the child requires close supervision during the period of metabolic recovery in the hospital. The desire and ability of the child to resume normal activities return rapidly as the nutritional status improves. During this critical period of nutritional repletion, activity patterns which resemble those of normal children are instituted as early as is feasible in the hospital. It is impractical to adjust food intake to compensate for random variations in energy output. Consequently, every effort should be made to maintain as constant as possible the daily activity pattern and also to approximate closely the weekend pattern to that of week days. To attain that objective, it is extremely important that the child be up and about at the same time each day and that a definite pattern of activity be established for the entire day -- morning, afternoon, and evening. After the early morning insulin injection and before breakfast, the child should be out of bed, washed, and dressed. Children in our hospital have two 1-hr periods daily of supervised, intensive physical activity in a playground or gymnasium. They attend school in another part of the hospital for 3 hr in the morning and 2 hr in the afternoon. Study and ward recreational periods are structured according to the age of the child. Bedtime is at 9:00 or 10:00 p.m. The parents of preschool-aged children are requested to help standardize the daily activities of their child. The caloric content of the prescribed meals or snacks are gradually increased as the child becomes stronger and more active during the recovery period. The daily activity pattern, however, is kept as constant as possible. During the nutritional repletion period, children are usually ravenous and willing to eat a wide variety of foods. It is preferable to satisfy the child's appetitie but to restrict the total caloric intake so the child readily eats all of the food offered in the meals and snacks. This also provides an opportunity for the child to learn to eat a wide variety of foods, for the child will more likely eat something less familiar, but available at meal times, to satisfy his appetite if just the right amount of food is provided.

After the insulin maintenance requirement has been established in the hospital and the child returns home, the insulin dosage should be kept as constant as possible from day to day. To compensate for variations in physical activity, the patient usually should then increase or decrease the intake of food rather than modify the type and dosage of insulin. Emphasis is placed on increasing food with more exercise to avoid insulin reactions, but it is equally important to decrease caloric intake with less exercise to avoid hyperglycemia and glycosuria.

In children who do not have diabetes, insulin levels decrease precipitously at the beginning of exercise and rise again rapidly after exercise (1, 2). Also, blood glucose levels usually remain stable in the nondiabetic child during shorter periods of exercise and may decrease to quite low levels during prolonged exercise (2, 3). Because the diabetic receives a certain dose of insulin based on predicted food intake and activity, subsequent changes in activity cannot be accommodated by changing the amount of insulin. To avoid hypoglycemia during and after a period of increased exercise, a change in food intake is needed for two reasons: 1) Diabetics who are in good metabolic control tend to have higher insulin levels during exercise than nondiabetics (4) because the insulin was injected earlier in the day and absorption will continue, regardless of metabolic need. To counteract this situation, more calories will need to be available during this period to prevent hypoglycemia. 2) The caloric distribution in the basic meal plan is structured to provide the requirements for usual daily activities. Extra activity implies increased energy usage. If more energy (food) is not provided during times of increased need, the body will have to revert to using its own stores (glycogen, protein, and fat) to a greater degree. This results in a gradual, overall deficit of body-building and energy-releasing materials available to the system and may cause an eventual negative balance with weight loss.

It is impossible to predict specific adjustments of food intake for a given child for a particular period of activity or inactivity. The parents and child must learn by experience and reliable daily urine tests or blood glucose monitoring how to adjust food intake by trial and error. The need for adjusting food usually begins the first day home from the hospital, when invariably there is a change in the physical activity pattern. At each office visit, this phase of management is reviewed and a program is gradually evolved to fit the pattern of each child's life. In general, it is preferable to change food intake for exercise with in-between-meal snacks rather than with meals.

For most American youngsters there are more social activities on weekends than during the week. The child may not only be more active in the early hours of the evening but may also retire at a later time. These variations in the physical activity pattern require some adjustment in food intake. The parents and the child are advised to use judgment in varying the time of the evening snack according to the various situations that might develop. If the evening program involves intensive physical activity for a relatively short period of time (as, for example, when participating in a short sports event, dancing or skating for an hour) we suggest either a larger evening meal or a double-portion snack, depending on which is more convenient and more in keeping with the eating habits of the peer group. However, if the program primarily varies from the usual by retiring at a later hour, it would be more appropriate for the child to take an additional small snack such as 4-8 oz of milk before going to bed.

As discussed in detail in Chapter 5B, the insulin requirement of children who receive prompt physiologic insulin replacement usually is less than 0.4 U/kg/day, indicating that they are only partially insulin-deficient. Consequently, during the early months or even years after stabilization, they are able to secrete some endogenous insulin to metabolize wider variations in food intake. They are also able to suppress insulin secretion to varying degrees during periods of increased physical activities. This fact gives the diabetic in partial remission a wider margin of safety during exercise than the total diabetic.

In planned increases in exercise, (e.g., swim team practice) appropriate increases in food intake need to be planned to avoid emergencies in energy depletion (hypoglycemia). Several factors need to be taken into account before a reasonable decision can be made in regard to selecting extra food before, during, and after periods of prolonged strenuous exercise.

1. What is the rate of absorption and metabolism of different types of food?
2. How long is the exercise period, and what is its tempo (continuous or intermittent) and intensity?
3. During what time of the day does the exercise take place?
4. What is the physical fitness and metabolic state of the child?
5. How do various modifications in food intake affect blood sugar levels during and after a specific physical activity for a given child?

Prior to effective use of any of these factors, determining insulin and food needed for usual activity is essential. If the child is maintained in good overall metabolic control, the blood sugar levels are generally quite predictable. This makes it easier for the essential preplanning needed to ensure as near normal blood glucose levels during exercise as possible. Also, with good overall metabolic control, there are fewer and less drastic fluctuations in blood glucose throughout the day (especially if the child is only partially insulin-deficient). Any changes in blood glucose which might occur due to exercise are more predictable and less fluctuant under these circumstances.

Considering the first variable, the rate of digestion, absorption, and metabolism of different types of food, fats are the slowest to be absorbed and cause the lowest increase in blood glucose of the three major food groups. However, they do affect the rate of absorption of other foods and provide a prolonged, low level of energy which can be used during exercise. Protein and complex carbohydrates are digested and absorbed at an intermediate rate and cause a gradual elevation in the blood glucose levels. In constrast, simple carbohydrates, especially when ingested without other foods in liquid form, are absorbed very rapidly and cause a rapid rise in the blood glucose level.

All three types of food are useful for maintaining normal blood glucose levels during predicted periods of decreased or increased activity. In order to decide what type of food to select and how much and how fast to eat, the second consideration becomes essential. How long and intense is the exercise period? If the increased activity is intensive and relatively short, 30 min or less, use of extra food with quick-acting properties is more appropriate. If the exercise is less strenuous but longer, 1.5–2 hr or more, use of foods which are absorbed at intermediate rates are preferable. Also, if the exercise period is intensive and prolonged, more calories (energy) will be used and so the total number of calories consumed should be increased proportionally. When the exercise period is quite prolonged, a second or third snack may be more effective and better tolerated. Again, the composition and size of these snacks depends on the expected duration of exercise.

Some athletes find they do not perform physically as well when they have eaten a large snack before they participate in a sport. An alternative to eating more food before exercising is eating frequent small amounts of simple carbohydrates during a prolonged period of intensive exercise. One effective way to do this is to drink 2–4 oz of orange juice or eat orange sections at 15–30 min intervals during exercise.

Dextrosol tablets also have been used effectively. Each Dextrosol tablet contains about 10 calories of dextrose. The rate of absorption is very predictable. The tablets are somewhat expensive, but many families prefer them because they are designated for a special use (exercise). Plain hard candies can also be used, but most children find it desirable to avoid eating concentrated sweets as they find it difficult not to eat them at other times.

The tempo of the exercise is also important. The previous recommendations work well for continuous exercise, e.g., swim team practice. If the exercise is intermittent over a long period of time, loading with food prior to the time of exercise may cause hyperglycemia when not exercising. A swim meet where a child may only participate two or three times in 1.5 hr is a good example. To compensate in this situation, it makes more sense to eat extra food when it is needed and which will be quickly available. Drinking fruit juice or eating a few Dextrosol tablets just before the event without any extra food between events work well.

The intensity of the exercise is also an important variable. Intense but short spurts of exercise (a sprint) are unlikely to cause hypoglycemia, while prolonged exercise (over 2 hr) which is less intense but steady is more likely to cause hypoglycemia. Also, different sports require differing amounts of energy, as in the comparison between bowling and basketball. Generally, increased intensity for a given period of time requires more calories.

Hypoglycemia is still a possibility hours after an exercise period. This after-exercise tendency for hypoglycemia increases as the duration and intensity of the exercise increases and may be accumulative over days. To avoid this problem, extra food is needed for the next meal or snack after the period of increased activity. Blood glucose levels or urine testing must also be monitored carefully for the next 24 hr or so until the diabetic child and his family see a pattern which indicates safety. The third consideration is the time of day the exercise takes place. Exercise which is done between supper and bedtime has a greater likelihood of causing hypoglycemia during the night or early the next morning. This fact makes it imperative to eat more food than usual before going to bed and to give close attention to the blood glucose and/or urine tests the next morning. If the blood glucose levels are too low, then the amount of food ingested the night before was not adequate for the amount of exercise done the night before. When this same exercise takes place at another date, the diabetic child should eat more food to compensate. If the next morning's blood glucose is too high, either the food eaten the night before was too much or there was a rebound caused by an earlier hypoglycemia resulting in a later rebound hyperglycemia. In this situation, it is wise to get an extra blood glucose measurement between midnight and 3:00 a.m. Food adjustments then can be made accordingly. If a relatively short exercise period is to directly follow a meal or snack, the extra food for the activity may be added to that snack or meal. Do not assume that the usual food eaten at these times will compensate more activity than usual. The meals were planned for usual activities and will not be adequate for increased activities. If the extra activities do not occur within 30 min of the last meal or snack, an extra snack should be given prior to the exercise.

Increased exercise in the midafternoon is also a time of high risk for hypoglycemia. An early morning injection of NPH insulin continues to provide a relatively high insulin level in the midafternoon. Consequently, we advise the child to always eat a snack in the afternoon before undertaking strenuous activities. Many students have gym class, band marching, or other sports activities at this time. If extra food is not eaten to compensate for these activities, excessive hunger or even hypoglycemia may be present for the after-school snack. Many children wait until they get home from school for their afternoon snack. Because of the preceding facts, an extra snack or changing the afternoon snack to before the activity is to be encouraged. Much of the inability of a diabetic student to control after school snacks may be due to this lack of adequate calories during mid- to late-afternoon activities. This produces very low glycogen stores, if not true hypoglycemia. The appetite can be quite active in either situation and will make it difficult to maintain a consistant afternoon snack pattern. Often the food intake is too great, resulting in high blood glucose levels before dinner. This may prompt the individual to increase the NPH given at breakfast, but this will just worsen the problem.

The fourth consideration is related to the nutritional status of the child and what the blood glucose level is just before beginning exercise. The physical fitness and nutritional state of the diabetic child is a major factor influencing toleration to increased energy output. The well-nourished child has more glycogen stores and lean body mass to form glucose and protect against hypoglycemia. The nondiabetic child begins exercise with a normal blood glucose level, and we may assume that this is the optimal metabolic state for activity. Many diabetic children have experienced insulin reactions during and after periods of increased activity. Consequently, they believe that a positive urine test or elevated blood glucose will avoid this problem. Unfortunately, beginning intensive exercise with a high blood glucose level (200-300 mg/dl) causes an exacerbation of hyperglycemia frequently and may induce ketosis. This is especially true of intense, short bursts of activity because of the acute stress placed on the body and the lack of subsequent muscular activity to effectively utilize blood glucose. This problem of exacerbation of the diabetic state during exercise with hyperglycemia also makes it unwise to undertake short periods of intense exercise to lower an already elevated blood glucose level.

The fifth consideration is important for two reasons:

1. It emphasizes the individual needs of each child for each type of activity. The same activity varies in intensity from child to child, so metabolic needs also vary. The physician or dietitian can suggest what to eat prior to exercise based on the factors presented here. It is up to the parents to determine whether or not that recommendation worked best for their child. As previously stated, changes need to be made on a trial-and-error basis for each child.
2. It also emphasizes the need for frequent and accurate urine tests and for older children and adults, appropriately timed blood glucose measurements. The best way to find out whether the extra food or number of glucose tablets was adequate is to actually check the blood glucose levels. Only then can more rational changes in food intake be made. If the exercise is relatively short and of less intensity, the usual timing of urine tests and/or blood glucose measurements are adequate most of the time (i.e., before meals and at bedtime).

The availability of home blood glucose meters now makes it possible for parents and older children to make accurate and rapid measurements of blood glucose levels at home. Home glucose monitoring is especially useful for older children who are totally insulin-deficient and especially for adolescents who need to learn how to modify their treatment plan in keeping with their changing life-styles. Older children, during their growth spurt, also require large amounts of exogenous insulin and have much greater variability in their activities from day to day. They can quickly learn by frequent blood glucose measurements how important it is to adhere to the instruction they have been given by their parents and the diabetes health team. After the adolescent has performed blood glucose measurements under similar circumstances several times and has adjusted food intake to maintain euglycemia, the number and frequency of blood glucose measurements may be decreased. It is recommended, however, that blood glucose be measured before and after exercise periodically, even for familiar but increased activity.

Since the diabetic who participates in sports or other activity does so at his best when the blood sugar is as normal as possible, it is important that he plan ahead for each engagement as much as possible. It may be unwise to depend upon the pool or school concession stand to provide the right types and amounts of food which will be needed. Most of the time it is better to bring the extra food along to the engagement.

There are two other types of exercise to consider. The first is unexpected excercise. In this situation, prior preparation with appropriate amounts and types of food is not possible. If nothing is done to compensate, this type of exercise will cause hypoglycemia as readily as any other type of exercise. Ingestion of glucose containing food frequently during this type of exercise is one way to avoid hypoglycemia during this period. This makes it mandatory that the diabetic child have with her a supply of fast-acting food. Dextrosol tablets rolled in the sock top or hard candy in the pocket during playtime is one easy method of carrying extra food. Also remember that the next snacks and meals may need to be increased to avoid latent hypoglycemia.

Hidden exercise, the second type, is another source of rapid changes in blood glucose for the diabetic child. Some examples of this are walking to another bus stop or going on a field trip instead of sitting in school that day. The main way to be prepared for this type of exercise is to watch for it and provide food which is appropriate. Just as it is with unexpected exercise, hidden exercise has the same potential to cause problems as the planned exercise.

We encourage the parents of younger children with diabetes (over 8 years of age) to consider having their child attend a camp for diabetic children for at least one or two summer sessions. A well-organized camp can provide: 1) a safe place for the parents to leave the child so they can have a vacation without the responsibility of his daily care; 2) an opportunity for the child to become more aware that many other children also are diabetic; 3) a setting to reemphasize the basic instructions they have been given; 4) an opportunity for the child to be more responsible for his own care and to gain increased insight in adjusting food intake for wide variations in physical activity; and 5) a chance to learn that diabetes need not be a hindrance to participation in vigorous and often extremely difficult physical and mental activities.

Selection of staff and children for a camp for diabetic children should be made carefully to provide a wholesome psychosocial environment. We believe that well-adjusted adolescent children with diabetes who have had previous experience in a camp for children with diabetes can then attend summer camps with nondiabetic children. Identifying with healthy children overcomes feelings of being handicapped. Older children with diabetes having such camping experiences make excellent counselors for younger children.

Overall, exercise in the diabetic child is encouraged. Metabolic problems which might occur can be prevented if the child and her family make the effort to plan ahead for it whenever possible. Also, because not all exercise is planned, the child should be prepared with some sort of sugar-containing food at all times and instructed as to its usage. It is also important that the child tell the parents of any extra exercise so that more food can be made available at subsequent meals.

Although exercise is good for the diabetic child, it is recommended for the same reason that exercise is recommended for nondiabetic children. Exercise promotes health and well-being, as well as an opportunity for socialization. Exercise should not be used to substitute or compensate for other parts of diabetic care. In other words, doctors do not prescribe a set amount of exercise because the insulin or food intake is not being well regulated. Normal exercise which is appropriate for the age group will help develop physical strength and self-reliance for all children.

REFERENCES

1. Vranic, M., Kawamori, R., Pek, S., Kovacevic, N., and Wrenshall, G. A.: The essentiality of insulin and the role of glucagon in regulating glucose utilization and production during strenuous exercise in dogs. *J. Clin. Invest.* 56:245-255, Feb. 1976.

2. Krzentowski, G., Pirnay, R., Pallikaradis, N., Luyckx, A., Lacroix, M.. Masora, F., and Lefebure, P.: Glucose utilization during exercise in normal and diabetic subjects: The role of insulin. *Diabetes* 30:983-989, Dec. 1981.

3. Felig, P., Cherif, A., Minagawa, A., and Wahren, J.: Hypoglycemia during prolonged exercise in normal men. *N.E.J.M.* 306(15):895-900, April 1982.

4. Holm, G., and Bjorntord, D.: Metabolic effects of physical training. *Acta Ped. Scand.* 283 (Suppl.): 9-14.

G. INSTRUCTIONS FOR CARE OF THE CHILD DURING AN INTERCURRENT ILLNESS

Robert L. Jackson, M.D.

Parents should be taught what to do in case the child has an intercurrent illness. The parents and child are given detailed written instructions as part of their basic education and the nurse and dietitian spend as much time as they deem necessary to explain the instructions. This phase of management is again reviewed before the child is taken home and at each subsequent office visit. The parents must maintain close observation to prevent ketoacidosis, especially when the child has a febrile illness. During illness the child's food intake should be decreased and it is often necessary to use liquids or semisolid foods as small snacks at frequent intervals. A modified food plan is given to the parents for that purpose (see Table 6.4B). Basal caloric intake should be decreased about 20% during illness because physical activity should be decreased. Usually the child's appetite is poor, and vomiting is more likely if large quantities of food are eaten at one time. Food should be given at regular intervals as three meals and three snacks or even as more frequent smaller feedings.

The insulin requirement usually increases during a febrile illness, provided the child continues to ingest and absorb his food. In addition to needing slightly larger doses of insulin in the morning and evening, the child may also require supplementary doses of regular insulin at noon and late in the evening. When the child is old enough to understand and cooperate, we do at this time advise obtaining a double-voided specimen. If there is 3% or more glucose (without acetone) in the second-voided urine specimen before lunchtime, a dose of regular insulin, equal to about one-sixth of the morning dose, should be given. If acetone is also present, a dose of regular insulin equal to one-third of the morning dose is given. If 3% or more glycosuria without acetone in the second-voided specimen is observed in late evening (about 11:00 p.m.), an additional dose of regular insulin should be given, the dose being one-fourth of the evening dose. If both 3% glycosuria *and* acetonuria are present, a dose of regular insulin equal to one-half of the evening dose is given. In such a case, the child also should be given 4–8 oz of fruit juice about 30 min after giving the supplemental insulin. In addition, *the parents are advised to have their family physician examine the child if the symptoms and signs of the infection are progressing so that antibiotic therapy can be given early when indicated.* If ketonuria persists, we often advise the mother to offer the child four or six small meals at 6- or 4-hr intervals and to give only *regular* insulin about 30 min before each of the small meals. We rarely have had to rehospitalize a diabetic child who has responsible and informed parents. Children managed by such parents rarely have ketosis even during infections.

Although most children need increased insulin doses during illness, there is an occasional child who does not, especially when he has periods of vomiting and diarrhea. If the child is vomiting or having diarrhea, food cannot be retained or effectively absorbed. This is essentially the *only* time that the insulin dosage needs to be decreased during illness. When this occurs, we advise giving only two-thirds of the usual dose of insulin in the morning and evening and to recheck the urine as often as possible and then give additional small doses of regular insulin at midday and late evening as previously described. If the child is vomiting or has an upset stomach, we advise offering small quantities (1-2 oz) of a sweetened, carbonated beverage such as ginger ale about every 5-10 min and then to alternate with 1-2 oz of diluted sweetened fruit juice as soon as the child is retaining foods. Popsicles, hard peppermint candy, or afterdinner mints also may be used with small sips of water. One must, therefore, individualize treatment during illness and carefully monitor the urine glucose and acetone frequently, adjusting the dosage of insulin and intake of food as necessary. As the infection subsides and the urine becomes glucose-free, the child's insulin and food requirements will return rapidly to the maintenance level.

H. OFFICE VISITS (CONTINUITY OF CARE AND EDUCATION)

Robert L. Jackson, M.D.

When children with diabetes leave the hospital after their initial stabilization, they are requested to return for their first office visit in about 10 days-2 weeks. During this initial period of home care, the parents are advised *to notify a member of the health team at once if they are in doubt about how to cope with an unexpected problem.* Children with recent onset are in the honeymoon or partial remission phase of their disease, so they require very little exogenous insulin and it is easily possible to have all urine specimens free from glucose with little likelihood of the patient's having even a minor insulin reaction. The initial office visit is very important to assure the parents and child that they can control the diabetes at home when the child resumes a normal pattern of life. At the time of the first office visit, they are reinstructed in adjusting the child's food intake to varying degrees of physical activity and in modifying insulin dosage. The parents also are advised to consult their family physician for treatment of other health problems. The time interval for subsequent clinic visits is individualized. As soon as the parents are secure and the diabetes remains under good control, the interval between visits is increased. Ultimately, most of our patients return to the office at 3- to 6-month intervals. More frequent visits are desirable for those with special problems and those in their growth spurt.

I. SUMMARY

The regimen proposed is desirable and attainable. This flexible plan of treatment teaches the parents and child how to control the diabetes and how to manage periodic illnesses. Good metabolic control over the years conserves the child's health for the future. Each family finally reaches a compromise between that which is prescribed and that which the home environment makes possible. If the child is a member of an unstable family, a greater compromise must be made -- to the child's disadvantage.

Until more knowledge about the pathophysiology of juvenile diabetes is available, good control is the only known means of delaying or averting degenerative changes. Recent advances in research are encouraging. We are learning much more about human genetics, as well as the various environmental factors that influence the course of diabetes. Basic studies are elucidating the mechanism of synthesis and release of insulin from pancreatic beta cells. Interrelationships of insulin with other endocrine and humoral factors are being clarified. Advances in transplanting islet cells from normal animal pancreas to diabetic animals may ultimately have application for human beings. The need for injecting insulin may be eliminated by the availability of automatic delivery systems designed to maintain physiologic control of blood glucose levels throughout the day.

Early identification of subclinical diabetes provides an opportunity to observe the natural pattern of development of the disease and to evaluate different measures that may alter its progression. We look forward to the day when we will know the cause of diabetes and how to prevent it. Until then, it is important for physicians to maintain an optimistic outlook in caring for children with diabetes.

APPENDIX A CLASSIFICATION OF DIABETIC KETOACIDOSIS*

Severe

1. Venous $HCO_3 < 15$ or $pH < 7.2$
2. Severe dehydration > 10%
3. Blood glucose > 400, glycosuria, ketonuria
4. Kussmaul's respirations (deep, rapid breathing), acetone odor to breath
5. Depressed or altered level of consciousness (i.e., combative or sleepy)
6. Unable to take oral solutions (due to unconsciousness or vomiting)
7. Glycosuria and ketonuria, large

Moderate

1. Venous $HCO_3 > 15$
2. Moderate dehydration 5-10%
3. Blood glucose > 300
4. Kussmaul's respiration (acetone odor may be absent)
5. Alert
6. Vomiting
7. Glycosuria and ketonuria, moderate

Mild

1. Venous $HCO_3 > 18$
2. Mild dehydration < 5%
3. Blood glucose < 300
4. Kussmaul's respiration, no acetone odor
5. Alert
6. Not vomiting, able to take oral solutions
7. Mild glycosuria and no ketonuria

*Look for infection as precipitating cause. Clinical appearances in children may be deceiving, especially if in chronically poor control.

APPENDIX B PROTOCOL FOR MANAGEMENT OF MODERATE DIABETIC KETOACIDOSIS

1. Fluid and electrolyte therapy. Intravenous fluid therapy is essential for all children with moderate DKA.
   a) Assume 0-5% dehydration (may not be necessary in mild DKA) and infuse at a rate to provide maintenance plus correction of the deficit in 12 hr.
   b) Use one-fourth to one-half normal saline with 40 mEq KCl/L and 5% glucose.
   c) May be possible to rehydrate orally if child is hungry and not vomiting. In moderate ketoacidosis, start four equal meals at 6-hr intervals using 30 cal/kg/day for the pubertal and postpubertal patient, respectively. (The small prepubertal child may require six small meals beginning at 40-60 cal/kg/day and gradually increase to 60-80 cal/kg/day in keeping with the appetite.)
2. Insulin.
   a) Give insulin subcutaneously *30 min before meals* starting at 1-2 U/kg/day. Use the lower dosage for mild ketoacidosis.
   b) Adjust the insulin dosage at each 4- or 6-hr interval by assessing either semiquantitative urine glucose performed on each urine or reflectance meter blood sugar 30 min before each meal.

      The goal is negative-trace urines without hypoglycemia or blood sugars between 80-150 mg/dl. The insulin dosage is increased or decreased at each 6-hr interval to achieve this goal. The amount of increase or decrease depends upon the degree of hyperglycemia, ketoacidosis, and total body weight of the child but should be based upon a percentage of the previous dosage rather than an arbitrary dosage for a given blood sugar (sliding scales are dangerious in younger small diabetics). Roughly, the increases should not be greater than 20-30% of the dosage for urines or blood sugars above the limit. The dosage should be cut in half for significant hypoglycemia requiring repeated or IV treatment or by 20-30% for mild hypoglycemia. Small alterations may require the use of diluted insulin, U50, U25, U10.

c) Once the goal of negative urines or blood sugars between 80 and 150 mg/dl is achieved for several successive 4- or 6-hr periods, the patient's total daily dosage can be calculated by multiplying the dosage for a 6-hr period by 4. This total dosage will provide a close approximation of insulin need and can be used as a guide to switch to a two- or three-shot regimen using mixtures of long, intermediate, or short-acting insulin if the caloric intake correlates with the insulin distribution. For example, diabetics who have two-thirds of their total caloric intake at breakfast, lunch, and midmorning and midafternoon snacks will require approximately two-thirds of their insulin dosage 30 min before breakfast in a split-mixed 2:1 NPH:regular regimen and one-third of their insulin 30 min before dinner. As their pancreatic function improves, exogenous insulin will need to be lowered.

APPENDIX C PROTOCOL FOR MANAGEMENT OF SEVERE DIABETIC KETOACIDOSIS BY CONSTANT IV INSULIN INFUSION

1. Expand plasma volume. If hypotensive, the patient should receive a pump primer, such as:
   a) Normal saline or lactated Ringer's at 360 ml/m^2 for the first 30 min (15-20 ml/kg/hr).
   b) Repeat above step (a) if hypotension persists.
   c) If patient is in shock, initial treatment with albumin, plasmanate, plasma, or blood may be required.
2. Fluid and electrolyte therapy.
   a) After first hour use one-half normal saline solution (final concentration) at a rate to replace one-half of estimated fluid deficit over next 8-10 hr. Assume a 10% dehydration in severe ketoacidosis; plus maintenance fluids with one-half normal saline at 1500/m^2/day (or 6-8 ml/kg/hr).
   b) $NaHCO_3$ may be added if $HCO_3 < 15$ mEq/L or pH < 7.2. Calculate either to replace one-half of estimated base deficit over next 8-10 hr or to increase serum bicarbonate to 15 mEq/L over next 3-4 hr. May calculate using pH nomogram or serum bicarbonate.

mEq bicarbonate to be given over 8 hr = $\frac{1}{2}$ correction x base deficit x 0.3 body distribution x weight in kg

mEq bicarbonate needed to raise serum bicarbonate to 15 to be given over 4 hr = $\frac{1}{2}$ correction x (15-patient's bicarbonate) x 0.3 x kg

To be given at a rate not to exceed 1 mEq/kg/min

Discontinue when serum HCO_3 15 mEq/l. Make sure that the final IV solution is not greater than one-half to three-fourths normal saline after adding $NaHCO_3$. (Adding $NaHCO_3$ to one-half normal saline will yield isotonic or hypertonic saline in some cases.) Diabetics need free water. Note: Bicarbonate is incompatible with KPO_4 and insulin; also preferable that insulin not be mixed with KPO_4.

$$\underset{(35\ \text{mEq Na})}{\tfrac{1}{4}\ \text{NS}} + \underset{(40\ \text{mEq Na})}{40\ \text{mEq Na } HCO_3} = \underset{(75\ \text{mEq Na})}{\tfrac{1}{2}\ \text{NS}}$$

c) Add K (40 mEq/L) after normal urine output is demonstrated and serum K $<$ 5 mEq/L. Add one-half of K as KH_2PO_4 to correct hypophosphatemia that may accompany correction of ketocacidosis. Higher concentration of K in IV solution may be necessary to keep serum K above 2.5 mEq/L. Remember serum K will fall rapidly after giving insulin and after correction of ketoacidosis, which reflects the depletion of total body K. 20 mEq/L of K^+ is safe when T waves on EKG are peaked or normal. If low or flat T waves 40 mEq/L K should be used. May use up to maximum 60 mEq/L; K should be monitored by EKG and laboratory values.

d) Add 5% glucose when blood sugar is $<$ 250 mg% or Clinitest is negative.

e) Maintenance fluids after 8–10 hr of hydration or repletion of deficit given as 0.45% normal saline (3-6 ml/kg/hr, 40 mEq/L KCl, and 5% glucose.

f) When oral intake is tolerated, start four equal meals and four shots of regular insulin. Discontinue IV and insulin and glucose infusions. Notify dietitian 3–4 hr in advance; soft diet, advance as tolerated. Provide adequate potassium, calcium, and phosphate. Insulin dose is started between 1 and 2 U/kg/day depending on their nutritional status. Vitamin B complex should be included as part of parenteral therapy for the undernourished patient in severe DKA.

3. *Method A* : Mixing insulin for infusion:

   a) Regular insulin in normal saline with concentration of at least 0.1 U/ml (place 100 U U100 regular insulin in 1 L of 0.9% (normal saline)

b) Flush tubing with at least 50 cc of the insulin solution to saturate nonspecific insulin-binding sites.
c) Administer at a rate to give 0.1 U/kg/hr or at a rate of 1.0 ml/kg/hr. *Total maximum dosage 6.0 U/hr or 60 cc/hr.*

Method B: For those requiring careful volume replacement (cardiac or renal disease).

a) Regular insulin in normal saline with 0.5% albumin by constant infusion via four-way stopcock at rate of 0.1 U/kg/hr; *total maximum dosage 6.0 U/hr.*

   3 ml of 25% albumin are added to 250 ml of normal saline (the albumin will minimize the binding of insulin to tubing). Put 100 ml into volutrol and add 100 U of regular insulin.

This yields a final concentration of insulin:
0.1 U = 0.1 ml.

   Infuse at 0.1 U/kg/hr or 0.1 ml/kg/hr *total maximum dosage 6.0 U/hr* (6 ml/hr of insulin drip at this concentration).

b) Continue until blood sugar < 250 mg% and/or acidosis is corrected, then institute four equal meals and four shots of regular insulin if patient is alert and hungry. (See protocol for mild ketoacidosis)
c) Mix insulin fresh every 6 hr.

If treatment is delayed, give loading dose of 0.1 U/kg IV over 5 min.

4. Monitoring.
   a) Initial lab - CBC, UA (culture and sensitivity), electrolytes, BUN/creatinine, pH, glucose, ketones, CA/PO_4, Mg.
   b) Accurate in/out, may need to catheterize if unresponsive.
   c) Clinitest and Acetest urine *every* 30 min.
   d) Glucose or reflectance photometer blood sugar every 60 min. Reflectance meters allow quantitative blood sugar measurement by fingerstick and avoid lag time in laboratory determination.
   e) EKG -- continuous monitor for hyper- or hypokalemia.
   f) Check electrolytes at least every 2 hr or more frequently if problems with K.

g) Check PO_4 at 2-3 hr.
h) Vital signs every hour until stable.

Complications to look for during and after treatment for DKA (19, 20): 1. hypovolemic shock; 2. cerebral edema; 3. vascular occlusions; and 4. infection. Diabetic ketoacidosis carries increased morbidity and mortality.

1. Shock due to hypovolemia. Monitor closely and be sure fluids in exceed fluids out, may neeu volume expansion initially; stay ahead of the massive diuresis that occurs.
2. Cerebral edema: check neurologic signs. Cerebral edema may occur for unexplained reasons during treatment. It generally occurs at 4-6 hr when patients are generally improving in state of alertness. Be aware of headache, sleepiness, or decrease in level of consciousness at this time. Early signs include: obtundation, lower pulse from vagal stimulation, and raised blood pressure to keep cardiac output same. The cerebral edema may be irreversible if progression takes place; treat with mannitol 0.5-1.0 g/kg IV push if suspicious. Papilledema is a late diagnostic sign.
3. Vascular thromboses, myocardial infarction, or strokes due to the following:

<u>Impaired blood flow</u>	+	<u>Hypoxia</u>
dehydrated		↑$HgbA_1c$
↑viscosity		impaired O_2
↓CO due to acidosis		delivery

<u>Hypercoagulable state</u>
adhesive platelets
factor VIII
↑fibrinogen
↓fibrinolysis

However, the main causes for vascular thromboses may be iatrogenic:

a) Sudden lowering of serum blood sugar lowering the osmotic effect and thus further decreasing the intravascular and extracellular fluid volume. This decreases cardiac output and precipitates hypovolemic shock and thrombogenesis.

b) Quick correction of acidosis by insulin and bicarbonate therapy unmasks the abnormal oxyhemoglobin dissociation of low 2,3-DPG (which at normal levels promotes delivery of oxygen from hemoglobin to tissue). Patients remain at risk for days until RBC 2,3-DPG returns to normal.

c) Infection: check for infections as precipitating causes for DKA by fever, UA, CXR, thorough physical exam, review of systems, nuchal rigidity, abdominal pain, etc.

Chapter 7

EDUCATION OF PARENTS

Robert L. Jackson, M.D.

The example given by parents is the basic model that children use in developing their attitudes about health practices as well as their future life-style; therefore, the education of the parents as to why and how to maintain optimum health of their child with diabetes is of fundamental importance. The success of treatment and the ultimate prognosis are dependent upon the ability of the parents to continue management after the child has regained an optimal state of health from intensive care in the hospital.

Shortly after the child is admitted to the hospital, the parents are given the introductorv section of a manual prepared for their instructions (1). We have found this practice very helpful in meeting the immediate needs for answering the usual questions asked by parents about diabetes and how it will affect the future health of their child. For example, the first two paragraphs of the manual read as follows:

This information has been prepared to help parents learn what you should know about diabetes and how to control it so your child can enjoy an excellent state of health. It is important for both of you to realize that your child's diabetes is not due to anything either of you have or have not done. It is not your fault or that of anyone else. We realize how greatly concerned you are and should be about your child's welfare, but be thankful that we know what the trouble is and how to control it.

Everyone in the hospital will do everything possible to rapidly restore the health of your child. Although treatment of the child with diabetes requires expert knowledge and skill on the part of the doctors, dietitians, and nurses, *YOU ONLY HAVE TO LEARN A FEW THINGS WELL TO TAKE GOOD CARE OF YOUR CHILD. YOUR INSTRUCTIONS WILL BE SIMPLE AND WE SHALL MAKE SURE YOU KNOW WHAT TO DO AND HOW TO DO IT BEFORE YOU TAKE YOUR CHILD HOME.* Do not be afraid to ask any questions.

After the parents have had some rest and the child's condition is improved, a conference is held with them by the doctor and the nurse specialist. At this time the reasons for the length of hospital care are explained and any other questions which they have are answered in much greater depth. The doctor also defines the role of each member of the health team, which consists of the doctor, house officer, nurse specialist, dietitian, and medical social worker. The nurse then proceeds to make appointments and to introduce the parents to the other members of the health team.

The remaining sections of the teaching manual are given to the parents in an appropriately timed sequence by the nurse and dietitian. Teaching aids are used and include movies, videotapes, slide-tape programs, and many actual practice sessions in mixing insulins, giving insulin injections, testing for glucose and acetone, as well as planning and preparing the child's meals and snacks. By long experience we know that shorter teaching sessions are essential over a period of weeks and that longer sessions crowded into only a few days are ineffective.

Detailed social information also needs to be obtained by an experienced medical social worker to evaluate the family as well as the community resources. If the child is to make a good adjustment, not only the family but also the community need to be educated through whatever local resources are available or can be developed.

It is not surprising that the diagnosis of diabetes in a child results in a state of psychological crisis in a family. Four different stages of transition are discernable in each of the parents and in older children. During the *first stage* of *shock,* they try to deny what has happened. Life seems chaotic and the parents and child are not too receptive to information although they may appear superficially relatively calm. This first stage usually is short in a stable family but may persist and recur in an immature or unstable parent or an adolescent. The *second stage* is one of *recognition* and this is often characterized by feelings of guilt. Most often this stage also is quite transitory but varies widely depending upon many factors, such as family history of diabetes, health practices of the parents before and during gestation; care and feeding during infancy (breast vs. bottle feeding) and the care, incidence, and severity of infections during the preschool years. The *third stage* is characterized by *objectivity* where the parents as well as the child gradually accept the reality of the situation. Only then are the parents and child ready to proceed to the *fourth stage,* which is *reintegration.* Relapses into previous stages are common. It is not until a parent and child enter the third stage that they are ready for more intense and structured instruction. It is imperative for all members of the health team to work closely together in helping the parents reach this stage of reintegration. Input from all members of the health team is required to determine when each member of the family is ready for effective instruction. The medical social worker can play a major role in helping the parents and child attain the stage of objectivity by guiding them in making sensible immediate and long-term plans for the care of their child and family. The younger child's acceptance is directly related to the parents' acceptance and understanding and the older child's acceptance also is closely interrelated with that of the parents.

It is imperative that the parents and the child understand clearly the plan of treatment, including the need for insulin as soon as possible, and that they face the reality of the situation. Responsibility for management will rest with them; the physician and health team should instruct and help qualify them. As soon as the child is old enough, she should be similarly trained. The parents ultimately need to know about the nature of the disease, the theory of management, and recognition and treatment of complications. During the initial period in the hospital, they should be given as much practical information as they can understand and the physician and health team can impart.

It is necessary and important to instruct both parents and have each participate in the care of the child. Although the child should gradually assume more responsibility for his own care, it is undesirable and unrealistic to expect younger children to assume primary responsibility for that care.

Other factors that affect the learning process are individual differences in abilities and educational experiences. Instruction must be adapted to various cultural backgrounds and economic levels, so individualized instruction sessions are usually much more effective and practical than group sessions.

Most parents are exceedingly apprehensive about giving injections to their child. Mothers are also insecure and skeptical about their ability to plan meals and monitor their children's intake of food. Once they have received basic information and daily repeated practical experience in these aspects of diabetic management, only then are they psychologically ready for additional factual information and for learning other skills.

In general, it is better to teach only basic management during the time the child is in the hospital. More advanced concepts can be presented during future office visits in accord with the parents' (and child's) growing interests and capacities.

All members of the immediate family of the child with diabetes need to understand that the patient's meal plan is reasonable for each of them. *We repeat, one of the most effective ways to help the child is for family members also to establish regularity in meal patterns, avoid the use of poor quality foods, and adopt the same basic food plan advocated for the child who has diabetes.* Parents should be given anticipatory guidance in how to deal with siblings' resentment which may stem from their perception that they are being deprived of both their parents' attention (because of involvement with management of diabetes) and of the need for them to modify their eating habits which most often included excessive intake of sweets. Education and adherence to proper nutritional principles can benefit all members of the family and will greatly diminish the patient's feeling of being different.

Assuming responsibility for adjusting food intake and insulin dosage are worrisome for all parents. They are understandably fearful of the possibility of an insulin reaction, and they are concerned about how they will care for the child if she becomes sick. We give the parents detailed written instructions for maintaining control of the child's diabetes during an intercurrent illness. They are encouraged to call us whenever they have doubts, but with experience, most parents soon gain confidence and become capable of managing the diabetes even in the event of an intercurrent illness. The nurse and/or dietitian keep in contact with the parents by phone during the early weeks or even months after the child returns home.

The easiest time to attain compliance is at the onset of the disease. Unless both parents participate actively from the beginning, it becomes increasingly difficult to get one or the other involved. Often an intelligent older child learns the basics more easily and rapidly than do the parents, but then there is a tendency for the parents to shirk responsibility. The parents should not be dependent upon the child to teach them. Both parents should have at least as much basic information as the child before they assume responsibility for home care.

In general, we like to have the mother assume primary responsibility for planning the food, the father and mother for checking or supervising urine and blood tests, and the child for collecting urine specimens and learning how to adjust food intake for varying degrees of physical activity. When the child is about 9 or 12 years of age she should know how to measure and give insulin, but we suggest that one of the parents continue to give the larger morning dose of insulin into an area of the body not easily reached by the child. Supervised by one of the parents, the child can begin injecting the evening insulin dose into easily accessible sites.

The physician should use all facilities and personnel available in evaluating and educating the family. Ideally, the physician, nurse, dietitian, and social worker should periodically meet with the family as a team. Each member of the team provides unique expertise on some aspect of the management of diabetes mellitus.

Attainment and maintenance of a high level of control is contingent upon the ability to apply the learned principles to solve day-to-day problems in management of the diabetes. However, the cognitive level and knowledge base that is required for the development of problem-solving skills and the exercising of judgments and insights may be beyond the potential of some parents and children. Individuals vary widely in attributes such as education, health, perceptual ability, and motivation, which modulate reading ability and learning ability. It is important for all members of the health team to recognize this and to modify the educational content and sequence accordingly. *Keep in mind that the parents and child only have to learn a few skills but that mastery of these skills is essential. Mastery will only occur if sufficient time is allotted for repetition and practice of basic skills.* By focusing on only that content that they will need to know in order to solve day-to-day problems in management, the health professional will avoid overburdening and confusing the learners with complex concepts which are beyond their understanding at that time. Each member of the health team should avoid trying to impress the parents and child with all they know about diabetes.

Parents whose knowledge base and/or cognitive level is lower than is required for mastery of specific content will need to have close, even daily, supervision and guidance for each step of the diabetes management during the first weeks at home. Illiteracy or low reading comprehension ability impose an additional challenge for the educator. There is a need to increase the span of time allowed for comprehension of visual and verbal information and to intensify the learning sessions. For example, sample menus may be sent home if the parent is not able to plan meals accurately because of deficits in reading or math skills.

A good relationship between the physician and other members of the health team and the child (and other members of the family) is essential in obtaining compliance to the regimen of therapy. A healthy relationship is based on cooperation and understanding, with the common desire for the child to be well and able to lead an active life. All members of the health team must be willing to accept the child and parents with their limitations. Members of the team should avoid derogatory and threatening comments and should realize that at times the child will view them as she does her parents (whether this be positively or negatively). When discussing possible future complications, the physician should always maintain optimism without distorting reality.

At subsequent office visits, the physician, as captain of the health team, should always review how well the parents and child are carrying out instructions. Varying food intake with variation in physical activity, rotating injection sites, diluting and mixing insulins, and measuring doses correctly are skills that should be evaluated by a member of the health team at each office visit.

Adjustments of insulin and food intake must be individualized; they cannot be made without parental understanding of all aspects of diabetic management, including routine care and illness. Accurate, reliable home records are very helpful. They are used for recording daily insulin doses, urine and blood tests, remarks about food intake with exercise, emotional stresses, and symptoms or signs of insulin reactions. Detailed review of the information is the best means of teaching the child and parents the interrelationships of insulin, food, exercise, emotions, and infections in the management of the disease.

Parents should be given enough instructions so that if the child's appetite and demands for food and insulin increase rapidly (as in certain periods of growth), both food intake and insulin dosages can be increased appropriately without consulting physician, nurse, or dietitian. That is possible only when the parents understand the treatment plan, and their understanding depends upon their ability to learn and how well they have been instructed. How well the parents are able to apply what they have learned in a new situation is a measure of the effectiveness of a large part of the teaching. The ability to recall and apply principles is dependent upon how well the underlying concepts are understood. This understanding will be facilitated if the instructional activities incorporate extensive opportunities for repetition and practice. Written and/or illustrated instructions are essential.

The prognosis is much more dependent upon the daily home care of the child than upon variations in the severity of the disease. Each family ultimately reaches a compromise between that which is advocated and that which the environment makes possible. Most parents will do much more for their children than they will do for themselves. However, with an unstable family, compromises have to be made to the child's disadvantage. Our present knowledge makes it not only possible but practical to maintain a high degree of diabetic control for children living in well-adjusted families.

REFERENCES

1. *The Child with Diabetes (Manual for Parents and Child).* The University of Kansas, Department of Pediatrics, Section of Endocrinology.

Chapter 8

GROWTH AND MATURATION OF CHILDREN WITH INSULIN-DEPENDENT DIABETES MELLITUS*

Robert L. Jackson, M.D.

INTRODUCTION

Growth is a manifestation of life in the young and its rate and quality are related closely to the general health and nutrition of the child. Before the discovery of insulin in 1922, children with overt diabetes became severely undernourished

---

*This chapter is a modification of a previous publication, "Growth and Maturation of Children with Insulin-Dependent Diabetes Mellitus," by R. L. Jackson, E. Holland, I. D. Chatman, D. Guthrie, and J. E. Hewett, published in *Diabetes Care,* Vol. 1, No. 2, March - April, 1978. Reproduced with permission from the American Diabetes Association, Inc. Also as modified and published in *Pediatric Clinics of North America,* W.B. Saunders Co., June 1984. Reproduced with permission of *Pediatric Clinics* and the American Diabetes Association, Inc.

and usually lived for only a few months. During the early years after insulin became available, when a restricted diet and one or two doses daily of regular insulin were given, diabetic children were spared an early death but diabetic dwarfism resulted. Most studies published since 1930 and in recent years indicate that retardation of growth and maturation continue to be relatively frequent in children with insulin-dependent diabetes mellitus (1-12). In 1973, Tattersal and Pyke reported that in all but one of 12 pairs of identical twins in which one twin developed overt diabetes before puberty and the other did not, the affected twins treated by conventional methods were much shorter than the nonaffected twins. These authors concluded, "When we speak of 'good' or 'satisfactory' or even 'adequate' control of insulin-deficiency diabetes, we are deluding ourselves," and, "When assessed by critical indices, we see that the conventional criteria for diabetic control are almost always poor -- sometimes fairly poor, sometimes very poor -- but hardly ever good" (13).

In 1946, Jackson and Kelly (14) developed the Iowa growth charts and found that children with overt diabetes receiving physiologic replacement of insulin and maintained in good control (minimal transient glycosuria) grew and matured at normal rates; children in fair control (varying amounts of glycosuria some of the time) grew at essentially normal rates, but some of them matured at a slightly older age. Only those children in fair to poor control (varying amounts of glycosuria most of the time) failed to grow and mature at normal rates.

In 1978, we plotted and evaluated accurate height and weight measurements of children with diabetes under continuous care at the University of Missouri (Columbia).

SUBJECTS

Research records, including individual growth charts, overall control ratings, and socioeconomic classifications, of 252 children with overt type I diabetes were included in the study. Each of the children included in the study were observed at about 3- to 4-month intervals for more than 3 and up to 17 years (mean 5.7 years). Seventy-two percent of them were under continuous observation since time of onset of overt diabetes.

Figure 8.1 depicts the age of time of onset of overt diabetes in the 131 girls and 121 boys included in the study. Note the wide variation in age of onset of both sexes.

Figure 8.2 reflects the socioeconomic classifications of the 252 children with diabetes included in this growth study. The socioeconomic classification was based on a detailed social evaluation of the family by an experienced medical social worker at the time the child was admitted to our diabetic research program and from repeated interviews at subsequent clinic visits. *Note that most of the children maintained in higher degrees of control were from middle and lower-middle income families and that only a very small percentage of them were from unstable families.*

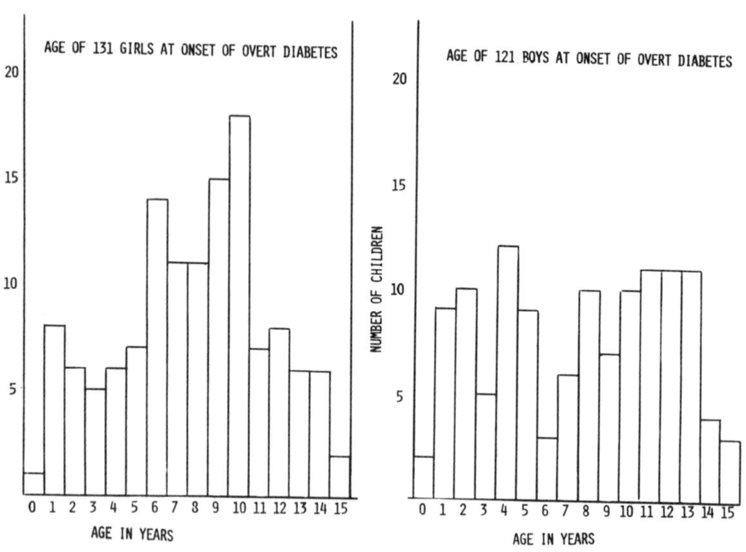

FIGURE 8.1 Ages of 131 girls and 121 boys at time of onset of overt diabetes.

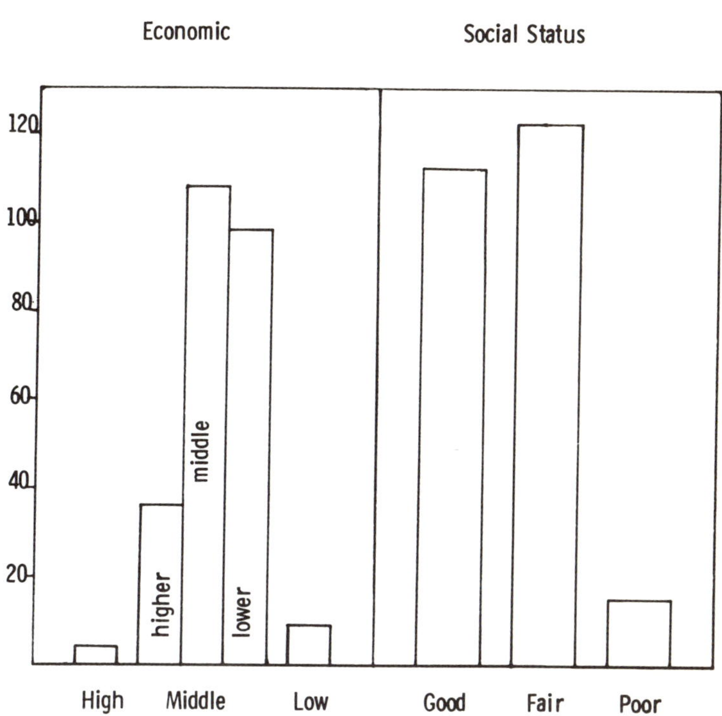

FIGURE 8.2 Economic and social status of the families of 252 children with overt diabetes maintained in higher degrees of control.

METHOD

Accurate height and weight measurements were made and plotted on an Iowa growth chart at each clinic visit. Interpolated height and weight measurements at 5, 8, 11, 14, and 17 years of age were used as bases for evaluating growth. Height and weight values at these age periods were derived by connecting the recorded points made 3-4 times a year.

An overall rating for diabetic control based primarily on the insulin requirement per unit of body weight and the frequency and degree of glycosuria was made for the time period between each clinic visit. The criteria used for rating overall diabetic control are found in Table 8.1.

OBSERVATIONS

The overall diabetic control rating and the size of the subgroups in higher degrees of control were: good -- 20%; good to fair -- 64%; and fair -- 16%.

Figures 8.3 and 8.4 depict the number of subjects and mean interpolated heights and weights of girls and boys in higher degrees of diabetic control. A study of the data indicated that *there were no differences in the growth patterns of the children in good, good-to-fair, and fair control.*

Figures 8.5 and 8.6 depict the mean $\pm$ 1 SD height values and the 16th, 50th, and 84th percentile weight values for the 131 girls and the 121 boys with diabetes in higher degrees of control plotted on Iowa growth charts. As can readily be seen, the linear growth of the combined groups of diabetic girls and boys maintained in higher degrees of control is almost identical to the Iowa norms. By chi square tests, the girls were significantly heavier ($p < 0.001$) than the Iowa norms by 8 years of age and the boys also were significantly heavier ($p < 0.001$) than the Iowa norms by 11 years of age. By physical examination, the increase in body weight of most of the girls and a few of the boys was on the basis of varying degrees of obesity; although many of the boys were outstanding athletes with increased muscle mass.

Figures 8.7 and 8.8 depict the 25th, 50th, and 75th percentile height and weight values for these 131 diabetic girls and 121 diabetic boys plotted in the 1976 National Center for Health Statistics (NCHS) growth charts. Using the NCHS growth charts, we observed that these diabetic girls and boys have an almost identical linear growth pattern as nondiabetic American children of the same generation. However, the obesity known to be present on the basis of physical examinations in many of the girls and some of the boys is no longer evident.

TABLE 8.1 Control Rating Criteria

I. "Good": All patients in this group had:
1. Been under continuous observation in our clinic from time of onset of overt diabetes, received early insulin treatment, and remained in partial remission with total insulin requirement less than 0.5U/kg/day for 1-4 years after onset;
2. Good understanding and execution of meal planning;
3. Reliable and relatively complete daily home records;
4. Remained essentially aglycosuric during the entire period of partial remission and subsequently had only minimal transient glycosuria in no more than one of three or four daily urine specimens;
5. No known ketonuria and very infrequent mild insulin reactions; and
6. Essentially normal postprandial blood sugar values at periodic clinic visits, and normal or only slightly elevated A1c hemoglobin values (less than 7.3%) when tested.

II. "Good to fair": Most patients in this group had:
1. Been under continuous observation in our clinic shortly after the time of onset of diabetes and remained in partial remission (total insulin requirement less than 0.5 U/kg/day) for about 1 year after onset;
2. Relatively good understanding and execution of meal planning;
3. Quite reliable and fairly complete home records;
4. Only transient glycosuria (on an average of less than one of 3 or 4 daily urine specimens);
5. No more than occasional transient ketonuria during an intercurrent infection and only occasional mild insulin reactions with very infrequent reactions of moderate severity; and
6. Variable but often normal or moderately elevated postprandial blood sugars at clinic visits, and only moderate elevation of A1c hemoglobin (less than 8.0%) values when tested.

TABLE 8.1 Control Rating Criteria (Cont'd)

III. "Fair":

1. Most children in this group were total diabetics at the time of admission to our clinic, i.e., their daily insulin requirement was 0.8 to 1.0 U/kg/day. These patients had:
2. Good, but more variable execution of meal planning;
3. Less complete and reliable home records;
4. Varying amounts of sugar in many urine specimens tested;
5. Ketonuria known or suspected at times and infrequent insulin reactions of varying severity; and
6. Postprandial blood sugars at clinic visits usually high (300 $\pm$ 150 mg%) and elevated A1c hemoglobin (less than 10%) values when tested.

IV. "Fair to poor": All patients had:

1. Fair or poor compliance most of the time;
2. Failure to keep regular clinic appointments, more often seen for emergency situations;
3. Meager and questionable home records;
4. Glycosuria of varying degrees in many urine specimens tested;
5. More frequent and severe insulin reactions; and
6. A1c hemoglobin values grossly elevated when tested. (All greater than 10% and most greater than 11%.)

All children coming under our care, after being in lower degrees of control for greater than 25 months after diagnosis, invariably had accelerated growth during early months after attaining and maintaining improved glucose control. Of the 252 children in the study, only 19 (8%) were considered to have delayed maturation (on the basis of clinical evaluation and Tanner classification of sexual development). None of these 19 children were seen at the University of Missouri Medical Center until more than 2 years after onset of overt diabetes. All of them experienced accelerated linear growth during the early months after attaining a higher degree of control and subsequently continued to grow at a normal rate and were included in the study. An additional 179

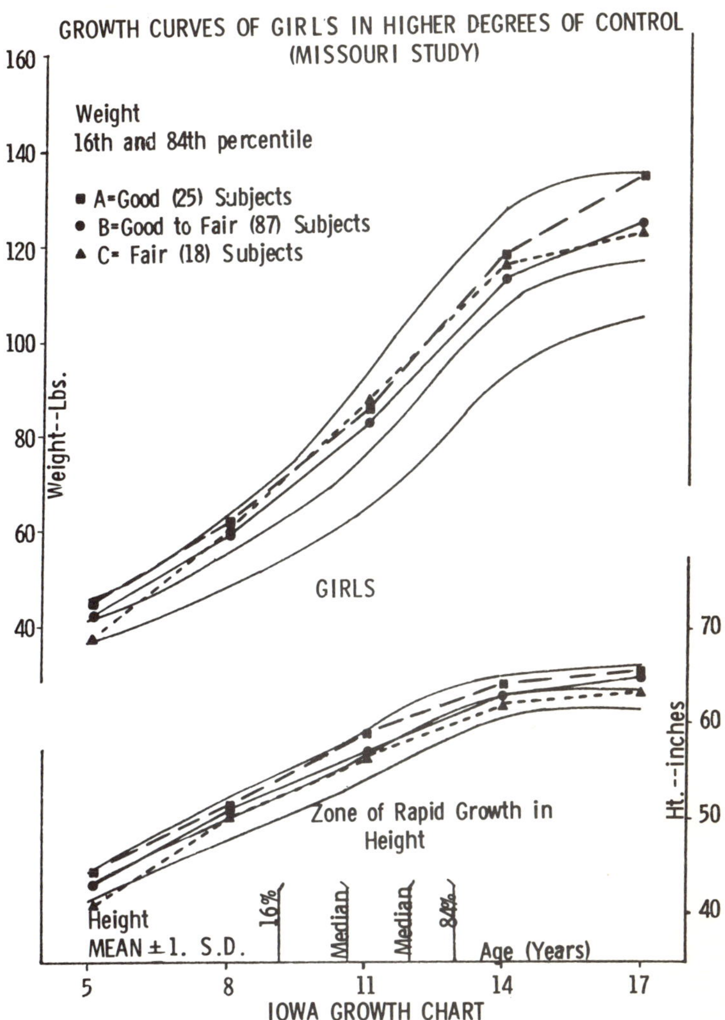

FIGURE 8.3 Mean height and weight and number of diabetic girls in varying higher degrees of metabolic control.

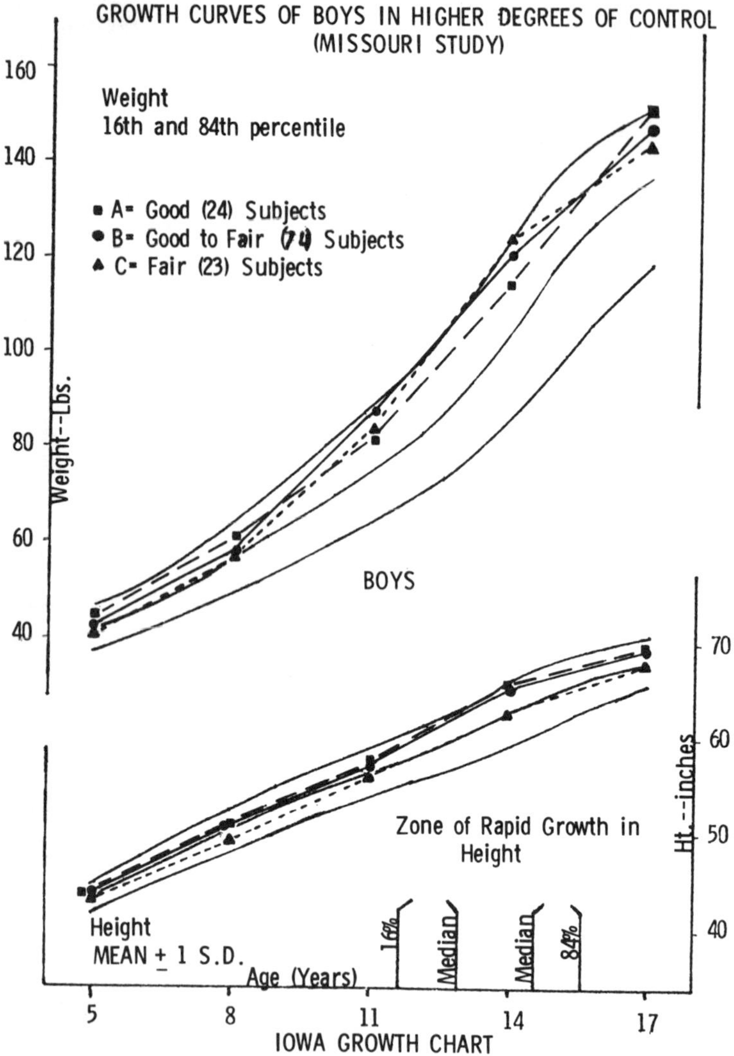

FIGURE 8.4 Mean height and weight and number of diabetic boys in varying higher degrees of metabolic control.

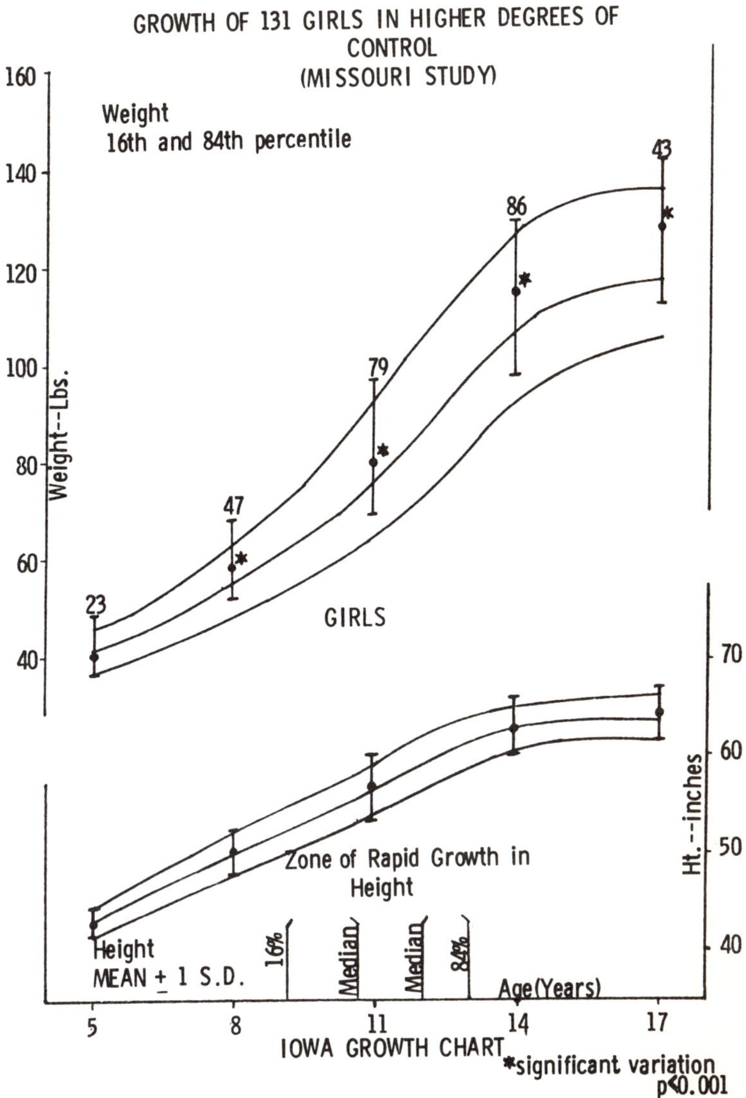

FIGURE 8.5 Mean ± 1 SD interpolated heights and 16th, 50th, and 84th percentile interpolated heights of the 131 diabetic girls maintained in higher degrees of metabolic control, plotted on an Iowa growth chart.

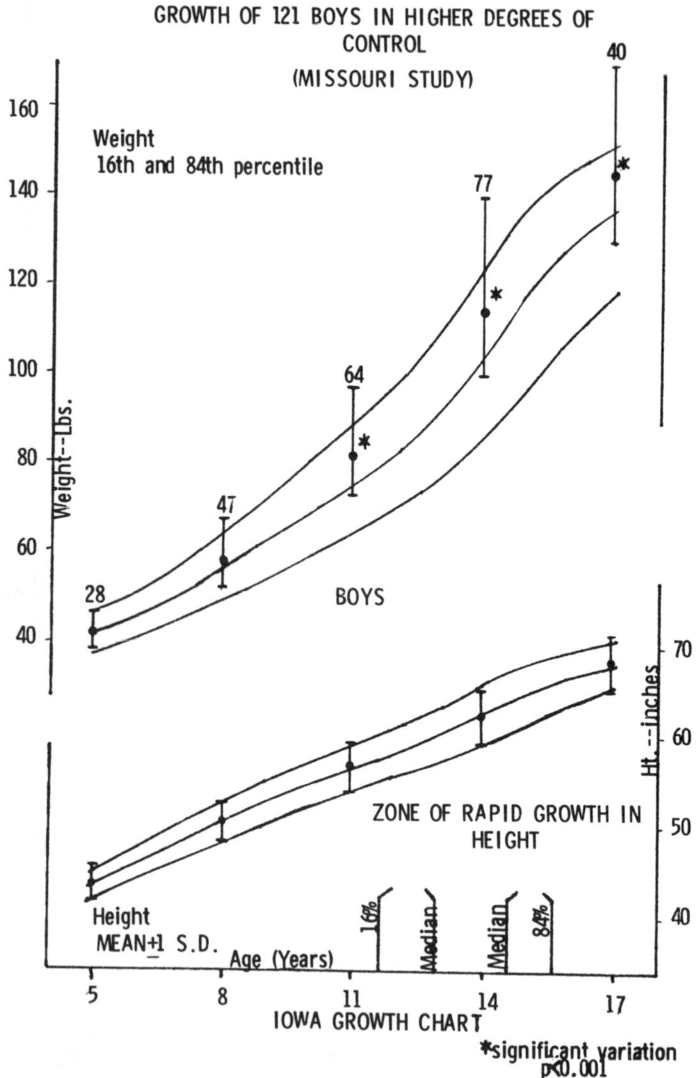

FIGURE 8.6 Mean $\pm$ 1 SD interpolated heights and 16th, 50th, and 84th percentile interpolated heights of the 121 diabetic boys maintained in higher degrees of metabolic control, plotted on an Iowa growth chart.

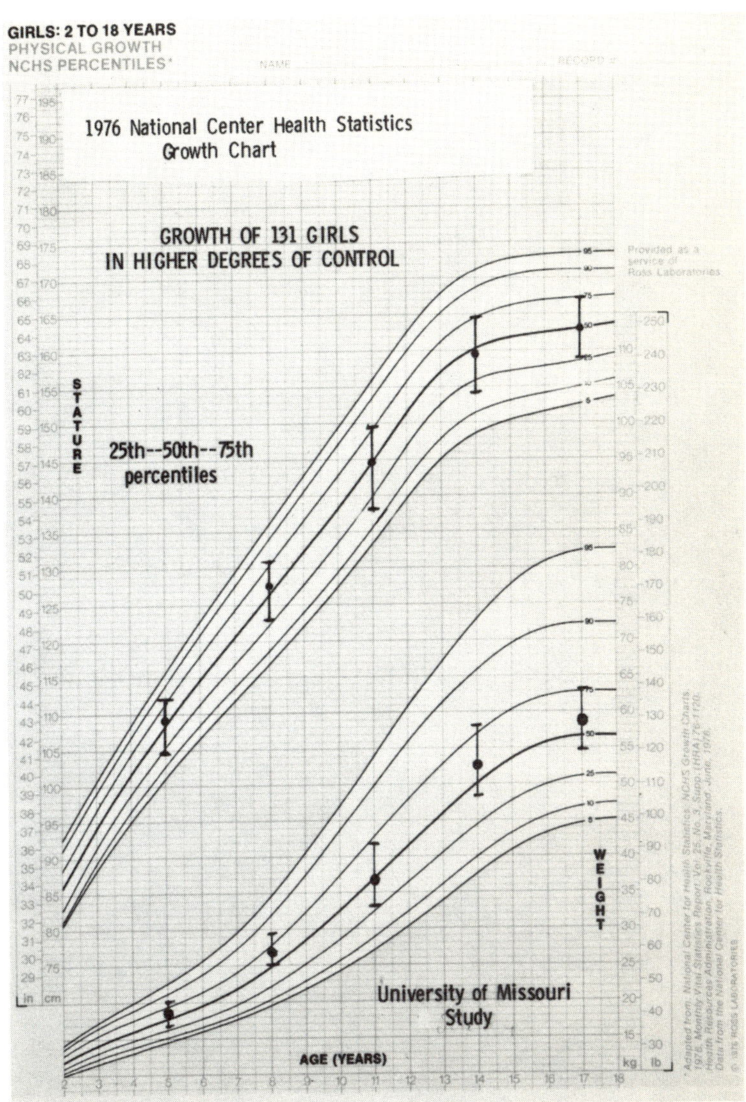

FIGURE 8.7 The 25th, 50th, and 75th percentile interpolated heights and weights of the 131 diabetic girls maintained in higher degrees of control plotted on an NCHS growth chart.

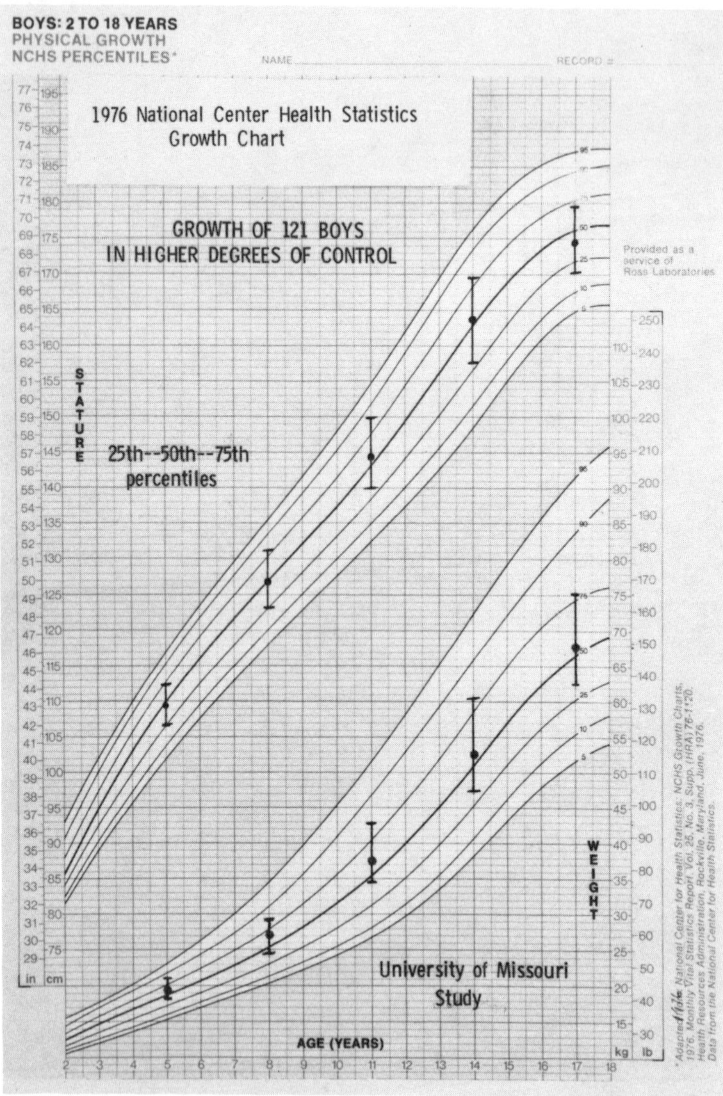

FIGURE 8.8 The 25th, 50th, and 75th percentile interpolated heights and weights of the 121 diabetic boys maintained in higher degrees of control plotted on an NCHS growth chart.

children with overt diabetes also were under observation in the clinic during the same time period. These children were excluded from the growth study, as 78 of them had recent onset and were observed for less than 3 years, 88 had incomplete growth records or were postpubescent at the time of admission to our clinic, and the remaining 13 had additional health problems. Most of the 78 children with recent onset were in a state of partial remission and all of them were growing at normal rates. Fifty-six of the 88 patients with incomplete growth records were from lower socioeconomic families and many of them were in lower degrees of control with delayed growth and maturation.

Figure 8.9 reflects the positive relationship between the control rating of the children and economic level of their families. Figure 8.10 reflects an even greater positive

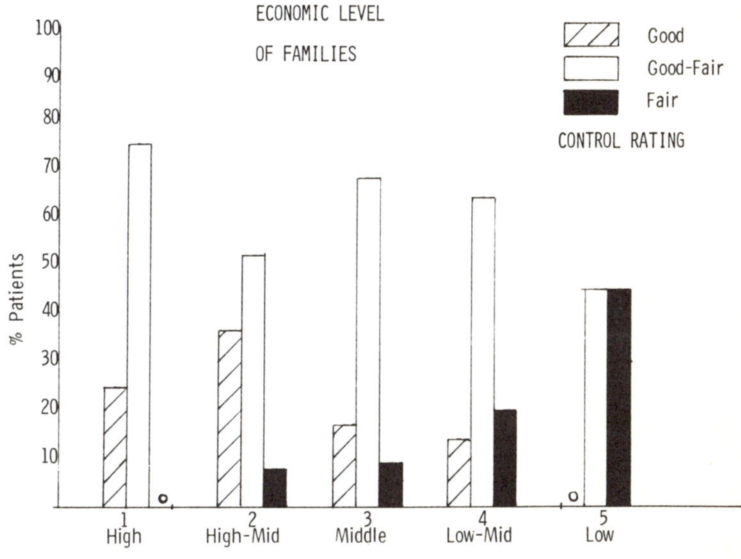

FIGURE 8.9 Interrelationship between the economic level of the families and control ratings of the 252 diabetic children.

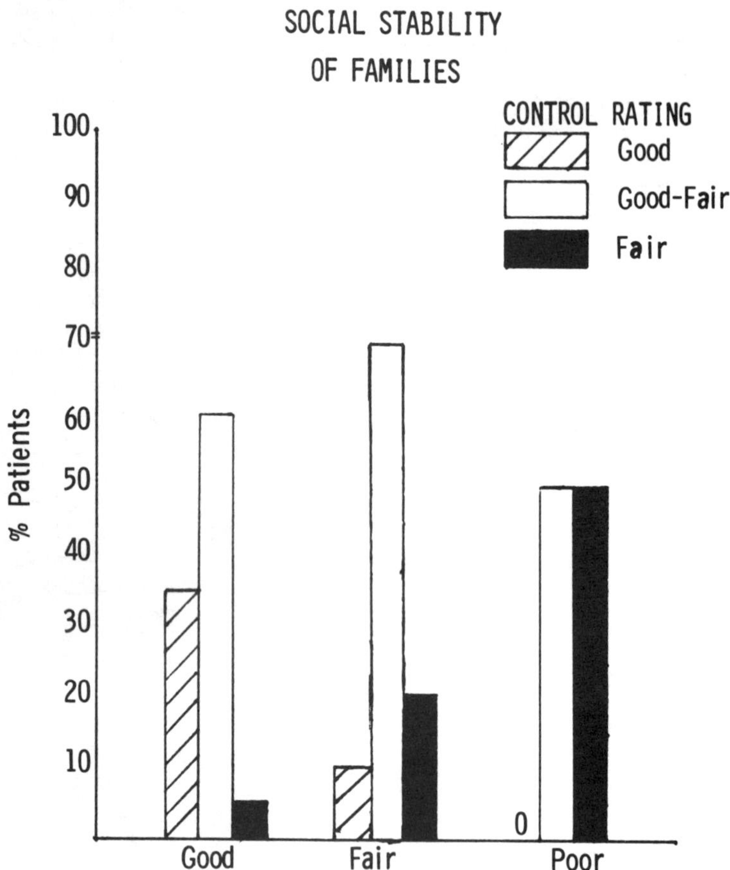

FIGURE 8.10 Interrelationship between the social stability of the families and the control rating of the 252 diabetic children.

correlation between the level of control and the social stability of the family.

None of these 252 children had any joint contractures as described by Grgic et al. (15). In fact, we have not observed definite joint contractures of thickened, adherent skin of hands in the small number of stunted children coming to our clinic or diabetic camp who had been in fair-to-poor control by our criteria for prolonged periods of time.

DISCUSSION

Advances in nutritional knowledge, refinements in the treatment of acute complications such as acidosis and coma, introduction of purified and longer acting insulin preparations, and the discovery of antibacterial agents with which to combat intercurrent infections have made it possible to improve the treatment of the disease. The result is a prolonged life expectancy of the child with diabetes mellitus.

Inasmuch as children with diabetes under our care are supervised more closely with regard to good nutritional practices than most nondiabetic children, it is likely that the quality of the nutritional intake of the children with diabetes was superior to that of the healthy children from whom the growth norms were derived. However, the Iowa growth charts were based on measurements of healthy normal children who were "well-born" and received good environmental care, including professional nutritional guidance. These charts became national and international standards for children who approached optimal growth patterns. It is of considerable significance that the heights and weights of the healthy Iowa girls and boys reported in 1945 (16) were essentially the same as those reported by Meredith in 1952 from a comparable higher socioeconomic group (17). The 1976 NCHS growth charts also indicate that the secular trend for linear growth in children from higher socioeconomic groups has remained essentially the same in the past 35-50 years. However, the greater and higher weight range of these 1976 charts clearly indicate that a higher percentage of American children have become heavier in recent years, which suggests that more of our American adolescent population, especially girls, are becoming obese.

In 1955, we published a study indicating a close interrelationship between the changing insulin requirement and physical growth (18). We found that the ratio of insulin requirement to ideal body weight increases only slightly. During the pubertal growth spurt, there was a sharper rise in insulin requirement, and control was more difficult to maintain. After puberty, the insulin requirement was found to decrease and remain relatively constant during adulthood. We did not find that age at onset of the disease significantly influenced the insulin requirement per unit of ideal body weight. (It is, therefore, important to know and be able to predict the insulin requirement of a given child as a result of increase in body weight.) As adulthood approaches, it also is very important that the insulin dosage and caloric intake be reduced gradually to the adult requirement. As confirmed in this study, it is well-known that the adolescent diabetic girl is especially prone to become obese if her insulin dosage and caloric intake are not adjusted to a lower requirement in keeping with her decelerated growth and physical activity pattern.

A knowledge of insulin requirements and growth rates at varying age periods of well-controlled diabetic children helps in the prediction of insulin and nutritional requirements for maintaining good control of the disease and a normal growth pattern (Figure 8.11). *Young children gain only about 2-3 kg/year, and even if they are total diabetics, their insulin requirement increases only about 2-3 U/year.* Consequently, to measure and give accurate insulin doses it is necessary to use U25 insulin when the total daily requirement is less than 15-20 U and to use U50 insulin when the daily requirement is less than 30-40 U. Up to 10 years of age, the growth patterns of girls and boys are quite similar, in contrast to the great differences after that age. The insulin requirements of girls and boys reflect the periods of similarity and differences in the sexes and clearly show a relationship of insulin requirement to growth. The insulin requirement of girls increases rapidly after age 10, concomitant with their growth spurt, and it decreases gradually as adulthood is reached. The insulin requirement of boys increases about 2 years later, as does their growth spurt. When the child's insulin requirement increases with growth, many parents may fear that the disease is becoming more severe, unless they have been informed that the increase is to be expected.

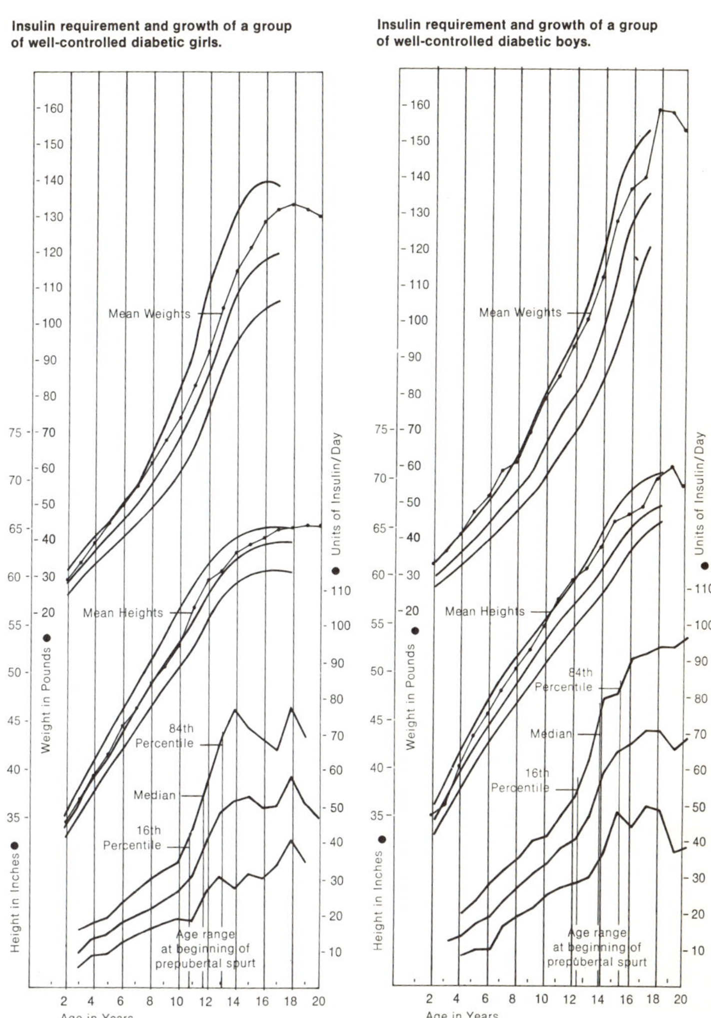

FIGURE 8.11 Insulin requirement and growth of children with well-controlled diabetes. The lower set of curves in each graph represents the mean insulin requirements and a range of 1 SD from the mean. The other two sets of curves are the mean heights and weights of the group, plotted in relation to the Iowa growth charts.

In 1956, we reported on our studies of a group of 140 patients whose duration of juvenile diabetes ranged from 10 to 29 years (19). We found that the degree of control of blood glucose was the only identifiable factor that consistently bore a significant relationship to the incidence and severity of vascular complications.

An ever-increasing number of patients with juvenile-onset diabetes are becoming handicapped by progressive vascular disease in adult life. Controversy persists as to what extent the degree of diabetic control influences the insidious development of serious vascular changes. Additional well-controlled studies are needed and are in progress to further clarify the interrelationship of metabolic control to vascular changes. Most internists and ophthalmologists are now convinced that a higher degree of control is desirable in an attempt to delay or prevent the vascular changes. On the other hand, some pediatricians and family physicians remain skeptical. Those who treat only a few diabetic children do not see the insidious development of complications, as the vascular changes develop slowly over many years and are not detectable clinically until early or midadult life.

The age of onset of diabetes in children varies considerably, and *for reasons not understood, detectable microvascular changes rarely occur in children until growth and maturation have essentially been completed.* These observations help explain why there is a poor correlation between duration of diabetes in young adults with onset during childhood and the time of appearance of vascular changes. The data also account for the earlier development of vascular changes in girls as compared with boys.

These data confirm our previous observation that only children in lower degrees of control, by our criteria, have delayed growth and maturation. Inasmuch as there were no significant differences between the growth rates of children in higher degrees of control, delayed linear growth or maturation of a child with diabetes indicates that, by our criteria, the degree of metabolic control of the child, at best, is fair to poor or poor.

From these observations we conclude that: 1) current knowledge makes possible a high degree of metabolic control for children with insulin-dependent diabetes; 2) all diabetic children who maintained higher degrees of control grew and matured at normal rates regardless of the age of onset or duration of the diabetes; 3) all diabetic children in lower degrees of control had accelerated growth initially after attaining a higher degree of control; 4) there was a close interrelationship between the level of diabetic control sustained and the socioeconomic condition of the child's family; 5) as cessation of growth is approached it is important, especially in girls, to reduce the insulin dosage and caloric intake to avoid obesity; and 6) microvascular changes rarely occur in children until growth and maturation have essentially been completed.

REFERENCES

1. Boyd, J. D., and Kantrow, A. H.: Retardation of growth in diabetic children. *Am. J. Dis. Child.* 55:460, 1938.

2. Wagner, R., White, P., and Bogan, I.: Diabetic dwarfism. *Am. J. Dis. Child.* 63:667, 1942.

3. Fischer, A. E., Mackler, H. S., and Marks, H. H.: Long-term growth of diabetic children. *Am. J. Dis. Child* 64: 413, 1942.

4. Beal, C. K.: Body size and growth rate of children with diabetes mellitus. *J. Ped* 32:170, 1948.

5. Sterky, G.: Growth patterns in juvenile diabetes. *Acta Ped. Scand.* 177 (Suppl.):80-82, 1967.

6. Larsson, Y., and Sterky, G.: Long-term prognosis in juvenile diabetes mellitus. *Acta Ped. Scand.* 51 (Suppl. 130): 27-45, 1962.

7. Craig, J. O.: Growth as a measurement of control in diabetic children. *Postgrad. Med. J.* 46:607-610, Sept., 1970.

8. Weil, W. B., Jr.: Skeletal maturation in juvenile diabetes mellitus. *Ped. Red.* 1:470, 1967.

9. White, P.: The child with diabetes. *Med. Clin. N. Am.* 49:1069, 1965.

10. Pond, H.: Some aspects of growth in diabetic children. *Postgrad. Med. J.* 46(Suppl.):616, Sept. 1970.

11. Drash, A.: Diabetes mellitus, a review. *J. Ped.* 8:919, 1971.

12. Jivani, S. K. M., and Rayner, P. H. W.: Does control influence the growth of diabetic children? *Arch. Dis. Child.* 48:109, 1973.

13. Tattersal, R. B., and Pyke, D. K.: Growth of diabetic studies in identical twins. *Lancet* 2:1105, 1973.

14. Jackson, R. L., and Kelly, H. G.: Growth of children with diabetes mellitus in relationship to level of control of the disease. *J. Ped.* 29:316, 1946.

15. Grgic, A., Rosenbloom, A. L., Weber, F. T., Giordano, B., Malone, J. I., and Shuster, J.: Joint contractures: Common manifestation of childhood diabetes mellitus. *J. Ped.* 88:584-588.

16. Jackson, R. L., and Kelly, H.: Growth charts for use in pediatric practice. *J. Ped.* 26:215, 1945.

17. Meredith, H. V.: Change in the stature and body weight of North American boys during the last 80 years. In: *Advances in Child Development and Behavior,* Vol. 69, New York, Academic Press, L.P. Lipsitt and C.C. Spiker (Eds.), pp. 290, 1952.

18. Kelly, H. G., Rao, T. R., Jackson, R. L.: Insulin requirements of children with diabetes mellitus maintained in good control. *Am. J. Dis. Child.* 89:31, 1955.

19. Hardin, R. C., Jackson, R. L., Johnston, R. L., and Kelly, H. G.: The development of diabetic retinopathy: Effects of duration and control of diabetes. *Diabetes* 5:397, 1956.

Chapter 9

PSYCHOSOCIAL ADJUSTMENT AND COMPLIANCE OF CHILD WITH DIABETES

A. PSYCHOSOCIAL ADJUSTMENT

Robert L. Jackson, M.D. and
Diana Guthrie, Ph.D.

There is no doubt that diabetes imposes an emotional stress on both the child and the family. Good relationships are strained; unstable ones are threatened, especially if communications among family members are interrupted. It is a cruel delusion which proposes that control of the disease can be attained only at the expense of emotional health. The self-discipline upon which good control depends actually can serve to make the child and parents better adjusted and strengthen family ties.

The emotional status of any patient with diabetes profoundly affects the regulation of the disease. *The emotional health of the child reflects the emotional health of the parents; consequently, the physician must help parents as much as, or more than, the child.* It is very important that the child and parents see the truth about the disease clearly as soon as possible and that they face the issue squarely. All must admit that the child has a disability for which at present there is no known cure; nevertheless, the condition is one that need not interfere with a useful, happy life. The truest type of sympathy for the child is that which helps him to meet the situation bravely. Sympathy of any other type will harm, not help. The child who is emotionally well at the time he develops diabetes usually has little difficulty in accepting the condition and in maintaining a high degree of control.

The child with diabetes, like other children, needs security, affection, and praise as well as discipline. To be happy, the child must learn to assume responsibility appropriate for a child his age. As with all children, the child with diabetes will on occasion do something he knows is wrong or will neglect to do something he should do. When that occurs, punishment should be given immediately. Equally important, parents should forgive and forget once the punishment has been administered. The emotional pattern of a child becomes fairly well established during the early years of life. With increasing age, it becomes more difficult to alter the patterns. To be happy, the child must learn how to use help and guidance from others to gain self-control without losing self-esteem.

Parental reaction to the child's diabetes will influence the child's adjustment because children take their cues from their parents. *Parents who satisfy the child's need for security, praise, affection, and discipline help the child develop the confidence and self-esteem necessary for eventual self-management of diabetes.* A younger child in a stable family, with established habits of self-discipline and trust in authority figures (e.g., parents, teachers, physicians) almost always makes a good adjustment to the insulin injections, meal planning, urine and blood tests, and office visits required for maintaining a high degree of control. A parent who is excessively sympathetic encourages the child's dependency and tendency to manipulate. A parent who denies the child's illness is likely to be indifferent about medical management, and the child is then likely to become negligent about his health.

Although diabetes imposes emotional stress on both the child and the family, the stress can be incorporated into the child's own life-style. Supportive and constructive intervention should come from a number of avenues. The parents need to encourage the use of objective statements regarding routine care. "It is time for your injection" — no asking, demanding, questioning -- the procedure is related to time and should be completed firmly and in a loving manner. The parents need to help the child develop socialization skills by giving consistent discipline and providing external structures and limitations. Consequences for infringements should be direct and immediate. It is important to set limited, short-term goals for the purpose of establishing good habits and to decrease the frequency of failures. Deal with fears directly by separating the imagined from the real. Fear of an insulin reaction can be ameliorated by the use of self-monitoring of blood glucose levels and ingestion of appropriate foods with varying types of physical activities. Creative relaxation also is useful and can be learned. Useful and enjoyable daily physical activities need to be developed in keeping with the child's personality, as well as quiet relaxation periods which enhance the ability to function more creatively. It is the responsibility of the physician and health team to help the family and child realize that with physiologic insulin replacement it is now possible to fully restore health and attain normal growth and maturation. In addition, learning self-discipline upon which good control of diabetes depends also will lead to improved mental health and social adjustment.

It is essential that all members of the health team have behavioral orientation, as psychosocial and behavioral stresses are major factors influencing day-to-day metabolic control. However, it is imperative that all members of the health team also have in-depth knowledge about physiologic management of insulin-dependent diabetes. Our experience indicates that it is preferable for bonding to occur with only one or two members of the team. There are predictable stresses and transitional periods when psychosocial interactions are most effective. For example, an experienced medical social worker can be very effective in helping the parent and child at the initial critical transition period -- the crisis of accepting the diagnosis (as discussed in detail on p. 60).

The physician should act as a liaison between the diabetes center and the family physician, who can provide badly needed emotional support for the parents and other members of the family; the social worker should act as liaison between the family and community systems; the nurse between the family and the school. Parent-to-parent programs which connect experienced families with newly diagnosed families have proved very helpful, as adjusted parents of children with diabetes can help families anticipate stresses and in modeling innovative coping strategies.

One of the primary responsibilities of each member of the health team is to help the parents and child move from dependence to independence. The *gradual* transfer of the responsibility from the team-parent complex to the team-child complex must begin early and proceed in a guarded, orderly fashion. Clear delineation of responsibilities at all stages of development must be made. It is wise to avoid giving adult responsibilities to children and thereby deny the child the normal and desirable freedoms of childhood.

Emotional reactions such as anxiety, fear, anger, and depression directly affect the secretions of the various hormones that regulate glucose and fat metabolism. Emotional reactions can also affect regulation indirectly. The child with diabetes may express feelings of frustration, rejection, and inferiority by breaking or disregarding the principles of treatment. He may have dietary indiscretions, alter or omit insulin doses, or refuse to do urine or blood tests. By reporting spurious test results he can manipulate the parents and the physician, thereby affecting the regulation of the diabetes. It is easy to understand why children doing their own tests are tempted to report false-negative results. In doing so, they avoid having to account for positive tests and possible criticism from parents and doctors. Omission of testing or ignoring positive results (by parents or child) may represent a basic denial of the disease. On the other hand, some children may report false positive tests to gain added attention from their parents.

Severe insulin reactions effect the emotional adjustment of parents and child. A few young children referred to our clinic have experienced severe hypoglycemia and have developed seizure disorders from central nervous system damage. In addition to insulin, they then require anticonvulsant therapy. A serious insulin reaction, especially in public or during the night, can leave an indelible impression. The parents and child understandably become very anxious about the possibility of another reaction. Parents then frequently overcompensate by giving too little insulin or too much food. If the child's friends witness an insulin reaction, they may become fearful about being with him because they are insecure about how they would react in the event of a recurrence. To guard against feelings of helplessness or embarrassment, other children may begin to avoid the diabetic child. That avoidance can result in the patient's developing a feeling of inferiority and in a lower degree of diabetic control.

Adolescence can be an especially difficult time for the child with diabetes. If unwholesome relationships exist between the child and the parents, they become exaggerated during adolescence, when self-discipline is difficult. To a great extent, problems can be prevented if opportunities for self-direction are given as soon as the child shows the capacity to handle them. When the child reaches senior high school, it is desirable that he gradually assumes independence in management of the disorder. The teenager with diabetes has the same emotional needs as the nondiabetic youngster and has as much capacity for acquiring self-direction. The adolescent desiring an even greater degree of independence from parents will be resentful if the parents must assume the responsibilities of directing insulin doses or testing urine or blood. Adolescence normally involves changes in the development of the personality, such as the need for a greater degree of independence and self-expression and a greater need for peer approval. The parents, therefore, should be prepared to expect changes in the behavior patterns of the stable diabetic child as he reaches adolescence.

The adolescent reevaluates diabetes in relationship to new perspectives. He takes greater liberty in varying the amount and kind of foods eaten, the frequency of checking urine or blood specimens, or altering the timing or dose of insulin injections. Most adolescents are sensitive about having new friends become aware of their diabetes. Others may use their disorder to become the center of attention or as an excuse for failure. Priorities shift: basketball practice or a class party are much more important than eating a snack or taking the next dose of insulin on time. In view of this possible change in behavior, the physician must periodically review with an adolescent his expectations concerning diabetic control and management. The patient must be made more aware of the reasons for timing injections and using good judgment about when and what to eat.

Experimentation, characteristic of adolescents and a manifestation of their strivings for independence, can be used by doctors to encourage the child to use his own judgment in varying the kind and amount of food to be taken depending upon his activity pattern. The child, like all of us, must learn by trial and error -- and there will be errors. If there is a question regarding reliability, it is better to give the adolescent the benefit of the doubt and not forget to praise him for what he has done or is doing correctly. The health team must be willing to make major expenditures of time and effort if they are to meet the needs of the patient and the family adequately.

Areas of conflict between parents and child become exaggerated during adolescence, but they can be diminished somewhat by understanding members of the team. More frequent visits to the office are desirable for that reason when the child reaches the period of rapid growth and development. An adolescent involved in independence-dependence conflicts with the parents will at times rebel and use indiscretions as a way of expressing independence. On the other hand, the adolescent may seek a dependency position. Carelessness about following the medical regimen is one way that the adolescent can force a takeover of diabetic management by the parents. The most idealistic, self-critical age is that of the teenage years; some depressed adolescents adopt an apathy about proper care as a means of punishment for themselves or their parents.

When overt diabetes develops during adolescence, the patient has greater difficulty accepting the reality of the situation. The teenager has a greater degree of understanding than does the younger child. He is concerned about the possible consequences of the disease and worries about the effect diabetes might have on his career or marriage. He should feel free to ask questions of his parents and physician and expect to be given honest answers.

The physician and other health professionals need to establish an understanding relationship with both the adolescent and the parents so they feel free to ventilate their conflicts and frustrations. It is important to listen to the problems as seen by the child as well as the parents.

Particular strivings that are natural for the adolescent seem (at least to the individual) to compete with sound medical management of diabetes. The adolescent seeks to broaden social and recreational life. The timing of insulin injections and meals and the inconvenience of testing urine specimens are resented, these restrictions regarded as interfering with the right to greater freedom.

Teenagers have a strong natural desire to identify with their peers and seek their approval. To avoid rejection, ostracism, or criticism from their peers, the adolescent is reluctant to admit that he has diabetes. With behavior such as eating sweets, they may try to demonstrate that they are not really diabetic. There is then the temptation to omit testing and to record false-negative tests.

Many diabetic youngsters will try to convince themselves, their parents, and their physicians that they are able to evaluate their blood-glucose level by how they "feel," their pattern of urination, and their appetite and weight changes. Such criteria are not reliable. Every effort should be made to encourage resumption of regular testing or urine and blood specimens each day or at a minimum, two daily profiles during the week and one on the weekend.

The health team can best attend to the emotional needs of the child with diabetes and the family by encouraging and expecting *parents* to:

1. Accept responsibility for management of the diabetes and gradually give responsibility to the child.
2. Avoid making the patient the focus of excessive attention in the family.
3. Discipline, *praise,* and punish the diabetic child and other children in the family fairly and equally.
4. Allow the child to lead a life as close to normal as possible; avoid unnecessary physical and social restrictions.
5. Provide a flexible insulin and meal plan so the child can participate in usual activities of his peer group.
6. Regard the diabetic team as a counselor whenever parents or child need emotional support, education, advice, or help in modifying the treatment plan to regain control.

The conscientious family physican or pediatrician can do much to alleviate the emotional problems of diabetes, if an emotional disorder in the child or family interferes with diabetic management or affects the social, cognitive development of the child, early referral for more intensive psychosocial care is indicated.

INTELLECTUAL DEVELOPMENT

The normal child who develops diabetes and is given good physical and emotional care will continue to have normal intellectual growth. Children with diabetes in a lower degree of control are likely to have frequent periodic illnesses resulting in absence from school and academic difficulties. Frequent, mild hypoglycemia can cause the child to be inattentive and can seriously interfere with the ability to do well at school. More directly, severe prolonged insulin reactions, especially in infants and preschool children, can cause irreparable damage to the central nervous system with varying degrees of mental retardation. The parents and members of the health team need to monitor closely the child's academic and social adjustment. The school provides a unique resource for early detection and evaluation of children's problems.

B. COMPLIANCE

Robert L. Jackson, M.D.

By compliance we mean the willingness and ability of the parents and child to act in accordance with the recommendations of the health team. A good relationsip between the health team and the parents and their child is essential to obtaining compliance. All members of the health team need to be in complete agreement so that instructions are consistent and not contradictory. To attain compliance, the plan of treatment must be flexible and adjusted to meet the individual needs of each child and family. The parents and ultimately the child must understand the rewards for maintaining metabolic control as well as the short- and long-term penalities for failure to do so. They also must understand that the rewards are for the child and not for the health team. When discussing possible future complications, the instructors should maintain optimism without distorting reality.

As documented in Chapter 5, most children with diabetes continue to produce varying amounts of endogenous insulin during the early months or years after the clinical onset of the disorder. Our experience indicates that the earlier the diagnosis is made, the lower the amount of exogenous insulin needed and the easier it is to attain and maintain metabolic control with little risk of hypoglycemia.

The preferred time to attain compliance is at the onset of the disease. It is of utmost importance that the child should remain in the hospital until nutritional repletion is complete, the maintenance insulin requirement is established, and the parents and child have the knowledge and security to continue the treatment at home. After stabilization, when the insulin requirement is low and the child feels and looks well, some parents and children begin to doubt if the insulin injections and the structured food intake are really necessary. Before the parents take the child home, the physician should emphasize the continued need for insulin replacement and dietary management to control the diabetes. The parents need to realize that maintaining excellent metabolic control (normal glycosylated hemoglobin levels) will help preserve the child's ability to make insulin and delay the need for increasing the insulin dosage. The parents also need to be informed that at each office visit laboratory studies will be done to determine if the insulin dosage should be modified.

After the stabilized diabetic child has maintained excellent control for many months or even years, the parents' and child's concept of good control is so well established that they often become concerned with even mild transitory glycosuria or occasional moderately elevated blood glucose levels. By their own experience, they will have learned that a high degree of metabolic control can be maintained, but that the insulin dosage has to be gradually increased to compensate for growth and/or maturation. They also will have learned that it gradually has become somewhat more difficult to keep the urine specimens sugar-free.

In contrast to the family who undertakes home management of a stabilized diabetic child, consider the frustrations of the family who is given the grave responsibility of home management of their child after only a relatively short period of rapid clinical improvement in the hospital (usually 7-10 days). During the next few weeks (period of metabolic recovery) the insulin and nutritional requirements are changing rapidly. Although the child is likely to have become asymptomatic with an improved dietary plan and a once-daily injection of an intermediate insulin, the metabolic control attained is usually at best fair and the insulin deficiency progresses and usually is complete within a few months. Increasing a once-daily insulin dosage often results in hypoglycemic episodes of varying intensities. It is not until this happens, when the insulin deficiency is essentially complete, that many children are referred for more specialized care. In contrast to the child with recent onset, the child with total diabetes (no endogenous insulin production) will not have a comparable recovery period. Reeducation of the parents of a child with total diabetes who previously has been maintained in only fair control is much more complicated. It is quite difficult for these families to accept the need for learning much more about regulating the diabetes because for a period of many months, it was relatively easy to keep their child asymptomatic without having to learn so much which seems so complicated and somewhat unnecessary to them. It is for these reasons that most children with diabetes have in the past received suboptimal care and find it so difficult to accept the discipline required to maintain metabolic control.

Compliance can be divided into direct and indirect measures. Examples of direct measures for a diabetic would include timing of insulin injections, meals, and snacks; frequency and reliability of doing and recording routine urine and blood tests; periodic determination of glycosylated hemoglobin levels; and accurate evaluation of growth and development. Indirect measures would include observations by the parents, schoolteachers, and health professionals as to the psychosocial adjustment of the child. It is important to obtain both types of measures at each office visit to identify potential or real problems as soon as possible so that corrective measures can be undertaken. A major disadvantage of using treatment outcome as the only measure of compliance or noncompliance is that a host of social and economic components contribute to the ability of the child to adhere to the treatment plan.

At each office visit the parents (and child) need to realize that the primary purpose of a meticulous review of what they are or are not doing is to help them to control the diabetes and not to find fault with how they are carrying out the instructions. On the basis of the information obtained or, if necessary, through home visits or phone calls, a decision must be reached to determine if their problems are those of noncompliance or pseudononcompliance. The term pseudononcompliant refers to those situations in which patient compliance is simply not a realistic possibility and refers to patients often considered to be in poor control due to noncompliance but in fact are in poor control due to a factor or factors previously unrecognized. We define the terms as follows:

Compliance: Adherence to a prescribed therapeutic plan for the management of a medical disorder such as taking a prescribed medication, following a structured meal plan, and making specific life-style changes.

Noncompliance: Intentional refusal or neglect to carry out a prescribed plan for the management of a medical disorder such as not taking prescribed medication, not following a dietary recommendation, and not making specific life-style changes.

Pseudononcompliance: Unintentional errors in adhering to a prescribed plan for the treatment of a medical disorder such as taking a prescribed medication, prescribed diet, or needed life-style changes due to previously unrecognized physiologic educational, psychological, or socioeconomic factors.

ATTAINING AND MAINTAINING COMPLIANCE

All too frequently the compliant child's family is taken for granted and not recognized and applauded for how well they have accomplished this difficult job. To sustain metabolic control, data collecting procedures for assessing potential problems also are important with these families. The child who has been historically compliant often has unrecognized needs which are not identified until an elevated glycosylated hemoglobin value indicates declining control. At the suggestion of Rapoff and Christophersen, of our department, we use questionnaires that ask both parents and children to rate on a five-point scale (5, very easy, to 1, very difficult) their responses to questions such as those depicted in Tables 9.1, 9.2, and 9.3. These types of questions will elicit specific ratings for different regimen components and help avoid putting the parents or child in a defensive position. Information obtained from these types of questions enables the health professionals to detect early problems with a compliant patient and to make an appropriate intervention.

TABLE 9.1 Diabetes Management Behavioral Inventory for Parents of Older Children or Adolescents*

		How often does this happen?					Is this a problem?	
		Never	Seldom	Sometimes	Often	Always		
1.	Child dawdles when getting a urine/blood specimen.	1	2	3	4	5	Yes	No
2.	Fails to perform blood/urine tests.	1	2	3	4	5	Yes	No
3.	Fails to take insulin at proper time.	1	2	3	4	5	Yes	No
4.	Fails to wait 30 min between injection and meal.	1	2	3	4	5	Yes	No
5.	Fails to weigh or measure food Circle meal: Breakfast Noon Supper Snack	1	2	3	4	5	Yes	No
6.	Fails to eat part of meal Circle meal: Breakfast Noon Supper Snack	1	2	3	4	5	Yes	No

7.	Takes other children's food at school lunch or recess.	1	2	3	4	5	Yes	No
8.	Leaves candy wrappers around home.	1	2	3	4	5	Yes	No
9.	Friends tease the diabetic child with food.	1	2	3	4	5	Yes	No
10.	Is given special privileges by parents because of the diabetes.	1	2	3	4	5	Yes	No
11.	Sleeps late on weekend days.	1	2	3	4	5	Yes	No
12.	Not asked to get together with friends.	1	2	3	4	5	Yes	No
13.	Hides diabetes from friends.	1	2	3	4	5	Yes	No
14.	Talks about death.	1	2	3	4	5	Yes	No

*This is not a complete form but are examples of the type of questions and scores.

TABLE 9.2 Diabetes Management Behavioral Inventory for Parents of Younger Children*

	How often does this happen? Never	Seldom	Sometimes	Often	Always	Is this a problem?	
1. We fail to give insulin on time.	1	2	3	4	5	Yes	No
2. We have trouble deciding dose of insulin to give.	1	2	3	4	5	Yes	No
3. Child fails to wait 30 min between injections and meals.	1	2	3	4	5	Yes	No
4. Child gives insulin injections.	1	2	3	4	5	Yes	No
5. Foods for meals and snacks are:							
planned	1	2	3	4	5	Yes	No
weighed	1	2	3	4	5	Yes	No
measured	1	2	3	4	5	Yes	No
estimated	1	2	3	4	5	Yes	No

6.	Child refuses to eat part of:							
	breakfast	1	2	3	4	5	Yes	No
	midmorning snack	1	2	3	4	5	Yes	No
	lunch	1	2	3	4	5	Yes	No
	midafernoon snack	1	2	3	4	5	Yes	No
	evening	1	2	3	4	5	Yes	No
7.	Child is unreliable about amount and kinds of food eaten.	1	2	3	4	5	Yes	No
8.	Child needs more than one reminder to obtain a urine specimen.	1	2	3	4	5	Yes	No
9.	We fail to record insulin dose.	1	2	3	4	5	Yes	No
10.	We fail to record urine/blood test results.	1	2	3	4	5	Yes	No

*This is not complete form but are examples of the type of questions and scores.

TABLE 9.3 Diabetes Management Behavioral Inventory for Adolscents*

		How often does this happen?					Is this a problem?	
		Never	Seldom	Sometimes	Often	Always		
1.	I need to be reminded to do urine/blood test.	1	2	3	4	5	Yes	No
2.	I neglect to do my urine/ blood test.	1	2	3	4	5	Yes	No
3.	I record urine/blood tests that I make up.	1	2	3	4	5	Yes	No
4.	I forget to take my insulin on time.	1	2	3	4	5	Yes	No
5.	I change my insulin dose when I increase or decrease my exercise.	1	2	3	4	5	Yes	No
6.	I take my insulin on time, but fail to wait 30 min before eating.	1	2	3	4	5	Yes	No

7.	I don't admit if I've eaten more than I should.	1	2	3	4	5	Yes	No
8.	I get teased about my diabetes.	1	2	3	4	5	Yes	No
9.	I sleep late on weekend days or vacation days.	1	2	3	4	5	Yes	No
10.	I smoke cigarettes.	1	2	3	4	5	Yes	No
11.	My friends don't ask me to do things with them.	1	2	3	4	5	Yes	No
12.	I am not doing my best in school.	1	2	3	4	5	Yes	No
13.	My mom and/or dad treat me special because I have diabetes.	1	2	3	4	5	Yes	No

*This is not complete form but are examples of the type of questions and scores.

Continuing education and review of basic information also are of vital importance at each office visit and are often overlooked with the compliant, well-controlled diabetic. It is to be stressed that during the early months and years when the child is in partial remission it is important to reassure the parents that a critical review of daily management is done to filter out anything they are doing or not doing which might be modified so as to make it easier or more effective for them to maintain a high degree of control and an optimal health level for their child. As mentioned previously, hyperglycemia has an insidious effect on the well-being of a diabetic. That is, the relative increments of pathologic change are individually small, but collectively great with time. This makes it difficult for the parents and child to assess health status unless objective measures (urine and blood glucoses and glycosylated hemoglobin levels) are utilized. *Understanding that there are varying degrees of wellness is a new concept for many parents.* In order to maintain a high level of health, the need for continuing education to attain self-management becomes more understandable and acceptable to the family. Their educational needs center around new developments, anticipated changes in the life-style of the child, previously erroneous or misunderstood information, and lack of recall of specific information.

Based on these categories there is always additional information that the parents and child can learn so they can alter their treatment plan and avoid unnecessary physical and social restrictions. An appropriate review regarding each aspect of care needs to be done by a member of the health team to praise the parents and child for what they are doing well. In order to increase the effectiveness of continuing education it is important to stress the changing needs of children with growth and maturation and to teach the parents and child how to modify insulin replacement and food intake to make it easier and more acceptable for the child as he becomes more independent and responsible (see Chapter 12). New information should be presented along with the understanding that it is difficult to retain all they have learned. Thus, some instructions may need to be reviewed, as well as new information provided during subsequent office visits or by phone conversations. The child as well as the parents should be able to explain why and how they have modified the treatment plan and identify the hurdles inhibiting compliance.

Before it is concluded that a patient is noncompliant, every effort should be made to identify factors that inhibit the child or parent from adhering to the prescribed treatment plan. Each family periodically should be evaluated to ascertain the diabetes knowledge base and the accuracy of their techniques for use in self-management of their diabetes. The following should be included:

1. A validated objective test over basic information related to insulin-dependent diabetes mellitus.
2. Detailed review of foods used for meals and snacks by the dietitian.
3. Evaluation of urine or blood testing procedures by qualified personnel who use a check-sheet of procedure steps to determine their competence.
4. Evaluation of insulin administration by having the child or a parent prepare insulin, draw it up into the syringe (reliability of measurement is checked by qualified personnel), and demonstration of the actual injection. The child or parent should explain the purpose of rotation and how they are rotating the injections.
5. Determination if the child and/or the parent are making appropriate food and insulin adjustments based on careful review of recorded blood and urine tests.
6. Evaluate the insulin dosage based on the expected daily requirement of ($<$ 0.3-0.7 U/kg for a child in partial remission to 0.8-1.5 U/kg for a completely insulin-dependent diabetic).
7. A thorough history based on home records (time structure of activities and food intake) for the previous week. This should be examined critically to determine if food intake and insulin doses are being properly adjusted for variations in the pattern of physical activity and to meet the insulin requirement.
8. A brief psychosocial history periodically should be done to identify social, economic, or psychological factors which might be interfering with the management.
9. Provide an opportunity for the child and each parent to ask questions or transmit confidential information. Often the parent or child wants to confess deviations in private and it is of utmost importance that confidentially be respected and given proper attention.

10. Determination of the glycosylated hemoglobin assay to objectively determine degree of metabolic control.

There is intense frustration experienced by the child and family when repeated attempts fail to improve metabolic control as reflected by glycosylated hemoglobin levels. Not only should an intervention be based on correcting errors identified in the aforementioned evaluation, but also on breaking the cycle of poor management of the diabetes. This recurring cycle results from the development of poor habits while attempting and failing to carry out daily self-management of the disease. Intervention must be aimed at correcting the errors and also changing the daily poor habits of self-management. This entails using a combination of education and behavioral strategies (as discussed in Chapter 7 and in the first section of this chapter).

BEHAVIORAL STRATEGIES

Behavioral strategies have been employed primarily with individuals on long-term regimens. We have always advocated self-monitoring. Unfortunately, all too often the families efforts to keep reliable records and share detailed information are not reviewed carefully and discussed by the health professionals at the time of their office visit. Time should be spent reviewing the records with the parent and child so that vital feedback can be given by interpretation of the results. In the instance where the intervention is aimed at correcting errors in record interpretation, weekly phone calls regarding mailed records will provide immediate feedback for the patient, thus correcting mistakes before they become a part of a poor habitual cycle. Records that are not critically reviewed become relatively useless to both the family and the professionals and soon become a superfluous burden. In the experience of the authors, when this happens the family refuses to keep the records or may go to the extreme of fabricating them.

Tailoring is the basic behavioral strategy needed in the care of the child with diabetes. This refers to the adapting the diabetic regimen to the personal life-style of an individual and his family. We wish to emphasize that the plan of treatment needs to be individualized and flexible. Too often children have been expected to fit into a so-called strict or rigid program rather than teaching the family and child how to modify the basic physiologic program to avoid unnecessary restrictions.

Prompts are behavioral interventions which direct or remind the parent or child to conduct a specific task, such as blood glucose monitoring. They can be very useful in getting the child and the family to comply with the recommended treatment. This can be done through increased supervision by a member of the health team or by a parent who has been educated and counseled on the use of prompts. An example might be more frequent clinic visits which provide a chance for the health professional to prompt adherence to the treatment plan. The frequency of visits can gradually be phased out and substituted with phone prompts. Subsequently, this form of prompting is faded and prompting becomes the responsibility of individuals in the child's natural environment.

A prompt known as glycosylated hemoglobin profile (Figure 9.1) has been used successfully to assist patients in conceptualizing their degree of control. This will provide vital feedback to the patient regarding the direction of his metabolic control and also serves as a prompt for maintaining compliance. Patients and their parents are directed to place the chart with the plotted profile in a place where it will be seen on a daily basis.

In the event behavioral problems of the child with diabetes and/or his siblings are identified, such strategies as token economies, time-out, and contracting can be used under the supervision of a qualified behavioral therapist.

PARENTAL SUPERVISION

Again we wish to emphasize that too often the older child or adolescent with diabetes is expected to assume full responsibility for his or her care. Many times, this insidiously occurs before the child is mature enough or has been properly educated. For the younger child, education usually comes in the form of bits and pieces from their parents, resulting in an adequate knowledge base for self-management of the disease. Complete responsibility obviously is the long-term objective for all adolescents but it must be individualized for each child and family. Rapoff and Christopherson recommend and

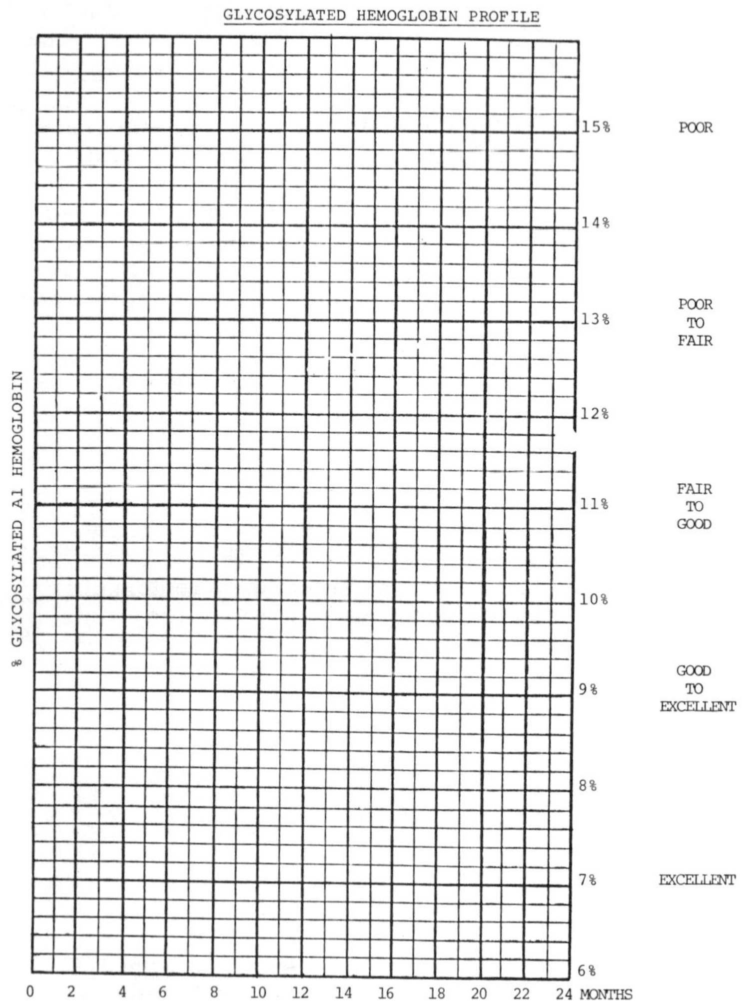

FIGURE 9.1 Glycosylated hemoglobin profile.

our experience confirms that the transfer of management must be a gradual process under the close guidance of the diabetic team.

All children and adolescents with diabetes need continued supervision even when they are successfully managing their disease. This is similar to the social support adult patients require not only from health professionals, but also from other significant persons in order to adhere to their diabetic regimen. Parents, health professionals, and other support persons such as teachers and classmates can provide positive reinforcement (a praise or hug) when the child or adolescent complies with their instructions. In addition, attention in the form of positive reinforcement should also be given for appropriate activities of daily living for both the child and his siblings. Many times children who are either pseudononcompliant or noncompliant are also experiencing behavior problems in their home. Appropriate behavioral strategies (positive reinforcement, time-out, etc.) can be provided to parents to enable them to deal with common behavioral proplems experienced with all children. Discipline should never be omitted for either the child with diabetes or his siblings. Lack of discipline may lead eventually from pseudo- to true noncompliance.

INTERVENTIONS WITH NONCOMPLIANCE

In the event there is true noncompliance, the same evaluation procedures are indicated that have previously been discussed. The same educational and behavioral strategies can be used for the noncompliant patient. Many noncompliance problems can be modified through this routine but in selected cases more intensive psychosocial care is indicated. The child or adolescent who is experiencing a psychiatric disorder is at high risk for noncompliance with his diabetic regimen. A psychiatric referral is indicated in all of these cases. Fortunately, this is not required for most children with diabetes whose families receive specialized care from the time of onset of their disease.

Social and economic factors are major determinants influencing compliance and are difficult to evaluate and modify. We have found that the time required for diagnosis and the duration of the period of partial remission is closely related to the socioeconomic status of the child's family. We also have found a close interrelationship between the ability of the parents to maintain a high degree of metabolic control and the economic status of the families and an even closer interrelationship to the social stability of the family (see Figure 8.2, Chapter 8). Consequently, it is important to have an in-depth social evaluation at the time of diagnosis and to provide as much help as possible in meeting the needs of each family.

Chapter 10

COMPLICATIONS

Richard A. Guthrie, M.D.
and Robert L. Jackson, M.D.

The major considerations in morbidity and mortality in diabetes mellitus are and will remain for the foreseeable future the vascular and neurologic problems associated with the disease. These problems are micro- and macrovascular disease and neuropathy. Since these problems usually take 10-15 years to become manifest, they are rarely seen by the pediatrician and are frequently ignored in the difficult practicality of day-to-day care (1). The long-term problems are of great concern to the internist and ophthalmologist, however, as they are becoming increasingly convinced of the need for improved control of the disease in childhood (2, 3).

Recent data indicate a "window of vulnerability" in the first 10-15 years of diabetes management, during which time there are functional changes which can be altered by improved control (4). After this time, however, if control has not been sufficient, the changes become structural, permanent, and irreversible (5). The burden of providing adequate control of the diabetic is therefore on the shoulders of physicians and allied health professionals managing the patients with diabetes during that all important first 1--15 years after clinical recognition of the disorder.

THE LONG-TERM COMPLICATIONS OF DIABETES

The complications of diabetes mellitus can be divided into three groups: short-term, intermediate, and long-term complications. Short-term problems are diabetic ketoacidosis (DKA) and hypoglycemia. Examples of intermediate problems are intercurrent infection, surgery, pregnancy, and psychosocial problems. The major long-term problems of children and young adults with insulin-dependent diabetes are vascular changes and neuropathy.

Vascular complications are of two types: small vessel disease or microangiopathy and large vessel disease or macroangiopathy. Neuropathy can involve the cranial and/or peripheral nerves, both sensory and motor, and the autonomic nervous system. We have recently observed what we believe to be involvement of the central nervous system as well. Neuropathy is rarely a problem in children except for sixth nerve palsies and occasional peroneal nerve palsy with foot-drop after short periods of extremely poor control.

Macroangiopathy in diabetes is not different from large vessel disease in nondiabetic persons. In adults with diabetes, the vascular changes of coronary artery disease, cerebral artery disease, and peripheral vascular disease, especially of the vessels of the legs, occur at a much earlier age than in persons without diabetes. Macrovascular disease is more commonly seen in older persons with DM II but also is seen in persons with DM I after 20-30 years of the disease if the person has survived the problems of microvascular disease and neuropathy. The etiology of macrovascular disease is complex, diabetes being only one of several risk factors which cause or accelerate the problems. The role of blood glucose in the development of macrovascular disease is poorly understood, but control of blood glucose and other metabolic factors seems prudent. The data for a close interrelationship between microvascular disease and diabetic control are better established.

PATHOLOGY OF MICROVASCULAR DISEASE

Microvascular changes in diabetes mellitus involve the small blood vessels of the body, especially the capillaries. The changes are generalized to all the capillaries, but the clinical manifestations are reflected in the eyes and the kidneys.

The changes in the eyes related to diabetes are many, including cataracts, proliferation of papillary vessels, and others. However, the primary and most serious manifestation of vascular damage is to the retinal vessels — diabetic retinopathy.

Retinopathy

Diabetic retinopathy begins with narrowing of retinal arterioles and dilatation of retinal veins. There is concurrently an increase in vascular permeability with leakage of small molecular weight proteins. The leakage can be assessed by observing the leakage of a fluorescent dye called fluorescein. Next, we see microaneurysms followed by exudates and hemorrhage. A particularly serious problem is edema of the macula. Finally, obstruction of the blood vessels of the retina results in ischemia of the retina followed by new vessel formation. This is called proliferative retinopathy.

Proliferative retinopathy is especially dangerous because of the possibility that the fragile vessels will break, causing hemorrhage into the retina and vitreous. Proliferating vessels along with fibrous tissue grow across the retina and eventually into the vitreous. When the fibrous tissue contracts between the vitreous and the retina, the retina can become detached, causing blindness.

Nephropathy

Diabetic nephropathy is initially manifested by enlargement of the kidney, with a paradoxical increased glomerular filtration rate (GFR) and creatinine clearance (CC) and the leakage of small molecular weight proteins into the urine. These proteins cannot be routinely detected and require special tests. As the disease progresses, larger molecular weight proteins such as albumin begin to leak into the urine. These proteins are detectable by routine laboratory tests such as urine dipsticks for protein. By the time the patient manifests detectable albuminuria, however, the damage is severe and relatively irreversible.

Early in the course of diabetes, the kidney size and vascular area increase. This results in a supranormal creatinine clearance which may be deceptive. The excess renal vascular blood flow may in itself be damaging. As the changes progress unchecked, GFR and CC begin to drop concurrent with the appearance of microproteinuria. Once GFR begins to fall, the rate of fall is predictable at the rate of 1 cc/min/month or 12 cc/min/year. After the GFR falls below 40–60 cc/min the decline is probably irreversible and can only be slowed. Slowing of the decline of GFR can be accomplished by meticulous control of blood glucose levels and especially by careful attention to control of the blood pressure.

Although both retinopathy and nephropathy can be treated with some preservation of life (dialysis and transplant), the treatment is difficult and some disability persists. Prevention of these problems is much more desirable than treatment. Can the problems be prevented?

THE CONTROL CONTROVERSY

As soon as people with DM I lived long enough (after the discovery of insulin) for long-term problems to develop, a controversy began. As the long-term problems have become more evident, the controversy has increased. Controversy is, however, not all bad. Controversy means that not all the data are yet in and leads scientists back to the drawing board to obtain the data. Such research is occurring today in diabetes mellitus and new data are rapidly becoming available.

The controversy regarding the relationship between control of diabetes mellitus and the development of long-term vascular and neurologic problems involves two opposing concepts. These concepts are: 1) The vascular and neurologic lesions of diabetes mellitus are a genetic *concomitant* of the disease unrelated to blood glucose, blood insulin, or the metabolic events of the disease (1). 2) The lesions are a *complication* of the disease somehow related to the metabolic events of the disease, i.e., blood glucose, blood or tissue insulin, serum lipids, etc. (2).

Those who take the first position argue that since the problems are a genetic concomitant of the disease, they are therefore inevitable and unalterable by control. The theory, then, is that one should not attempt to impose restrictions on the life of the child with diabetes that would be needed to achieve physiologic control, most often referred to as "tight" control, as such attempts may cause hypoglycemia or psychological damage to the child. These physicians have reasoned that it is not only difficult but of questionable value to attempt tight control because it will risk potential physical or psychological damage to the child (1).

Perhaps the best data to support this position comes from two sources: clinical studies (6, 7) and the muscle biopsy data of Siperstein et al. (8, 9). Many clinical studies have been performed in order to prove that good control would lessen complications. These past studies were reviewed by Knowles (10) in 1964 and all were found to have defects. None could prove that improved control had a beneficial effect on the incidence or prevalence of complications. More recent clinical studies have been better performed.

In 1968, Siperstein et al. (8) published data from muscle biopsies measuring the capillary basement membrane thickening (CBMT) of muscle capillaries. These data seemed to support the concept that microvascular disease was genetically predetermined and even preceded the onset of carbohydrate intolerance. In 1972, Kilo et al. (11) published data dissimilar to those of Siperstein. The controversy was enjoined and continues (9-12).

Until 1972, the available data seemed to support the first concept, i.e., control was not a major factor in vascular disease in diabetes. There was, therefore, a tendency to relax control, especially in children with diabetes, for fear of hypoglycemia and psychosocial maladjustment (13). Many clinics assumed that tight control would exact a discipline which would cause psychological damage (2); however, our observations indicated the opposite (14).

Pediatricians especially have tended to advocate control techniques utilizing the simplest management possible, with the least restraint upon the child and family. Not seeing the complications since they develop later in life, this control was deemed adequate if growth and development was considered satisfactory and the child was reasonably happy and well adjusted to home and school (13).

Accumulated data indicate the need to reassess this former position and to maintain as physiologic control as possible from the beginning to teach the patient self-management and to avert complications (15-17).

THE WINDOW OF VULNERABILITY

In a recent lecture on this subject, Dr. Daniel Mintz (18), diabetes investigator at the University of Miami School of Medicine, drew a timeline for diabetes. His timeline indicated a period of 10-15 years after the clinical diagnosis of diabetes mellitus when *functional* changes occur, during which the ultimate course of the vascular and neurologic damage could be modified. During this prolonged initial period, the diabetes patient may perceive little or no physical impairment. If metabolic control remains poor during this period, a state of *structural,* irreversible damage ensues which could no longer be stopped or reversed even if control is improved. Dr. Mintz calls this early period the window of vulnerability. Data now show that during these early years changes do insidiously occur in the tissue of persons with diabetes, but the initial changes are to a considerable extent functional (i.e., without structural damage to the tissues) and reversible. Changes seen during this earlier period are those of loss of vascular integrity (4), protein leakage by capillaries all over the body including the kidney (19), increased renal size and GFR (20), and reduced nerve conduction times in the motor and sensory nerves (21). These functional changes are reversible (4, 20-22) by improving of control of the blood glucose. If control is not improved, however, the functional lesions progress to structural lesions (5, 21-29) familiar to us as the chronic vascular and neurologic complications of the disease (retinopathy, nephropathy, and neuropathy). These structural changes (microaneurysms, hemorrhage, exudate, retinal vessel proliferation, glomerulosclerosis, and clinical neuropathy, especially autonomic neuropathy) are probably not reversible lesions. Indeed, data with insulin pumps suggest that tightening control quickly in a long-standing, poorly controlled diabetic with background retinopathy may *temporarily* accelerate the retinopathy with proliferation and hemorrhage (30). This is not to indicate that appropriate and more gradual blood glucose control should not be undertaken, as this problem stabilizes in a few months.

THE TRIANGLE

No individual study or group of studies to date definitely prove that physiologic control of blood glucose and other metabolites will prevent the vascular and neurologic problems of the disease. The data taken together are, however, mounting and do indicate that improved control will at least delay the complications of the disease. There are three avenues of approach to the problem, which taken individually will not completely clarify the problem, but which taken together support each other as sides of a pyramid support each other to make a whole. One side or even two sides of a pyramid will by itself or themselves not stand, but three sides together support each other in a way to make a structure infinitely stronger than even the sum of its parts. The same is true with new diabetes research data relating to the control problem. The three areas which support each other are: 1) more definitive clinical studies; 2) data from research animals; and 3) biochemical data on the mechanism of the structural and functional changes.

Clinical Studies

Early clinical studies of the relationship between vascular disease and metabolic control in diabetes mellitus were fraught with many problems. Most studies have been retrospective. Control in these studies was poorly defined and the end points were not very sensitive. Perhaps the largest and most conclusive of the new studies published to date is that of Pirart (26). This study from Belgium was a prospective study of 4400 persons followed for 25 years with multiple tests for degree of control and for vascular and neurologic disease. The conclusion of the study was that small vessel disease (nephropathy and retinopathy) and neuropathy correlate very well with blood glucose levels and diabetic control, but no such correlation could be found for large vessel disease.

Recent clinical studies of Mauer (27) demonstrating the development of nephropathy in transplanted kidneys from *nondiabetic donors* also support the concept of a metabolic basis for the lesions. The studies of Job (28) and Tchobroutsky (29, 30) demonstrated a relationship of retinopathy to control of blood glucose, and recent studies of Williamson and Kilo (31), Jackson et al. (32), and others (33, 34) have demonstrated an effect of control on the primary lesions of microvascular disease -- CBMT. These studies and others demonstrate conclusively that capillary basement membrane changes do not precede the onset of carbohydrate intolerance but rather develop gradually after the onset of diabetes (11, 31-34). Capillary basement membranes are universally normal at the onset of definitive diabetes and thicken with time (11, 32, 35). The very recent publications of Jackson et al. (36, 37) indicate that the speed of thickening of the basement membranes is influenced by the blood glucose level and that the early lesions (thickening) are reversible. Measurements were made of muscle CBMT in 95 normal boys and girls and 167 postpubescent insulin-dependent diabetes. Of 110 diabetics in whom higher degrees of metabolic control were maintained, only two had increased CBMT values. Of 57 diabetics in whom lower degrees of metabolic control were maintained, 26 had increased CBMT values. Two or more muscle biopsies were done in each of 65 diabetic subjects. Mean CBMT values of 24 subjects with higher degrees of metabolic control for 2-9 years remained within the normal range; values of 23 subjects with lower degrees of metabolic control for only 1-3 years increased from 858 ± 142 A° to 1155 ± 227 A°; values of 13 subjects who had been in lower degrees of control decreased from 1255 ± 232 A° to 869 ± 135 A° after maintaining improved metabolic control for about 1 year. In postpubescent children with diabetes, the CBMT is labile and progresses or regresses depending upon the degree of metabolic control.

CBMT also was measured by our laboratory in an additional 56 boys and girls with diabetes for 8 or more years. These subjects had received conventional therapy in other clinics and had been in fair-to-poor metabolic control by our criteria. Increased CBMT was found in only one of 11 prepubertal children, an 11-year-old stunted diabetic boy. Thirteen (10 girls more than 14 years of age and three boys more than 16 years of age) were postpubescent (Tanner stages V or VI). All of this group had increased CBMT, except for one girl with onset of diabetes after puberty and who had diabetes for only

1 year. The remaining 32 (17 girls and 15 boys) were 12-16 years of age at the time of their biopsies. Nine of the 17 girls had delayed linear growth, and eight of these nine also had delayed bone age values. Eight of the 17 were considered to be stunted. Eleven of the 15 boys had delayed bone ages and eight also had delayed linear growth. Six of the eight were also considered to be stunted. Seventeen of the more mature subjects (Tanner stages V and IV) had thickened capillary basement membranes. The remaining 15 had normal CBMT. These 15 adolescents without CBMT had longer duration of diabetes with delayed growth and bone ages and were in earlier stages of maturation.

The age of onset of diabetes in children varies considerably and *for reasons not understood, detectable microvascular changes rarely occur in children until growth and maturation have essentially been completed.* These observations help explain why there is a poor correlation between duration of diabetes in young adults with onset during childhood and the time of appearance of vascular changes. The data also account for the earlier development of changes in girls as compared with boys.

Concurrently, retinal studies were done in 181 postpubescent, insulin-dependent diabetic patients who developed diabetes before the age of 20 (36). Retinal studies included serial direct ophthalmoscopic examinations, stereoscopic fundus photography, and fluorescein angiography. At the time of retinal studies, muscle biopsies also were done to measure CBMT as an index of early microvascular changes in skeletal muscles. Assessment of clinical metabolic control, interpretation of retinal findings, and CBMT were done independently. No retinopathy was detected in patients observed continuously and known to have been in higher degrees of control. Twenty-five patients in lower degrees of control for extended periods had retinopathy. As stated before, CBMT was found to be labile and to progress or regress within a year depending upon the degree of control. All patients in lower degrees of metabolic control with retinopathy had increased CBMT, but if they subsequently attained and maintained a high degree of metabolic control for a year, then CBMT diminished and there was no progression of retinopathy. These studies demonstrate that a high degree of metabolic control delays and may prevent microvascular changes. It also confirms other studies indicating that most postpubescent, insulin-dependent diabetic patients will develop retinopathy within 15 years unless a relatively high degree of control is maintained. These data are entirely consistent with the biochemical data on the mechanism of the development of CBMT, i.e., enzymatic and nonenzymatic glycosylation of basement membrane proteins.

Perhaps the most telling of the clinical studies are the evidences of reversibility of the lesions (4, 5, 20–22, 27, 36, 37). While there is disappointment that advanced changes cannot be reversed even with insulin pump therapy (5, 23, 24), there are now ample data to support the concept that the early lesions of microvascular disease and neuropathy are reversible (21, 38).

Several investigators have demonstrated that slowed nerve conduction time (the earliest measurable lesion of diabetic neuropathy) is reversible with improved glycemic control. This is true at least before clinical neuropathy develops (39). Clinical neuropathy is less reversible but may improve or at least slow its progression when control improves (40).

The earliest functional lesion of retinopathy so far demonstrated is that of vascular leakage of protein and dye (41). Fluorescein is used in this test and its leakage into the vitreous can be measured by vitreous photofluorometry (42). Studies by Waltman (4) have demonstrated reversal of this lesion by improved metabolic control of the diabetes.

Studies on the kidney are less clear-cut. However, several studies do indicate that early renal lesions are also reversible. There are isolated reports of transplant of diabetic kidneys into normal individuals with improvements of the nephropathy (43). There are also early reports of a decrease in renal size, the exaggerated GFR of early diabetes, and albuminuria (20, 22, 44). The problem in the earlier reports that renal disease in diabetes was nonreversible is that the methods of measurement of functional changes in the kidney are insensitive. The kidney is such a resilient organ that most of its function can be lost before our crude tools can detect problems. As we develop more sensitive tools such as radioimmunoassay for microprotein molecules in the urine (a sign of early or functional damage before creatinine, BUN, CC, or GFR are affected), we should see the emergence of new data on the relationship of renal damage to control and the reversal of early functional lesions.

Finally, the recent data of Jackson et al. (36, 37) on CBMT in children and adolescents with type I diabetes and of Raskin (45) on adolescents and young adults are clear. They not only show prevention of CBMT by control but also demonstrate reversal in a relatively short period of time of what is a definite anatomic lesion.

What is thought to be the definitive clinical study is currently being planned. This study to be conducted in 21 centers by the National Institutes of Health (NIH) will study prospectively large numbers of children and young adults for several years. These persons will be randomized to either conventional insulin therapy using a one-dose/day or a two-dose/day split-mixed regimen or to an intensified regimen using either four doses/day of injectible insulin or to an insulin pump. Many end-point parameters will be studied serially to arrive at a final conclusion of whether control of blood glucose levels influences vascular changes. If the answer to this question is positive, the NIH study will attempt to answer the question of what level of blood glucose control is needed to prevent vascular disease. This study, while perhaps definitive, will take probably 10 years to complete. In the meantime, we cannot allow thousands of children to pass the window of vulnerability into permanent damage.

Animal Data

Critics of the concept that physiologic control would prevent vascular disease initially stated that data from experimental animals did not support the concept. It was stated that animals made experimentally diabetic did not develop vascular and neurologic lesions (8); therefore, the lesions in humans must be genetically determined. This statement is no longer true, as over 50 papers involving several species of animals with experimental diabetes and developing diabetes-type vascular and neurologic lesions have now been published. Some of the first papers were published by Bloodworth and Engerman (46, 47) in dogs. These investigators induced diabetes in dogs with no predisposition to diabetes. Littermates were kept as controls. The diabetic dogs treated with a single injection of NPH insulin per day developed CBMT, cataracts, retinopathy, and neuropathy very similar to human disease. Furthermore, a group of dogs made similarly diabetic (littermates) but kept in better diabetic control with multiple-dose insulin therapy developed very few or no lesions of diabetic vascular disease. Capillary basement membranes were not thickened in the well-controlled diabetic dogs.

Mauer (27, 48, 49) has done similar studies in rats and has demonstrated that not only are the lesions preventable by controlling blood glucose levels and insulin but also that early lesions even in the kidney can be reversed when blood glucose is normalized. Mauer has crosstransplanted kidneys from diabetic to normal and from normal to diabetic animals and can reproduce the results at will, i.e., when the kidney is in an abnormal insulin-glucose environment, it develops lesions of diabetic glomerulopathy, and when put back on a normal milieu, it begins to heal the lesions. These investigators have similar data on transplanted kidneys in humans indicating that the animal data are applicable to humans as well (27).

Data from other animals are similar and confirm that the lesions of diabetic vascular disease and neuropathy can be experimentally induced by the hyperglycemia-hypoinsulinemia state in nearly every species of animal even when there is no genetic susceptibility in the animals. This is not surprising. Even though the lesions are not absolutely identical to those seen in humans, the lesions are similar enough to be specific for diabetes and to be consistent with the theory that glycosylation of proteins from hyperglycemia causes the tissue damage in diabetes.

Biochemical Data

Three mechanisms have been proposed for the development of small vessel disease and neuropathy in diabetes: 1) the polyol pathway, and 2) the enzymatic and 3) nonenzymatic glycosylation of protein. The polyol pathway is perhaps the least important and is limited to only a few tissues such as the lens of the eye and to nerve tissue. In all these biochemical mechanisms of disease, one central fact emerges as the piece of information that ties them all together. This fact is that only tissue which is permeable to glucose without the presence of insulin is damaged in persons with diabetes. Such tissues as the lens of the eye, vascular tissue, nerve tissue, etc., all have this permeability in common. Muscle tissue, fat tissue, etc., require insulin for the entry of glucose into the cell and are not damaged by hyperglycemia. This fact is important because it points directly to abnormal glucose homeostasis as the critical factor in the damage and is consistent with the glycosylation of protein hypothesis causing damage.

Glucotoxicity

The hypothesis of glycemic damage to tissue (glucotoxicity) is that tissue, permeable to glucose without insulin, accumulates glucose intracellularly to a level equal to the ambient extracellular glucose level. Since the intracellular environment cannot tolerate a high glucose level for long, secondary to osmotic and perhaps other factors, the cell must then dispose of the glucose. Since the normal glycolytic pathway of glucose via the Krebs cycle is insulin-dependent and insulin is deficient in diabetes which is poorly treated, this path (normal glycolysis) is at least partially blocked. The cell must then choose *alternate pathways* of glucose disposal, such as the polyol pathway, enzymatic glycosylation of basement membrane protein, and nonenzymatic glycosylation of other tissue proteins. Each of these pathways will be briefly discussed.

The Polyol Pathway (Figure 10.1)

When glucose is present in excess in tissues containing aldose reductase, glucose can be changed to its alcohol, sorbitol (50, 51). Some tissues also contain the enzyme sorbitol dehydrogenase which can change sorbitol to fructose. Certain tissues (muscle, etc.) can then phosphorylate fructose and reactivate the normal glycolytic pathway. Other tissues, such as the lens of the eye and nerve tissue, cannot do this and sorbitol and/ or fructose become an end-pathway product which will accumulate in the tissue. The adverse effect of these slowly diffusible sugars is not well understood. Osmotic gradients with water entry and swelling may be a factor. In the Schwann cell and the axon, the accumulating sorbitol may prevent entry of a similar but vital compound, myoinositol (52). It may then be the myoinositol deficiency that may damage the Schwann cell or axon, preventing them from carrying out their functions (21). Diabetic neuropathy is the end result. In the lens of the eye, sorbitol accumulation has been demonstrated but may not be the primary cause of cataracts. Although glycosylation of lens fibers seems to be paramount,

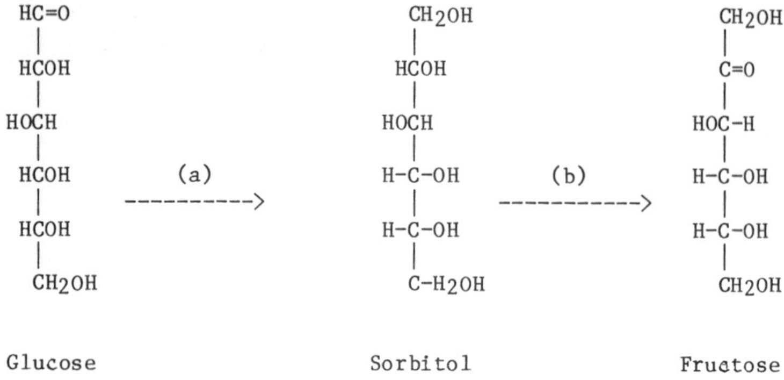

(a) Aldose Reductase

(b) Sorbitol Dehydrogenase

FIGURE 10.1 Polyol pathway.

the sorbitol accumulation may somehow create osmotic factors which facilitate the glycosylation process (53).

Enzymatic Glycosylation (Figure 10.2)

This mechanism of tissue damage was first demonstrated by Spiro (54) and has now been confirmed by others (55, 56). In both renal and retinal tissues, there are transferase enzymes which transfer glucose (or more specifically glucose and galactose disaccharide units) onto the proteins of the basement membrane (57).

Basement membrane material of capillaries consists of chains of glycoproteins which are laid down by the endothelial cell of the capillary. The membrane carries an electrical charge which is a major factor determining its permeability. The endothelial cell is exposed to the contents of the lumen of the vessel (blood plasma) and is permeable to glucose, as it must be to permit glucose to leave the vessel and enter the

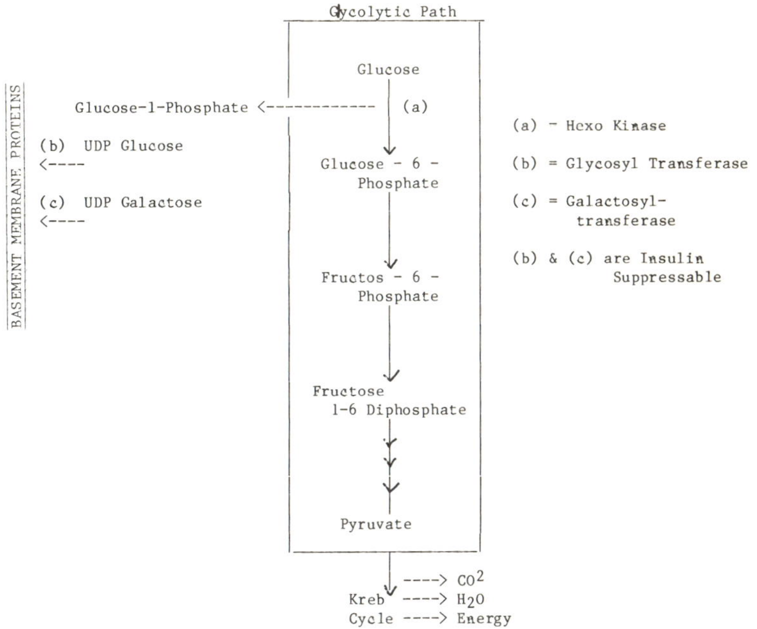

FIGURE 10.2 Enzymatic glycosylation.

extravascular tissue. The endothelial cell contains transferase enzymes (glucosyl- and galactosyltransferase) which can transfer the disaccharide units of glucose and galactose accumulating in the endothelial cell to the hydroxylysine molecules of the basement membrane (57). This glycosylation of the membrane proteins then alters the negative charge of the membrane, increasing its permeability to vascular proteins. The result is protein leakage (proteinuria is the earliest clinical sign of diabetic nephropathy).

Of most importance in this mechanism of vascular disease is the fact that transferase enzymes (glucosyl- and galactosyltransferase) are suppressible by insulin (57). In insulin deficiency, then, the substrates glucose and galactose (which is made from glucose) are available and the enzymes are active so the reaction can be expected to occur. What is necessary in the prevention of this chemical reaction is to keep the level of the substrate (glucose) low (blood glucose control) and the enzyme (transferase) suppressed. Enzyme suppression is best accomplished by 24-hr insulin delivery, something which usually cannot be accomplished in the absence of endogenous insulin by a single injection of insulin per day. This statement is true even in the face of the presence of some insulin in the blood for 24 hr from a single injection of NPH or Lente insulin since tissue insulin levels at the beginning (1-3 hr after injection) and ending (last 4-6 hr) are low. Adequate tissue insulin for glucose control and enzyme suppression are best obtained by delivering the insulin in a more physiologic manner mimicking as closely as possible that of endogenous insulin delivery, i.e., the maintenance of basal insulin in the blood stream continuously and the pulsing of boluses of insulin with feedings (see Chapter 6).

Nonenzymatic Glucosylation (Figure 10.3)

In 1912, Maillard (58) described a process in plants and in food whereby glucose became attached to certain amino acids

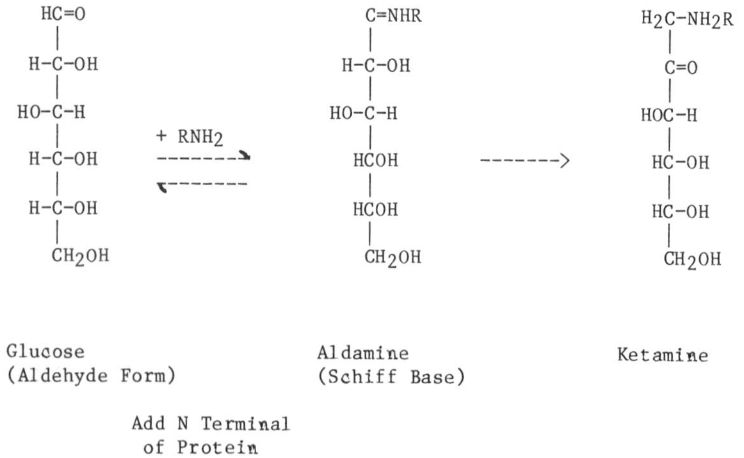

```
  HC=O                         C=NHR                    H2C-NH2R
   |                            |                          |
 H-C-OH                       H-C-OH                      C=O
   |                            |                          |
HO-C-H                       HO-C-H                      HOC-H
   |       + RNH2               |                          |
 H-C-OH   ------->             HCOH       ------->        HC-OH
   |      <-------              |                          |
 H-C-OH                        HCOH                       HC-OH
   |                            |                          |
  CH2OH                        CH2OH                      CH2OH

Glucose                      Aldamine                  Ketamine
(Aldehyde Form)              (Schiff Base)

         Add N Terminal
          of Protein
```

FIGURE 10.3 Nonenzymatic glycosylation.

of proteins. When the reaction is prolonged or intensified, the glycosylated proteins condense to form polymers which have a brown color, giving rise to the entity called the browning reaction. It is this process which causes the toasting of bread and the browning of meat when cooked and of peaches when removed from the freezer. The reaction is widespread in nature and can involve a wide variety of proteins, including those within the human body.

The Maillard reaction (nonenzymatic glycosylation) occurs between the number 1 carbon of glucose and the N-terminal amino acid of the protein (59). Initially, a reversible Schiff base (aldimine) reaction occurs. If the glucose level is sufficiently high to force (by the law of mass action) the glucose to remain in contact with the amino acid, then an internal rearrangement of the double bond from the first to the second carbon occurs. This is called an Amadori rearrangement. The end result is the formation of a ketamine compound with a carbon-nitrogen bond between the first carbon of glucose and the nitrogen of the protein. This bond is permanent (60). In most cases, the glycosylated protein then loses its biologic activity. This reaction in man was first described for hemoglobin (HbA_1C now used to document control), but has also been described for albumin, globulins, collagen, elastic tissue, basement membrane protein, lens of the eye, and myelin in nerve tissue (61-63). Nonenzymatic glycosylation is driven exclusively by the ambient glucose level to which the tissue is exposed and may be the primary process in vascular and neurologic disease associated with diabetes mellitus (64).

SUMMARY

Thus, glucose would appear to be a toxic compound [Dr. Peter Forsham (64) refers to the above process as glucotoxicity], which would explain why the body attempts (and succeeds in the nondiabetic person) to maintain the blood (and thus the tissue) glucose level in such a narrow range. Such persons virtually always avoid microvascular disease (63). It has been argued that none of the above studies are in themselves conclusive and no absolute proof exists that control of blood glucose will prevent microvascular disease (13). It also can be argued that such proof does indeed exist, not only from the data reviewed above, but also from an extraordinary experiment of nature. Persons whose pancreas functions normally and whose blood glucose level fluctuates within only very narrow ranges (60-140 mg/dl) even after high-carbohydrate meals or glucose loads virtually never develop the complications associated with diabetes mellitus, while persons whose control of blood glucose varies have a high frequency of these problems.

It is conceded that there is a high degree of variability in the development of the complications of the disease. Some persons, in spite of a reasonably high degree of metabolic control, may develop lesions early, while other persons in lower degrees of metabolic control seem not to develop lesions even after many years. These are the exceptions that prove the rule and probably do indicate some element of genetic susceptibility to the lesions. Nonetheless, the preponderance of evidence is that the primary factor remains glucose control (65). Until we have a marker that can detect the persons with diabetes mellitus that are genetically resistent to vascular damage, we must therefore attain and maintain the highest degree of metabolic control possible without causing serious hypoglycemia or undue psychological stress upon the individual (66). Means to accomplish this end (flexible, multiple-dose insulin schedules; self-blood glucose monitoring; HbA_1C measurements; diabetes education programs; insulin pumps; etc.) are now available to us.

The window of vulnerability (18) occurs all too often during the time pediatricians and family physicians are responsible for the diabetes care. We must turn this window of vulnerability into a "doorway of opportunity" to pass on to the internist not irreparably damaged, but healthy young people who will remain healthy, happy, and productive adults. With the tools we have, imperfect as they are, it is possible to accomplish this goal.

REFERENCES

1. Siperstein, M. D., Foster, D. W., Knowles, H. C., Levine, R., Madison, L. L., and Roth, J.: Control of blood glucose and diabetic vascular disease. *N.E.J.M.* 296:1060, 1977.

2. Cahill, G. F., Etzwiler, D. D., and Frankel, N.: Control and diabetes. *N.E.J.M.* 294:1004, 1976.

3. Ingelfinger, F. J.: Debate on diabetes. *N.E.J.M.* 296: 1228, 1977.

4. Waltman, S. R., Santiago, J., Krupin, T., Singer, P., Becker, B., and Bleecher, S.: Vitreous fluorophotometry and blood sugar control in diabetes. *Lancet* 2:1068. 1979.

5. Rand, L. I.: Recent advances in diabetic retinopathy. *Am. J. Med.* 70:595, 1981.

6. Knowles, H. C., Guest, G. M., Lampe, J. et al: The course of juvenile diabetes mellitus treated with unmeasured diet. *Diabetes* 14:239, 1965.

7. Malone, J. I., Hellrung, J. M., Malphus, E. W., Rosenbloom, A. L., Gorgie, A., and Weber, F. T.: Good diabetic control--A study in mass delusion. *J. Ped.* 88:94, 1976.

8. Siperstein, M. D., Unger, R. A., and Madison, L. L.: Studies of capillary basement membrane widths in normal subjects, diabetes and prediabetes patients. *J. Clin. Invest.* 47:1973, 1968.

9. Raskin, P., Marks, J. F., Burns, H. J. et al: Capillary basement membrane widths in diabetic children. *Am. J. Med.* 58:365, 1975.

10. Knowles, H. C., Jr.: The problem of the relation of the control of diabetes to the development of vascular disease. *Trans. Am. Clin. Climatol. Assoc.* 76:142, 1964.

11. Kilo, C., Vogler, N., and Williamson, J. R.: Muscle capillary basement membrane changes related to aging and to diabetes mellitus. *Diabetes* 21:881, 1972.

12. Williamson, J. R., Rawold, E., Hoffman, B. P., and Kilo, C.: Influence of fixation. Morphometry techniques on CBMT. Measurement data in diabetes. *Diabetes* 25:604, 1976.

13. Drash, A.: The control of diabetes mellitus. Is it achievable? Is it desirable? *J. Ped.* 88:1074, 1976.

14. Simonds, J. F.: Psychiatric states of diabetic youth matched with a control group. *Diabetes* 26:921, 1977.

15. Jackson, R. L., Hardin, R. C., Walker, G. L., Hendrick, A. B., and Kelly, H. G.: Degenerative changes in young diabetic patients in relationship to level of control. *Pediatrics* 5:959, 1950.

16. Hardin, R. C., Jackson, R. L., Johnston, T. L., and Kelly, H. G.: The development of diabetic retinopathy. Effects of duration and control of diabetes. *Diabetes* 5: 397, 1956.

17. Marble, A.: Relation of control of diabetes to vascular sequelae. *Med. Clin. N. Am.* 49:1137, 1965.

18. Mintz, D.: Complications--Overview. Lecture-Diabetes Seminar, University of Miami School of Medicine. January 18, 1983.

19. Osterby, R., and Gundersen, H. J. G.: Glomerular size and structure in diabetes mellitus. I. Early abnormalities. *Diabetologia* 11:225, 1975.

20. Morgensen, C. E., and Anderson, M. J. F.: Increased kidney size and glomerular filtration rate in untreated juvenile diabetes. Normalization by insulin treatment. *Diabetologia* 11:221, 1975.

21. Porte, D. J., Graf, R. J., Holter, J. B., Pfeifer, M. A., and Haloar, E.: Diabetes neuropathy and plasma glucose control. *Am. J. Med.* 70:195, 1981.

22. Viberti, G. C., Pickup, J. C., Jarret, R. J., and Keen, H.: Effect of control of blood glucose on insulin excretion of albumen and B_2 microglobulin in insulin dependent diabetes. *N.E.J.M.* 300:638, 1929.

23. Goetz, F. C., and Kjellstrand, C. M.: The treatment of kidney disease. *Diabetologia* 17:267, 1979.

24. Gundersen, H. J. G., and Osterby, R.: Glomerular signs and structure in diabetes mellitus. II. Rate of abnormalities. *Diabetologia* 13:43, 1977.

25. Seyer-Hansen, K., Hansen, T., and Gundersen, H. J. G.: Renal hypertrophy in experimental diabetes: A morphometric study. *Diabetologia* 18:501, 1980.

26. Pirart, J.: Diabetes mellitus and its complications: A prospective study of 4,400 patients observed between 1947 and 1973. *Diabetes Care* 1:168, 252, 1978.

27. Mauer, S. M., Barbosa, J., Vernier, R. L. et al: Development of diabetes vascular lesions in normal kidneys transplanted into patients with diabetes mellitus. *N.E.J.M.* 295:916, 1976.

28. Job, D., Eschwege, E., et al: Effect of multiple daily insulin injection on the course of diabetic retinopathy. *Diabetes* 25:463, 1976.

29. Tchobroutsky, G.: Relation of diabetic control to development of microvascular complications. *Diabetologia* 15:143, 1978.

30. Tchobroutsky, G., Charitanski, D., Blouqui, Y., Papoz, L., Soria, J., and Rosa, J.: Diabetes control in 102 insulin treated outpatients. *Diabetologia* 18:447, 1980.

31. Williamson, J. R., and Kilo, C.: A common sense approach resolves the basement membrane controversy and the NIH Pima Indian Study. *Diabetologia* 17:129, 1979.

32. Jackson, R. L., Guthrie, R. A., Esterly, J., Bilginaburan, N., James, R., Yeast, J., Sathoff, J., and Guthrie, D. W.: Muscle capillary basement membrane changes in normal and diabetic children. *Diabetes* 24:400, 1975.

33. Sheikholislam, B. M., Irias, J. J. et al: Carbohydrate metabolism and capillary basement membrane thickness in children. I. Gross sectional studies. *Diabetes* 25:650, 1976.

34. Sheikholislam, B. M., Irias, J. J., et al: Carbohydrate metabolism and capillary basement membrane thickness in children. II. Longitudinal studies. *Diabetes* 25:661, 1978.

35. Osterby, R.: Morphometric studies of the peripheral glomerular basement membrane--Early juvenile diabetes mellitus. I. Development of initial basement membrane thickness. *Diabetologia* 8:84, 1972.

36. Jackson, R. L., Ide, C. H., Guthrie, R. A., and James R. D.: Retinopathy in adolescents and young adults with onset of insulin dependent diabetes in childhood. *Ophthalmology* 89:7, 1982.

37. Jackson, R. L., Esterly, J., Guthrie, R. A. et al: Capillary basement membrane thickness in adolescents with diabetes mellitus. *J.A.M.A.* 282:2143, 1982.

38. Graf, R. J., Halter, J. B., Pfeifer, M. A., Haloar, E., Brozovich, R., and Porte, D. J.: Glycemic control and nerve conduction abnormalities in non-insulin-dependent diabetic subjects. *Ann. Intern. Med.* 90:298, 1979.

39. Gregersen, G.: Diabetic neuropathy, influence of age, sex, metabolic control and duration of diabetes on motor conduction velocity. *Neurology* 17:972, 1967.

40. Graf, R., Halter, J., Pfeifer, M., and Haloar, E.: The influence of glycemic control on nerve conduction abnormalities in diabetics. *Diabetes* 28:387, 1979.

41. Cunha-Vaz, J., Deabreau, J. R. F., Canipos, A. J., et al: Early breakdown of the blood-retinal barrier in diabetes. *J. Ophthal.* 59:649, 1975.

42. Waltman, S., Krupin, T., Hanish, S., Oestrich, C., and Becker, B.: Alteration of the blood brain barrier in experimental diabetes mellitus. *Arch. Ophthal.* 96:878, 1978.

43. Mauer, S. M., Steffes, M. W., and Brown, D. M.: The kidney in diabetes. *Am. J. Med.* 70:603, 1981.

44. Morgensen, C. E.: Urinary albumin excretion in short-term and long-term juvenile diabetes. *Scand. J. Clin. Lab. Invest.* 28:183, 1971.

45. Raskin, P., Pietri, A. O., Unger, R., Shannon, W. A., Jr.: The effect of diabetic control on the width of skeletal-muscle capillary basement membrane in patients with type I diabetes mellitus. *N.E.J.M.* 309:1546, 1984.

46. Bloodworth, J. M. B., Jr., Engerman, R. L., and Powers, K. L.: Experimental diabetic microangiopathy. I. Basement membrane studies in the dog. *Diabetes* 18:455, 1969.

47. Engerman, R., Bloodworth, J. M. B., and Nelson, S.: Relationship of microvascular disease in diabetes to metabolic control. *Diabetes* 26:760, 1977.

48. Mauer, S. M., Sutherland, P. E. R., Stiffes, B. W. et al: Studies of the rate of regression of the glomerular lesions in diabctic rats treated with pancreatic islet transplant. *Diabetes* 24:280, 1975.

49. Mauer, S. M., and Brown, D. M.: Is diabetic nephropathy preventable? *Metab. Ther.* 5:1, 1976.

50. Gabbay, K. H., and O'Sullivan, J. B.: The sorbitol pathway, enzyme localization and content in normal and diabetic nerve and cord. *Diabetes* 17:239, 1968.

51. Gabbay, K. H.: The sorbitol pathway and the complications of diabetes. *N.E.J.M.* 288:831, 1973.

52. Winegard, A. I., and Greene, D. A.: Diabetic polyneuropathy: The importance of insulin deficiency hyperglycemia and alterations in myoinositol metabolism in its pathogenesis. *N.E.J.M.* 295:1416, 1976.

53. Stevens, V. J., Rauzer, C. A., Monnier, V. M., and Cerant, A.: Diabetic cataract formation. Potential role of glycosylation and lens crystallins. *Prac. Nat. Acad. Sci.* 75:2918, 1978.

54. Spiro, R. G., and Spiro, M. J.: Affect of diabetes on the biosynthesis of the renal glomerular basement membrane. Studies on the glucosyltransferase. *Diabetes* 20:641, 1971.

55. Beiswenger, D. J.: Specificity of the chemical alterations in the diabetic glomerular basement membrane. *Diabetologia* 22:744, 1973.

56. Brownlee, M., and Spiro, R. G.: Glomerular basement membrane metabolism in the diabetic rat. *Diabetes* 28: 121, 1979.

57. Spiro, R. B.: The search for a biochemical bases of diabetic microangiopathy. The Claude Bernard Lecture. *Diabetologia* 12:1, 1976.

58. Maillard, L. C.: Action des acides amines sur les sucres, formation des melanoidines par voie methodologique. *C.R. Acad. Sci.* 154:66, 1912.

59. Bookchin, R. M., and Gallop, D. M.: Structure of hemoglobin A_1C. Nature of the N-terminal B chain blocking group. *Biochem. Biophys. Res. Commun.* 32:86, 1968.

60. Bunn, H. F., Haney, D. N., Gabbay, K. H., and Gallop, D. M.: Further identification of the nature and linkage of the carbohydrate in hemoglobin A_1C. *Biochem. Biophys. Res. Commun.* 67:103, 1975.

61. Day, J. F., Thorpe, S. R., and Bagres, J. W.: Non-enzymatically glucosylated albumin. *J. Biol. Chem.* 254:295, 1979.

62. Guthrow, C. E., Morris, M. A., Day, J. F., Thorp, S. R., and Bagres, J. W.: Enhanced nonenzymatic glucosylation of human serum albumin in diabetes mellitus. *Prac. Nat. Acad. Sci.* 76:4258, 1979.

63. Bunn, H. F.: Nonenzymatic glycosylation of protein: Relevance to diabetes. *Am. J. Med.* 70:325, 1981.

64. Forsham, P.: Glucotoxicity. Presented Mesa Lutheran Hospital Symposium, Mesa, Arizona, Oct 1983.

65. Skyler, J. S.: Complications of diabetes mellitus: Relationship of the metabolic control. *Diabetes Care* 2: 499, 1979.

66. Jackson, R. L., and Guthrie, R. A.: *The Child with Diabetes.* Current Concept Series, Scope Monograph. Upjohn Co., Kalamazoo, Mich., 1954.

Chapter 11

SPECIAL PROBLEMS

Richard A. Guthrie, M.D.

There are many special situations to be considered involving the young person with diabetes mellitus. Young persons with diabetes may need to have a surgical procedure, may have a serious infection, and may sometimes become pregnant. The physician caring for these persons must be prepared to handle these situations and others in order to prevent serious complications, which can occur rapidly. There are some similarities in dealing with each of these problems.

INFECTION

Minor infections in children and adolescents with diabetes are as common as they are for nondiabetics and usually pose no major problems. With minor infections, the glucose control usually is altered and the treatment of the infection is usually no different than for the person who does not have diabetes. Any drug indicated for a person without diabetes can be used in a person with the disease. Some of the common remedies such as cold medications carry warnings recommending that they are not to be used in persons with diabetes. They can be used but may raise blood glucose levels, and the insulin dose should be increased to compensate. Serious infections are fortunately not common but can pose difficult problems in management, which are dealt with in detail in Chapter 6.

There are frequent references in the literature to the increased incidence of asymptomatic bacteriuria and recurrent urinary tract infections in young people with diabetes. The increased incidence of infection reported in the literature is probably related to lower levels of glycemic control resulting in increased glucosuria. Glucosuria can create an excellent culture media for bacteria in the urinary tract. It is important, therefore, to maintain the urine as glucose free as possible in order to minimize this problem.

Other infections which commonly affect young people with or without diabetes are penumonia, strep throat, and various kinds of cellulitis. In older persons with diabetes and neuropathy, serious infections result from ulcers of the feet and legs, which can lead to osteomyelitis. These problems are very rare in children, although osteomyelitis can occur for the same reasons as in a nondiabetic. Meningitis and other serious infections should be handled in the same way as in a nondiabetic person, with appropriate attention to the insulin therapy as detailed in Chapter 6.

TRANSIENT HYPERGLYCEMIA

Transient hyperglycemia, sometimes associated with ketoacidosis and coma, can be seen with several conditions such as prematurity of infants, acute pancreatitis, central nervous system disease such as encephalitis, head trauma, heat stroke, tumor, or infiltrative process of the hypothalamus (1-3). Blood glucose levels may also be transiently elevated during periods of acute electrolyte imbalance, such as during dehydration with hypokalemia or hypernatremia (4, 5). The administration of certain drugs, especially the adrenocorticosteroids, may cause an elevation of blood glucose until the drugs are discontinued (6). It must be remembered that steroids will cause serious blood glucose elevations in persons with diabetes even when given into closed spaces such as the joints. Steroids elevate the blood glucose level by stimulating gluconeogenesis. Diuretics may elevate the blood glucose level by the production of hypokalemia. Hypokalemia, of whatever cause, results in a delay in insulin secretion (7, 8).

Severe stress such as burns, trauma (especially crush injuries), surgical procedures, severe infections, and general anesthesia may produce transient hyperglycemia, probably by the secretion of stress hormones such as steroids and epinephrine. Transient hyperglycemia may also be seen during the first 24–48 hr of IV hyperalimentation, where it may cause significant osmotic diuresis and dehydration (9).

Several conditions can produce an apparent or real glycosuria when the urine is tested for reducing substances. Renal glycosuria secondary to a very low glucose threshold will produce a real glycosuria by any test. Fanconi's syndrome and other renal tubular reabsorption syndromes may have accompanying renal glycosuria. These syndromes can be diagnosed by the presence of other substances such as amino acids in the urine. Some conditions such as aspirin intoxication, galactosemia, and pentosuria may cause reducing substances in the urine. These conditions can be differentiated from diabetes or transient diabetes by checking the urine with glucose oxidase strip or by determining blood glucose levels.

Transient hyperglycemia will usually abate when the prior condition, such as the burn, etc., is alleviated or treated. Such patients, however, should be followed carefully. It should be borne in mind that in the presence of stress in most individuals, the serum insulin level will increase, keeping the blood glucose level normal. In persons with transient hyperglycemia, serum insulin levels do not or cannot increase enough to compensate for the stress. This, then, may represent a defect in insulin secretion which may manifest as diabetes mellitus later in life or with a subsequent stress. If the hyperglycemia is mild, there may be need for no other treatment than for the underlying condition. If the hyperglycemia is severe or prolonged, the condition should be treated with insulin, which may be discontinued when the underlying condition is alleviated. When insulin therapy is initiated in such conditions, purified human or pork insulin should be the type of insulin used in order to reduce the chances of immune reactions sometimes seen with intermittent insulin therapy.

Small doses of regular insulin, 0.5-1.0 U/kg/day, may be given at 4- to 6-hr intervals.

HYPEROSMOLAR, HYPERGLYCEMIC, NONKETOTIC DIABETIC COMA

Sament and Schwartz (10) in 1957 called attention to a new medical emergency known as hyperosmolar diabetic coma. It has occurred primarily in older patients, some of whom were not known to be diabetic. Adult mortality is reported to be over 40% (11). Hyperosmolar coma in children with juvenile-onset diabetes is rare (12-14).

The syndrome is more likely to develop in association with a serious infection, such as encephalitis, and in the diabetic child who has been receiving medications such as thiazides or steroids. However, mismanagement of severe diabetic ketoacidosis by extremely rapid administration of fluids with excessive dextrose and electrolytes in conjunction with too little insulin can in itself cause hyperosmolar coma (15, 16).

The disorder is characterized by coma, severe dehydration, and marked hyperglycemia with minimal or no ketoacidosis. The child may present with focal or generalized seizures or with a focal neurologic deficit. Hyperosmolarity results from excessive hyperglycemia and, in many instances, from marked hypernatremia. Typically, the blood glucose level is 800 mg/dl or higher and the plasma osmolarity 325 mOsm/L or greater. The marked change in sensoria of affected patients is apparently due to intracellular dehydration of the central nervous system secondary to extracellular hyperosmolarity.

Marked hyperglycemia and dehydration without ketoacidosis may be caused by the presence of low but critical levels of circulating insulin at concentrations sufficient to inhibit lipolysis but insufficient to promote glucose transport into muscle. Zierler and Rabinowitz (17) have shown that the amount of insulin required to inhibit lipolysis is about one-tenth of that required for glucose transport. Studies of Passmore (18) and Gerich (19) suggest that dehydration and hyperosmolarity per se also exert antilipolytic effect on adipose tissue.

The principles of therapy for hyperosmolar coma are not significantly different from those for diabetic ketoacidosis.

Although the dose of insulin required for treatment of hyperosmolar coma is usually less than that for diabetic ketoacidosis, it is quite variable from patient to patient (20). Hyperosmolar coma has been reported to occur in a few adult patients with insulin resistance, and their insulin requirement may be very high (21, 22).

For treatment of the condition, the initial dose of regular insulin should be about 0.5–1.0 U/kg of body weight. Half of the initial dose should be given intravenously and the other half subcutaneously. About one-fourth of the initial dose should be administered every 2–4 hr after the beginning dose until the blood glucose level is decreased to about 200 mg/dl. Fluids and electrolytes should be administered as outlined for DKA in Chapter 6, section B.

CEREBRAL EDEMA

Transient elevation of CSF pressure has been observed during overzealous treatment of hyperglycemia. As a complication of the management of diabetic ketoacidosis or hyperosmolar coma in children, however, cerebral edema causing irreversible central nervous system damage or death is rare. Nonetheless, the diagnosis should be considered if the patient's condition improves over the first few hours of treatment, but suddenly the patient lapses into coma.

Cerebral edema, first described by Dillon et al. (23) in 1936, may be caused by increased volume of the brain, cerebrospinal fluid, or cerebral blood flow. Increased intracranial pressure in diabetic ketoacidosis is caused by:

1. Osmotic dysequilibrium: The blood-brain barrier permits easy passage of water but not glucose, ionic particles, and macromolecules. Too rapid correction of the plasma osmolarity during the treatment of ketoacidosis and hyperosmolar coma leads to the passage of water into the brain and causes cerebral edema (24).
2. Polyol pathway metabolism: In patients with diabetic ketoacidosis and hyperosmolar coma, hyperglycemia results in increased polyol pathway activity in brain cells, which contain aldose reductase (25). Since the membranes are not permeable to these formed sugar

alcohols, sorbitol accumulates in the brain cells. Again, too rapid rehydration results in a sudden shift of water into the brain cells and causes cerebral edema.

3. Cerebral hypoxia: As discussed in Chapter 6B, because of the low 2,3-DPG level in ketoacidosis, the sudden correction of acidosis may lead to cerebral anoxia. Cerebral anoxia is well known as a cause of acute cerebral edema, as is severe prolonged hypoglycemia (26).

Cerebral edema, once it develops, is very difficult to treat. Mannitol, glycerol, and steroids may help, as in cerebral edema in persons without diabetes. In diabetic persons, however, these agents are less effective. They should be utilized along with the monitoring of intracranial pressure through a burr hole transducer. Since therapy is not too effective, it is important to be alert to present its development during the treatment of DKA or hyperosmolar coma and to be alert for early signs of its development.

LACTIC ACIDOSIS

Although lactic acidosis is reported to occur in both diabetic and nondiabetic adults, it is not a major problem in children with diabetes. The condition usually occurs as a secondary phenomenon of circulatory failure (27) or in association with various medications (28). Excessive accumulation of lactate may occur as a result of either increased production of lactate or decreased utilization of lactate in the organism. Huckabee's studies indicate that widespread tissue hypoxia can cause lactic acidosis (29, 30). In fact, lactic acidosis in nondiabetic adults may be caused by certain diseases such as leukemia, severe anemia, circulatory insufficiency (cardiac or renal), gram-negative septicemia, and hepatocellular dysfunction. These diseases can cause tissue hypoxia and increased anaerobic glycolysis with subsequent elevation of lactate production, or they can inhibit the gluconeogenesis, which causes decreased lactate utilization. A number of chemicals also can cause lactic acidosis. These include phenformin, ethanol, barbiturates, salicylate, sulfonamides, certain adrenergic blocking agents, chlorpromazine, antihistamines, cyanide, and carbon monoxide. These compounds inhibit either tissue respiration or gluconeogenesis, with subsequent lactate accumulation and lactic acidosis. Another cause of lactic acidosis that occurs during DKA is inhibition of the enzyme pyruvate dehydrogenase.

In general, the onset of lactic acidosis is relatively acute. The patient is markedly weak and fatigued, exhibits Kussmaul's respiration, and develops stupor that progresses to coma within a few hours.

Lactic acidosis can be diagnosed simply by determination of the anion gap:

Anion gap = [serum Na^+ (mEq/L)] - [serum Cl^- (mEq/L) + serum HCO_3^- (mEq/L)]

The normal value is approximately 12 mEq/L. Accumulation of other anions such as lactate, B-hydroxybutyrate, salicylate, and formate will increase the value. A more definitive diagnosis should be made by direct measurement of serum lactate and pyruvate levels. In normal persons, fasting levels of lactate and pyruvate and the lactate/pyruvate ratio are, respectively: serum lactate, 0.40-1.40 mM/L; serum pyruvate, 0.07-0.14 mM/L; and lactate/pyruvate ratio, 10:1. A level of lactate greater than 7 mM/L or a lactate/pyruvate ratio of more than 10:1 indicates lactic acidosis.

Patients with lactic acidosis also have decreased serum pH and bicarbonate concentration; slightly elevated ketone levels in plasma and urine; increased concentration of serum lactate dehydrogenase, transaminases, and amylase; elevated blood urea nitrogen and serum creatinine levels; and an increased serum inorganic phosphate concentration.

Since anoxia and chemical compounds are the basic causes of lactic acidosis, it is important to detect the underlying problems and attempt to correct them as quickly as possible. The administration of alkali (bicarbonate) is indicated until the causes of the condition are recognized and removed.

CYCLIC EPISODES OF KETOACIDOSIS

A very small number of patients, most often adolescent, are admitted repeatedly to hospitals to be treated for ketoacidosis. Most of these children have severe emotional problems which, when acutely exacerbated, lead to rapid development of ketoacidosis. The mechanism has not been fully explained, but ketoacidosis may result from increased autonomic stimulation producing excessive release of catecholamines which mobilize free fatty acids and increase the concentration of blood glucose. An interesting approach to management of such patients was suggested by Baker and associates (31, 32). They reported a decrease in the need for frequent hospitalization when beta-adrenergic blocking agents were administered continually. We have used the Baker approach with doses of propranolol as high as 120 mg/dl with little or no success. We have abandoned the use of these drugs because of the many other effects which they have, including the masking of hypoglycemic reactions. The basic problem in emotionally induced ketoacidosis is psychosocial adjustment. For that reason, a more definitive approach to the problem is psychotherapy.

While most problems of cyclic DKA are psychosocial in nature, there are some cases where such causes cannot be found. Some patients seem not to have serious psychosocial problems or pseudononcompliance and the cyclic problem remains unexplained but usually goes away with time. However, the problem can be severe, life threatening, and costly while it exists. Some explanations of this problem have been subcutaneous enzymatic inactivation of insulin, poor insulin absorption, hypersecretion of counterregulatory hormones, peripheral resistance to insulin, and insulin resistence due to insulin-binding antibodies. All of these problems should be investigated and corrected if found. In our experience, most of these conditions are very rare and account for probably less than 1% of cases of cyclic DKA. In our experience, most cases of cyclic DKA (85% or greater) are psychosocial in nature, 5% perhaps will be pseudononcompliance problems, and most of the remainder are idiopathic metabolic instability. It is this latter group that we have found to respond best to the insulin pump. Usually after about a year of pump therapy the metabolic disturbance, whatever it is, will settle down, the pump can be discontinued, and therapy resumed with injectable insulin.

SURGERY

Much minor surgery can be performed on the diabetic youth as an outpatient using local anesthesia and a small dose of regular insulin prior to surgery. Another dose of regular insulin can be given before the next meal and the usual dose resumed in the evening. If general anesthesia is anticipated, we believe that persons with type I diabetes should be admitted to the hospital. Whenever possible, surgery should be on an elective basis and the person properly prepared for surgery. If the individual is in DKA when admitted for surgery (acute appendicitis is an example where this may be the case), the DKA should be corrected before the surgery, if at all possible. The most rapid method of correcting the DKA and preparing the person for surgery is with intravenous insulin as described in Chapter 6.

When DKA is not present and the surgery is elective, we prefer to admit the patient to the hospital on the evening before the surgery. Stress induced by administration of a general anesthetic or by a surgical procedure increases the blood glucose level to varying degrees. The primary objective of diabetic control during and after an operation is to avoid hypoglycemia and marked hyperglycemia. To accomplish this, an adequate amount of carbohydrate must be provided and balanced with appropriate small, repeated doses of insulin.

The total amount of fluid for maintenance therapy is calculated as 2000 ml/m^3 of body surface area/day (65-70 ml/kg). The fluid should be a multielectrolyte solution containing 5% dextrose. Early on the morning of surgery (usually about 6 a.m.) an IV is started of 5% dextrose in lactated Ringer's solution at an appropriate rate for the size of the child. When the IV is running, a small dose of regular insulin is given based upon the total daily dose. After surgery, the fluids should be changed to D5 and a hypotonic solution such as half-normal saline with appropriate addition of potassium. The composition of the electrolytes can be adjusted according to the serum electrolyte determinations. Intravenous fluids should be continued until adequate amounts of oral fluids are tolerated.

The amount of insulin to be given daily can be calculated on the basis of the patient's usual requirement and the clinical condition. If the patient is in DKA, the insulin requirement will be greater and should always be calculated on the basis of body weight.

Special attention must be given to the type of insulin used and to the route of its administration. Insulin may be given during and after surgery by one of three methods:

1. Addition of regular insulin to intravenous fluid.
2. Injection of regular insulin, intramuscularly or subcutaneously, every 4-6 hr. In most instances, this is the preferred method.
3. Subcutaneous injection of a mixture of regular and intermediate-acting insulins. This method should be reserved for patients undergoing minor elective surgical procedures when oral intake of food can be resumed quickly.

The specifics of management of the diabetic child who needs a surgical operation depend upon the patient's condition and on the type of procedure proposed.

Minor Surgery

If the surgical procedure is minor (e.g., abscess drainage or toenail extraction) and general anesthesia is not required, it may be done without any extraordinary attention to the diabetes. When indicated, a small supplementary dose of regular insulin can be given as outlined in Chapter 6.

Elective Surgery

For purposes of managing the child's diabetes, there are two types of elective surgery depending upon the expected duration of postoperative recovery in the hospital. If the patient's anticipated stay in the hospital is only a few days or if rapid resumption of oral intake is expected, it is desirable to maintain continuity in administration of intermediate-acting insulin. For that purpose, on the day of operation:

1. The operation is scheduled in early morning, preferably no later than 8:00 a.m.
2. The patient should not eat breakfast.
3. A multielectrolyte infusion containing 5% dextrose is started about 1 hr before the operation.

4. As soon as the IV infusion is begun, one-half of the patient's usual morning dose of insulin (given as a 2:1 mixture of NPH:regular) is administered subcutaneously.
5. As indicated by degree of glucose and acetone concentrations in the urine, doses of regular insulin are administered subcutaneously every 4-6 hr until the child can tolerate oral feeding.

Supplementary doses of insulin may be indicated depending upon results of urinalysis and blood glucose determination. If the patient's urine specimen contains more than 2% glucose but acetone is not detectable and the blood glucose level is < 250 mg/dl, one-fourth of the usual morning dose of insulin is given. If acetone is present or the blood glucose level is > 250 mg/dl, one-third of the usual morning dose is given.

For example, if the patient's usual total daily requirement of insulin is 60 U (40 U of a 2:1 mixture of NPH:regular before breakfast and 20 U of the mixture before the evening meal) he should be given 20 U of 2:1 NPH:regular insulin initially. He should then receive regular insulin every 4-6 hr, depending upon the degree of glycosuria and blood glucose level and presence or absence of acetone in the urine. If the urine glucose is 2% or more but no acetone is detectable and blood glucose is < 250 mg/dl, the patient should receive 10 U of regular insulin. If both acetone and a 2% (or greater) concentration of glucose are present in the urine and blood glucose is > 250 mg/dl, the patient should receive 13 U of regular insulin subcutaneously.

If, after the operation, the patient can tolerate oral feeding by afternoon, he may be given usual evening 2:1 NPH:regular insulin mixture 30 min before the evening meal.

If the patient undergoes a major surgical procedure and is expected to remain in the hospital longer than a few days, it is desirable to maintain therapy with regular insulin for some time before resuming treatment with the intermediate-acting form. Since the calories will be administered on a continuous basis for the next several hours, an appropriate system is to administer the insulin more or less evenly as well. This is done by dividing the usual daily dose of insulin into four equal doses of regular insulin given in 6-hr intervals. The first such dose is given in the morning before surgery. Blood glucose levels can be determined every few hours and the dose adjusted as needed to maintain blood glucose control using the previous day's insulin requirement as a guide. We feel that it is imperative to maintain glucose control during and after surgery to ensure adequate wound healing, to promote good white blood cell and immune system function to fight infection, and to reduce platelet adhesiveness in order to prevent thromboses.

After surgery, the four equal-dose regimen is continued until the patient is ready to take oral feedings. At that time the IV is slowed and eventually discontinued as oral intake increases. When oral feeding is begun, the calories will no longer be entering in a continuous basis so the insulin regimen must be changed to a proportional basis. At this point we change to the four-dose regimen, giving 35% of the total daily insulin before breakfast, 22% before lunch, 28% before supper, and 15% at about 1:00 a.m. The total daily dose is adjusted up or down depending upon the blood and urine glucose measurements but maintaining the four-dose schedule described previously. The "sliding scale" is never used. Blood glucose levels are determined at frequent intervals, preferably by fingerstick at the bedside, so that more frequent values can be determined and the values known quickly. Adjustments in insulin dosage can then be made on a rational basis as often and as quickly as necessary. Once recovery is complete, the IV is completely out, normal meals are reestablished, and the patient is ambulatory, the patient's previous insulin regimen can be reinstituted and adjusted as needed with the daily blood glucose profile.

Emergency Surgery

The most common indication for emergency surgery in children is an attack of acute appendicitis. By the time the diagnosis is made, the child may already be dehydrated and have mild ketoacidosis. The acidotic patient is a poor risk for surgery. It is better to delay the operation for a few hours until the conditions of acidosis and dehydration are corrected with intravenous fluids, electrolytes, and insulin. As soon as the patient is able to tolerate surgery, the operation may be done while the intravenous fluid (multielectrolyte solution containing 5% dextrose) is being infused. As described above, regular insulin should be injected subcutaneously every 4-6 hr thereafter if necessary, according to results of tests for urinary glucose, acetone, and blood glucose.

On the other hand, a child who has no dehydration or ketosis but who needs an emergency surgical operation (as in the case of injury, for example) may undergo the procedure after administration of intravenous fluid (multielectrolyte solution with 5% dextrose) is begun. Regular insulin should be given every 4-6 hr, depending upon the degree of glycosuria and ketonuria, and hyperglycemia.

Note that in discussing adjustment of insulin dosage based upon results of tests for glycosuria or blood glucose levels, we are not referring to the sliding scale for insulin administration. The sliding scale is a method of management in which an arbitrary dose of insulin is given for an arbitrary degree of glycosuria (i.e., an arbitrary number of pluses in the results of a given test for urinary glucose) or hyperglycemia. The presence of glucose in a given urine sample or a given blood glucose level actually indicates a need for insulin some hours in the past, and the degree of glycosuria or hyperglycemia is not an accurate indicator of the proper dose of insulin for the moment.

To illustrate the danger of the sliding scale method for adjusting dosage (in which no insulin is given for a 1+ urinary glucose test result), let us consider a child whose last dose of insulin will carry over to the next urine-testing period, thus causing a negative or 1+ reaction. If the usual insulin dose is then omitted in accordance with sliding scale practice, hyperglycemia will result as the prior dose of insulin wears off. (Regular insulin lasts only 6-8 hr.) The next urine sample then may show a reaction of 4+ or greater, and again the child will be given an unnecessarily high dose of insulin with a resulting "rollercoaster" effect on blood glucose. Sliding scales using blood glucose values have the same results.

Insulin doses may be adjusted depending upon results of tests for urinary and blood glucose, but they should be omitted or lowered beyond established maintenance requirements for the child. If regular insulin is used, four doses a day is the minimum frequency with which it can be given. We have been using the Biostator Glucose Controller-Monitor in a variety of surgical problems with great success as discussed in Chapter 12. Since the Biostator will control blood blood glucose levels within a very narrow range, the complication of high, low, or fluctuating blood glucose levels are avoided and the postoperative course is smoother. We believe we can shorten hospitalization with use of this machine.

PREGNANCY

Pregnancy in young persons with type I diabetes is a difficult and expensive affair and should always be planned. Evidence is rapidly accumulating that the congenital malformations so often seen in the infants of diabetic mothers are related to elevated blood glucose values in the mother during the first 12 weeks of the pregnancy (33). Unquestionably, the macrosomia and other problems seen in the newborn of the diabetic mother are related to elevated blood glucose levels in mid and late pregnancy. It is therefore important to attain good blood glucose control prior to pregnancy and maintain that control throughout the entire pregnancy (34).

Blood glucose control before and during pregnancy must be tighter than in the nonpregnant state in order to protect the infant (35). Such control can be accomplished by a variety of techniques (36). Recently we have favored the insulin infusion pump; however, adequate control can be achieved with injectable insulin as well. We prefer a four dose per day insulin schedule using regular insulin before each meal and NPH insulin at bedtime as the easiest and most flexible regimen to achieve the degree of control desired (35). Prior to, or as early in the pregnancy as we can begin, we establish glucose control with a minimum two dose per day split-mix insulin regimen. If control is not very soon established with this regimen or if control cannot at any time be maintained with this regimen, we immediately switch to a three- or four-dose regimen. Many pregnant women can be maintained into the midsecond trimester or later on three doses per day of insulin, but many need to go to a four-dose regimen. The proportions to begin are similar to the four-dose regular insulin schedule, although usually more NPH is needed at night and less regular will then be needed in the morning. The individual doses are adjusted by post- or preprandial blood glucose levels determined usually by self-blood glucose monitoring. It is important to control the fasting blood glucose value first in order to begin the day's insulin cycle at a normal blood glucose level. It will be easier then to control the insulin doses the remainder of the day. The fasting blood glucose level is controlled by adjusting the evening NPH insulin up or down until the value is in the desired range (60-110 mg/dl).

Once the fasting blood glucose value is in the desired range, the morning dose of regular insulin is adjusted to get the blood glucose values between breakfast and lunch into the normal range (80-130 mg/dl). Next, the noon dose of regular insulin is adjusted to control the noon-to-supper values, and finally, the supper dose of regular insulin is adjusted similarly to control the postsupper and bedtime glucose values. The patient must then determine the blood glucose level at least four times a day and the insulin doses are adjusted as often as necessary to maintain control.

Insulin requirements may fall slightly during the first trimester of pregnancy, then rise slowly during the second trimester, and rise rapidly during the third trimester. During the latter half of pregnancy insulin requirements may double and occasionally can triple. It is therefore important that the patient do daily self-blood glucose monitoring and that she be seen by the physician at frequent intervals. We usually see the patient monthly during the first half of pregnancy, every 2 weeks for the rest of the second trimester and weekly during the last 2 months. At each visit the home blood glucose records are carefully evaluated and adjustments in the insulin and diet are made. A glycosylated hemoglobin measurement is made each month to document that the patient is in control. If home blood testing indicated good control but the glycosylated hemoglobin value is elevated, the entire program, including the patient's education are reevaluated.

Throughout the pregnancy, the patient should monitor urinary acetone as a measure of the adequacy of the diet and the total calories and/or carbohydrate content of the diet adjusted to eliminate the ketones, as these substances are harmful to the fetus. The obstetrician and the diabetologist should stay in very close contact throughout the pregnancy and the termination date jointly planned. The termination date varies with the circumstances, the control during the pregnancy, and signs of fetal well-being, but in general we believe that, if control has been good, it should be possible to carry the pregnancy to term or near term even in teenage primagravida women. In our group of 96 patients, including teenagers, controlled as above over the last 3 years, there have been no major problems with the infants. Seventy-six percent were delivered at term (50% by vaginal delivery), were of normal size, and experienced none of the typical problems of the infants of diabetic mothers. The primary problem of this group of infants has been some mild and transient hypoglycemia. Control of blood glucose levels is possible during pregnancy and will prevent the devastating problems of the infant of the diabetic mother which remain all too common even today.

COMPLICATIONS OF INSULIN THERAPY

Lipodystrophy

The term lipodystrophy indicates either localized increase or, more commonly, decrease in sucutaneous fat (hypertrophy or atrophy, respectively). It typically but not exclusively occurs at injection sites and adjacent areas. Lipodystrophy is a benign condition, but the resulting cosmetic disfigurement is extremely disturbing to the diabetic child and the parents. Although it is seen most frequently in young women, one-fourth of the children and adolescents who are treated with insulin develop varying degrees of lipodystrophy. Trauma, coldness, acidity, and impurities of the insulin preparations have been considered the cause of the lipodystrophy. In fact, Calder and Watson were successful in filling the atrophied areas with injections of highly purified insulin (37). The incidence of lipoatrophy has markedly decreased since the introduction of neutral-regular and highly purified insulins.

The incidence and severity of lipohypertrophy can be decreased by rotating injection sites and lipoatrophy by using more purified and concentrated insulins (38). Injection of more purified insulin directly into the affected area has also been effective for treatment of lipoatrophy.

Insulin Allergy

Hypersensitivity to insulin is uncommon in children but may be manifested as a local reaction, generalized allergic reaction, and very rarely as anaphylactic shock. The problem is commonly seen in adults receiving intermittent insulin therapy.

Local skin reactions sometimes occur during the first or second week of insulin treatment. One-half hour to a few hours after the insulin injection, the child complains of a burning or itching sensation. Tenderness, induration, erythema, or a few urticarial wheals then may develop. These local manifestations gradually disappear completely within a few days to a few months.

Generalized insulin reactions such as hives, urticaria, or angioneurotic edema are seldom seen in children. These types of reactions usually appear within 30 min and tend to disappear in a few hours.

Treatment

Mild, local insulin allergies do not require any special treatment. Oral antihistamines can be used if local symptoms are more severe. Antihistamines may also be useful in the treatment of generalized skin reactions. In some cases, a hypersensitivity reaction can be treated by changing insulins. If the patient is sensitive to mixed beef-pork insulin, for example, one can try pure pork or pure beef insulin (39). The treatment of choice today is the use of a human insulin. For more resistant cases of insulin hypersensitivity, densensitization may be advisable. Kits are available for desensitization from pharmaceutical companies.

Insulin Resistance

True insulin resistance in the adult diabetic patient is defined as an insulin requirement in excess of 200 U/day for more than 48 hr in the absence of ketoacidosis, coma, or infection. In children, an insulin requirement in excess of 2.50 U/kg/day represents true insulin resistance and a requirement in excess of 1.25 U/kg/day represents insulin insensitivity (40). It probably occurs only in approximately every 5000 children with diabetes.

The main cause of insulin resistance is the development of antibodies to insulin. Most diabetic children develop some antibodies to insulin during the first 6 months of therapy. That number of antibodies remains relatively constant with a longer duration of the disease. An occasional diabetic child develops more antibodies, especially to beef insulin, with a concurrent rapid increase in insulin requirement (41).

Unresponsiveness of peripheral tissue to excessive plasma insulin (42) and binding of insulin by a protein different from insulin antibody can also cause the insulin resistance.

Treatment

Antibodies to beef insulin are produced more frequently than antibodies to pork insulin. In case of insulin resistance in a patient receiving mixed beef-pork insulin, it is advisable to change to a highly purified pork insulin (single-component pork insulin) (40, 41). The introduction of human insulin in 1983 made it the treatment of choice because it is the least immunogenic insulin available. Steroids may occasionally be needed but such treatment is rare in children.

SUMMARY

Maintenance of normal or near-normal blood glucose levels can be attained and maintained in the majority of young people with diabetes mellitus even during illness, surgery, pregnancy, and other stressful situations by the use of flexible multiple-dose insulin schedules. With proper control, the young people can be expected to recover from the episode as well as the nondiabetic person. There are multiple systems that can be used to accomplish the needed control. Some of the systems are previously outlined. Other algorithms for specific situations can be found in Chapter 6 on management and in Chapter 13 on insulins.

REFERENCES

1. Filler, R. M., and Eraklis, A. J.: Care of the critically ill child: Intravenous alimentation. *Pediatrics* 46:456, 1970.

2. Cawthorne, C. W. H., and Hobday, J. D.: Transient hyperglycemia, acidosis, and coma. A case report and review of nine similar cases. *Aust. Pediatr. J.* 9:208, 1973.

3. Fromantain, M., Gauthier, M., Beisselier, P., and Duriez, R.: Coma inaugural d'un diabete juvenile aigu avec glycemie a vingt trois grammes. *Diabetes* 17:91, 1969.

4. Gorden, P.: Glucose intolerance with hypokalemia. *Diabetes* 22:544, 1973.

5. Mandell, F., and Feller, F. X.: Hyperglycemia in hypernatremic dehydration. *Clin. Ped.* 13:367, 1974.

6. Glenn, E. M., Miller, W. L., and Schlagel, C. A.: Metabolic effects of adrenocortical steroids in vivo and in vitro. Relationship to anti-inflammatory effects. *Rec. Prog. Horm. Res.* 19:107, 1963.

7. Rapoport, M. I., and Hurd, H. F.: Thiazide induced glucose intolerance treated with potassium. *Arch. Intern. Med.* 113:405, 1964.

8. Chowdbury, F. R., and Bleicher, S. J.: Chlorthalidone-induced hypokalemia and abnormal carbohydrate metabolism. *Horm. Metab. Res.* 2:13, 1970.

9. Groff, D. B.: Complication of intravenous hyperalimentation in newborns and infants. *J. Ped. Surg.* 4:460, 1969.

10. Sament, S., and Schwartz, M. B.: Severe diabetic stupor without ketosis. *S. Afr. Med. J.* 31:893, 1957.

11. Danowsky, T. S., Nabarro, J. D. N.: Hyperosmolar and other types of nonketoacidotic coma in diabetes mellitus. *Diabetes* 14:162, 1965.

12. Ehrlich, R. M., and Bain, H. W.: Hyperglycemia and hyperosmolarity in an 18-month old child. *N.E.J.M.* 276:683, 1967.

13. Lotz, M., and Geraghty, M.: Hyperglycemia, hyperosmolar nonketotic coma in ketosis-prone juvenile diabetic. *Ann. Intern. Med.* 69:1245, 1968.

14. Kolodny, H. D., and Sherman, L.: Hyperglycemic non-ketotic coma in insulin-dependent diabetes. *J.A.M.A.* 203:461, 1968.

15. Umber, F.: Stoffwechselkrankheiten II. Der diabetes mellitus. *Munch. Med. Wochenschr.* 71:1324, 1924.

16. Root, H. F., and Leech, R.: Diabetic coma and hyper-glycemic stupor compared. *Med. Clin. N. Am.* 30:1115, 1946.

17. Zierler, K. L., and Rabinowitz, D.: Effect of very small concentrations of insulin on forearm metabolism. Persistence of its action on potassium and free fatty acids without its effect on glucose. *J. Clin. Invest.* 43:950, 1964.

18. Passmore, R.: On ketosis. *Lancet* 2:939, 1961.

19. Gerich, J. E., Penhos, J. C., Gutman, R. A., and Recant, L.: Effect of dehydration and hyperosmolarity on glucose, free fatty acid and ketone body metabolism in the rat. *Diabetes* 22:264, 1973.

20. Arieff, A. I., and Carroll, H. G.: Non-ketotic hyperosmolar coma with hyperglycemia: Clinical features, pathophysiology, renal function, acid-base balance, plasma-cerebrospinal fluid equilibria and the effects of therapy in 37 cases. *Medicine* 51:73, 1972.

21. Jackson, W. P., and Forman, R.: Hyperosmolar non-ketotic diabetic coma. *Diabetes* 15:714, 1966.

22. Saftel, H. C., and Goldin, A. R., Rubenstein, A. H.: Hyperosmolar nonketotic coma. *Lancet* 2:1042, 1967.

23. Dillon, E. S., Riggs, H. E., and Dyer, W. W.: Cerebral lesions in uncomplicated fatal diabetic acidosis. *Am. J. Med. Sci.* 192:360, 1936.

24. Clements, R. S., Prockop, L. D., and Winegrad, A. I.: Acute cerebral edema during treatment of hyperglycemia. *Lancet* 2:384, 1968.

25. Prockop, L. D.: Hyperglycemia, polyol accumulation and increased intracranial pressure. *Arch. Neurol.* 25: 126, 1971.

26. Marks, V., and Rose, F. C.: *Hypoglycemia.* Philadelphia, F.A. Davis Co., 1965, p. 317.

27. Rees, S. B., Krall, L. B., and Root, H. F.: Persistent lactic acidemia secondary to peripheral vascular failure in diabetic acidosis. Presented at the conference on Nonketotic Metabolic Acidosis in Diabetes Mellitus. New York, November 1972.

28. Tranquada, R. E., Bernstein, S., and Martin, H. E.: Irreversible lactic acidosis associated with phenformin therapy. Report of three cases. *J.A.M.A.* 184:159, 1963.

29. Huckabee, W. E.: Abnormal resting blood lactate. II. Lactic acidosis. *Am. J. Med.* 30:840, 1961.

30. Huckabee, W. E.: Abnormal resting blood lactate. I. The significance of hyperlactemia in hospitalized patients. *Am. J. Med.* 30:833, 1961.

31. Baker, L., Barcai, A., Kaye, R., and Hague, N.: Beta adrenergic blocade and juvenile diabetes. Acute studies and long-term therapeutic trials. *J. Ped.* 75:19, 1969.

32. Baker, L., Kaye, R., and Hague, N.: Metabolic homeostasis in juvenile diabetes mellitus. *Diabetes* 18:421, 1969.

33. *The Prevention and Treatment of Five Complications of Diabetes. Detection and Prevention of Adverse Outcome in Pregnancy.* National Diabetes Advisory Board, p. 13, 1984.

34. Ibid, p. 11.

35. Coustan, D. R., Berkowitz, R. L., and Hobbins, J. C.: Tight metabolic control in overt diabetes in pregnancy. *Am. J. Med.* 68:845, 1980.

36. Jovanovic, L., Peterson, C. M., Saxema, B. B., et al: Feasibility of maintaining normal glucose profiles in insulin-dependent prognant diabetic women. *Am. J. Med.* 68:105-112, 1980.

37. Calder, J. S., and Watson, B. M.: A treatment for insulin-induced fat atrophy. *Diabetes* 20:628, 1971.

38. Davidson, J. A., Wentwork, S. M., and Galloway, J. A.: The effect of concentration (volume) on absorption of subcutaneously administered insulin. *Diabetes* 22: (Supp. I) 317, 1973.

39. Davidson, J. A., Galloway, J. A., Petersen, B. H. et al: The use of purified insulins in insulin allergy. *Diabetes* 23:(Supp. I) 352, 1974.

40. Guthrie, R. A., Mrthy, D. Y. N., and Womack, W. N.: Insulin resistance in diabetes in juveniles. *Pediatrics* 40:642, 1967.

41. Murthy, D. Y. N., Guthrie, R. A., Womack, W. N., and Jackson, R. L.: Insulin binding in children with diabetes mellitus. *Pediatrics* 43:558, 1969.

42. Antoniades, H. N., Gundersen, K., Beigelman, P. M., Pyle, H. M., and Bougas, J. A.: Studies on the state, transport and regulation of insulin in human blood. *Diabetes* 11:261, 1962.

Chapter 12

RECENT ADVANCES IN DIABETES THERAPY

Richard A. Guthrie, M.D.

INTRODUCTION

In recent years there have been significant advances in the therapy of DMI. Some of these advances have been detailed in previous chapters. Speculations on the advances of the future will be discussed in Chapter 13, "Hope for the Future."

MONITORING OF GLUCOSE CONTROL

It is vital that various metabolic parameters be monitored, whatever the method of control or insulin regimen used in children with diabetes mellitus type I. In the past, only urine testing and intermittent blood glucose measurements in the office or hospital were available. Today glycosylated hemoglobin and self-blood glucose monitoring (SBGM) are added tools to assist in measuring parameters necessary to achieve physiologic control.

URINE TESTING

Although now replaced by blood testing for many older children and adolescents, urine testing still has a place in diabetes control. For children of school age (5-12 years) continued use of urine testing as the primary method of monitoring control is still recommended. Children in this age group have fairly low and relatively stable renal thresholds (165-185 mg/dl) and can collect urine specimens easily. On the other hand, they have more difficulty manipulating blood-testing equipment (especially at school) and have tender fingers, making frequent testing difficult.

New urine test strips (such as Chemstrip uGK), which measure urine glucose in percentiles, have facilitated the use of urine testing in the appropriate age groups when used to test first-voided urine specimens. If Clinitest is used for urine testing, the two-drop method should be used and the results recorded in percentiles. If any other urine method is used, results should always be recorded in percentiles, not in pluses. Pluses mean different percentages of glucose in the urine with different reagent strips and, therefore, cannot be interpreted without knowing the method used. Recording results in percentiles obviates this problem and makes results more comparable.

Urine testing has considerable value in children in middle childhood when performed by a stable method (two-drop Clinitest or Chemstrip uGK) on an appropriate specimen (first-voided specimen 3-4 times/day) and properly interpreted.

SELF-BLOOD GLUCOSE MONITORING

One of the most significant steps forward in blood glucose control in diabetes management is the ability of the parents or older child to determine their own blood glucose levels at home by SBGM, which is rapidly becoming utilized by the diabetic population for management of their disease (1). Specific persons within the diabetic population may receive greater benefit from SBGM than others. The pregnant diabetic and her fetus have much to gain from excellent diabetic control not easily attained without SBGM (2). The diabetic having an inaccurate renal threshold must resort to SBGM to achieve blood glucose control (3). Frequently, adolescent diabetics find urine testing so unpleasant that it is deleted from their schedule (4), however, many have accepted SBGM as an alternative form of testing.

Young children in whom the danger of hypoglycemia is more acute and threatening are also candidates for SBGM since the availability of the test provides security for the parents. Many persons can use the visually read strips (Chemstrip bG or Visidex II) without a meter. Unstable type I diabetics and diabetics with impaired vision or blue-green color blindness may find use of the glucose meter highly beneficial, if not imperative (5). Glucose meters may also be used by diabetics who have a problem discerning symptoms of hypoglycemia (6).

SBGM allows the potential for "fine-tuning" the balance of insulin, food intake, and exercise never before available to persons with diabetes (7). According to current research, fine-tuning blood glucose control leads to prevention and possibly amelioration of known diabetic complications (see Chapter 10). Meter accuracy, however, is of utmost importance to attain a high degree of metabolic control. Increments or decrements of the insulin dosage based on an inaccurate machine reading may lead to hyperglycemia, ketosis, or hypoglycemia. Besides accuracy and reliability, the meter must have ease of utilization, as increased complexity may lead to decreased monitoring (8). If SBGM is accurate, reliable, and easy to use, persons with diabetes may participate more actively in their own management, leading to an improved sense of well-being and frequently to improved compliance (9).

Studies in our clinic (10) have shown that properly cared for and properly used, the meters are accurate with a correlation coefficient of 0.99 when laboratory blood glucose measurements are 55-250 mg/dl. Meter values in the lower and higher ranges showed greater deviations from laboratory values. There are many meters on the market, and more are becoming available every few months. Some measure more accurately in the low range, and others are more accurate in the high range. Most measure within 15% of the laboratory value in the midrange (55-250 mg/dl) and are satisfactory for SBGM.

Selection of the proper strip and meter, therefore, is more a matter of personal taste than medical recommendation. Different clinics usually have different biases for the various strips and machines. Patients and families should be allowed to see and handle the various machines and select the one best suited for their personal use. Fox example, we have found that the Glucometer which reads Dextrostix and the Gluco-check II which reads Chemstrips bG are the easiest to use and the most accurate. We usually recommend these for home use. The Accu-Chek is another accurate machine; however, it is large, bulky, and often temperamental to operate. While less accurate, the Glucoscan II and Glucokey are smaller, fold easily to fit into a coat pocket, and are accurate enough for most uses. These meters are excellent for adolescents and young adults on the move who need greater flexibility and portable equipment. Therefore, the medical team should be familiar with all the meters and strips and adapt the method of SBGM (strip alone, strip plus meter, and type of strip and/or meter) to the individual who will be using it and to the life-style of the user. There will be better compliance and increased use.

There are many algorithms for use of SBGM. Some authors recommend postprandial blood glucose measurement, while others use premeal values. A flexible program of postprandial and/or premeal values adapted to the changing lifestyle of the individual is widely used. In an idealized situation to determine total daily insulin requirements and proper insulin distribution, it would be useful to have eight or more blood glucose values per day: one taken 1-2 hr after each meal (three/day), one before each meal (three/day), one at bedtime, and one or more in the middle of the night (3:00 a.m.). It is unrealistic to recommend that every patient (or any patient) do eight blood glucose measurements day after day. From what is ideal, there must be a compromise to what is practical. The minimum testing needed for reliability is four tests/day at least 2-3 times/week. A table (Table 12.1) of ideal and acceptable blood glucose values is provided to each patient or family for each time period (fastings and 1-, 2-, and 3-hr postmeal).

These are target blood glucose values we ask patients to attempt to achieve with SBGM. These targets are for older children, adolescents, and young adults and are achievable with a flexible insulin-food regimen and SBGM.

The patient or family is told to test as follows:

1. A 24-hr blood glucose profile with a fasting blood glucose and a postmeal blood glucose value sometime

TABLE 12.1 Ideal and Acceptable Blood Glucose Values for Self-Blood Glucose Monitoring

	Blood Sugars	
	Ideal	Acceptable
Fasting	70-100 mg/dl	70-120 mg/dl
Before meals	70-105 mg/dl	70-130 mg/dl
After meals (1 hr)	90-160 mg/dl	90-180 mg/dl
After meals (2 hr) and bedtime	100-120 mg/dl	100-150 mg/dl

after each meal daily during initial regulation or during illness or reregulation.

2. During pregnancy, when using an insulin pump, when ill, or when changing insulin doses to improve control, do a 24-hr blood glucose profile daily.
3. When control is good and insulin doses are stable, do a 24-hr profile 2-3 times/week with one of the sampling days being a weekday and one a weekend day.
4. Do additional blood glucose tests at times when hyper- or hypoglycemia is suspected.
5. Record all values along with the time they are performed so that values can be compared with the appropriate norms for the sampling time.

In the clinic, the blood glucose values obtained during times of illness are evaluated separately and the remainder of the values are averaged for each sampling time. Patterns of hyper- or hypoglycemia in addition to the overall averages are evaluated. Algorithms for response to individual blood glucose values during periods of poor control or illness can be found later in this chapter. Except during such periods, it is preferred to monitor blood glucose values over several days and respond to overall patterns of hyper- or hypoglycemia rather than responding to individual values. Frequently responding to every high blood glucose value can lead to overinsulinization, hypoglycemia, and rebound hyperglycemia. A postprandial or premeal blood glucose value measures the effect of the previous dose of insulin, the preceding meal, and the preceding activity. Response to an individual blood glucose value (a premeal value, for example) with extra or supplemental insulin is analogous to the old and obsolete sliding scale. An elevated premeal blood glucose value means that more insulin was needed at the *previous* dose, *not* at the present time. For example, if a person is receiving a mixture of regular and NPH insulin in the morning and has an elevated blood glucose value at noon, it is not appropriate to give an extra dose at noon except during illness. If the elevated noon value is persistent, it means more regular insulin was needed in the morning (or less food) rather than giving a noon supplement. Giving a noon supplement of insulin may cause hypoglycemia in the afternoon when the supplement overlaps with the peak of the morning NPH. A rebound hyperglycemia then could occur which might lead the unwary to give further insulin supplements (for example, at supper), creating a rebound rollercoaster of hypo- and hyperglycemia. The establishment of patterns by observing a few days of monitoring and then an appropriate adjustment of the insulin and food preceding the consistent hyper- or hypoglycemia will avoid this pitfall. Sometimes supplements of extra insulin are necessary as, for example, with illness or when control is very poor. Supplements will bring the blood glucose level closer to normal so that basal insulin requirements can be better determined. These supplements should be recorded as such and then added to the total insulin dosage as a part of the basic insulin schedule.

It is important to remember that blood glucose values in persons with DMI will have frequent fluctuations related to inappropriate matching of peaks and valleys of food, insulin, and activity. If the patient is adequately insulinized, these elevations of blood glucose will be rapidly self-corrected and need no response other than observation and correction of patterns with better monitoring and alteration of food and activity. The glycosylated hemoglobin test is a good measure to use with SBGM. If fluctuations in blood glucose are of such short duration as to exert no effect on glycosylated hemoglobin, they need not be corrected. Indeed, attempts at correcting these temporary glucose fluctuations may lead to overcorrection and hypoglycemia. If glycosylated hemoglobin values are elevated, then the elevated blood glucose values must be lowered and the fluctuations suppressed. Adjustments then must be made in insulin dosage and distribution. Remember that even with frequent SBGM the blood glucose sampling is very intermittent and does not measure the entire 24-hr period. Overresponse to individual values is to be discouraged. Response to overall patterns of hyper- or hypoglycemia are more appropriate.

GLYCOSYLATED HEMOGLOBIN

Glycosylated hemoglobin (usually referred to as HbA_1 or HbA_1C) is a test of longer term glucose control which takes advantage of the principle of glycosylation of proteins detailed in Chapter 10. Since the hemoglobin pool is in constant turnover with a life span of about 120 days for each red blood cell, the measurement of the percentage of total hemoglobin which is glycosylated at any point in time is a marker of the average daily blood glucose in which the cells are floating. HbA_1C, then, measures the mean daily blood glucose value of the past several (6-12) weeks. The advantage to the test is that: 1) it averages out the daily fluctuations in blood glucose, 2) it is independent of the blood glucose values at the time it is measured; 3) it can be measured anytime; and 4) it measures what has already happened and therefore cannot be altered acutely by the patient. HbA_1C becomes an excellent test of diabetes control over an extended period of time (11).

HbA_1C is an excellent test, but the values can vary considerably from laboratory to laboratory or even within a given laboratory. Present methodology has not been completely standardized so values between laboratories cannot usually be compared. For example, one laboratory may measure total HbA_1, which encompasses HbA_1A, HbA_1B, and HbA_1C. The norms will therefore be different than for HbA_1C alone. It is also important to know if the laboratory dialyzes the sample since, in an undialyzed sample, the early reversable Schiff's base compound (the aldimine) may be present. This compound varies with the blood glucose value, so that value must be known to interpret the results. Preferably, the laboratory should dialyze the specimen to remove the aldimine or unstable portion and leave only the ketamine which is stable and is a more reliable marker of glucose control. Finally, the test is quite temperature sensitive so that temperatures must be kept constant before values are stable and interpretable (12).

The normal values for an individual laboratory must be known before the interpretation of the degree of diabetes control can be assessed. In our Wichita laboratory, values have changed from an upper limit cut-off point of 8% in 1979 to 8.5% in 1981 (HbA_1) to 6.2% (HbA_1C) in 1983. At our Kansas City laboratory (KUMC), the upper limit of normal is 9.0% (HbA_1). Values must be compared within an individual program or laboratory over time and not be compared between labs or programs.

Table 12.2 defines the criteria of control in the KUMC program. In the Wichita program with an HbA_1 upper limit of normal of 8.5%, the criteria of Table 12.3 define control.

We have just begun to use the new HbA_1C values with an upper limit of 6.2% and are now attempting to redefine control criteria based upon these norms. Our current thinking (subject to future revision with more experience) is shown in Table 12.4.

TABLE 12.2 Hemoglobin A_1 Values — KUMC

Normal Values	6.0-9.0%
Diabetes	
Excellent control	< 9.0%
Good control	9.0-10.0%
Fair control	10.0-11.0%
Fair-to-poor control	11.0-12.0%
Poor control	> 12%

TABLE 12.3 Hemoglobin A_1 Values

Normal Values	5.5-8.5%
Diabetes	
Excellent control	< 8.5%
Good control	8.6-9.5%
Fair control	9.6-10.5%
Fair-to-poor control	10.6-12%
Poor control	> 12%

TABLE 12.4 Hemoglobin A_1C Values

Normal Values	3.2-6.2%
Diabetes	
Excellent control	< 6.2%
Good control	6.3-7.5%
Fair control	7.6-9.0%
Fair-to-poor control	9.1-10.5%
Poor control	> 10.5%

Anyone falling into the group with fair-to-poor control should have an intensive reevaluation of their program to see if the problem is 1) underinsulinization, 2) overinsulinization, 3) improper insulin distribution, 4) lack of compliance or pseudononcompliance, 5) psychosocial problems, or 6) miscellaneous problems (lack of insulin absorption, insulin resistance, etc.). Frequent SBGM should help to define the cause of the poor control and lead to appropriate measures such as reeducation; adjustment of amount and distribution of insulin, food, and activity; or help with psychosocial problems.

The use of SBGM and HbA_1C together provides the optimum parameters of monitoring for control. SBGM will determine the cause of the elevated HbA_1C and lead to adjustments for its correction. The HbA_1C, in turn, will determine whether fluctuations of blood glucose detected by SBGM are significant in overall control and whether steps should be taken for correction. SBGM is a very useful tool for diabetes control but should always be interpreted in light of HbA_1C since SBGM measures only momentary control, which is subject to so many momentary variables. HbA_1C smooths out these momentary variables and provides a better measure of overall control. Since HbA_1C is also a marker of total body glycosylation, it is therefore a better marker of developing vascular disease and neuropathy than are the momentary fluctuations of blood glucose. Both tests (HbA_1C and SBGM) are important and when used together are extremely useful tools to monitor physiologic metabolic control in diabetes mellitus type I.

INTENSIVE INSULIN THERAPY

Single-dose insulin therapy is outmoded and has been almost totally abandoned by diabetologists. Diabetes regimens today are based on the principle of physiologic insulin replacement, i.e., insulin replacement in such a way as to provide 24-hr basal insulin and a bolus after feeding. There are many ways to achieve physiologic insulin replacement. Conventional insulin therapy with the split-mix regimen has been explained in Chapter 6. We begin therapy with a conventional split-mix program and continue that regimen as long as control (as measured by blood or urine monitoring at home and HbA_1C in the office) remains satisfactory.

If control begins to deteriorate on conventional split-mix insulin therapy and psychosocial problems or noncompliance are not the cause, we then move to intensive insulin therapy using a variety of regimens tailored to fit the needs and problems of each individual. These programs and the indications for each will be described.

Introduction

There are certain times when it is helpful or necessary to alter the insulin dosage. These times are: 1) during illness; 2) during the beginning and end of the remission, or honeymoon period; 3) during periods of rapid growth, especially adolescence; 4) a few days prior to and during the menstrual period; and 5) during temporary increases or decreases in activity (i.e., a week-long ski trip, rainy weather, a weekend float trip, basketball or cheerleading camp, etc.).

Adjustment of Insulin Dosage

There may be other times when it is necessary to temporarily adjust the insulin dosage. The following section will explain when to increase and decrease insulin dosages and by how much.

This section will deal with the adjustment of insulin according to different insulin schedules. These schedules include:

1. *Two daily injections* of NPH mixed with regular insulin taken 30 min before breakfast and 30 min before

supper, approximately 12 hr apart (see Figure 12.1 and Chapter 6).

2. *Three daily injections,* the morning injection being a mixture of NPH and regular insulin taken 30 min before breakfast, with an injection of regular insulin taken 30 min before supper. The third injection is NPH insulin taken at bedtime (see Figure 12.2).
3. *Three daily injections,* the morning injections being regular insulin taken 30 min before breakfast, regular insulin 30 min before lunch, and a mixture of regular and NPH insulin taken 30 min before supper (see Figure 12.3).
4. *Three daily injections,* the morning injection being a mixture of regular and Ultralente insulin taken 30 min before breakfast. The noon injection is regular insulin only, taken 30 min before lunch. The third injection is a mixture of Ultralente and regular insulin taken 30 min before supper (see Figure 12.4).
5. *Four daily injections* consisting of regular insulin 30 min prior to each meal and one injection of NPH at bedtime (see Figure 12.5).
6. *Four daily injections* consisting of four doses of regular insulin given 30 min before each meal and at 1:00 a.m. (see Figure 12.6).

Definitions of Types of Insulin Changes

Basal Insulin Requirement

Once good control has been achieved, it should be possible to maintain by keeping food intake, energy expenditure, and insulin dosage relatively constant from day to day. This assumes the absence of illness or unusual psychological stress. The insulin dosage required to maintain blood glucose control is called the basal insulin requirement. The basal insulin requirement may vary during specific times of the week (e.g., with increased or decreased weekend activities), month (e.g., with ovulation and the menstrual period), or year (e.g., from summer to winter). It may also change as food intake and/or activity patterns change or with growth but is relatively constant.

Adjustment

In response to unexpected fluctuations in control it may be necessary to alter the basal insulin requirement. This alteration (increase or decrease) is called an adjustment. When making an adjustment, the normal dose is altered but no extra shots are given. The adjustment is made during good health when the patient is free from unusual stress and following a stable food and activity pattern.

Supplement

Unlike the adjustment, which is an altered amount of insulin that will remain altered for an extended period of time, the insulin supplement is used during times of illness, increased stress, or unstable food and/or activity patterns. The supplement may be an increase of the normally given dosage, or an extra shot given to decrease an abnormally high blood glucose. After the temporary situation has passed (e.g., illness, menses, etc.), the individual should resume taking the basal or normal insulin dosage. The supplement is, by definition, a temporary insulin dosage. There are two types of supplements as listed below.

Anticipatory Supplement

This is given in anticipation of a large meal (e.g., birthday or dinner party) or a time of decreased activity. It is given *before* the blood glucose rises to maintain a *normal* blood glucose. The patient should know when to anticipate a rising blood glucose due to menstrual periods or inactivity by watching for patterns in the previous blood glucose records.

Compensatory Supplement

This is given to decrease blood glucose found to be excessively high for unanticipated reasons or due to illness. It is given to decrease the blood glucose. Sometimes compensatory supplements may become frequent or permanent, in which case they should be added to the basal insulin as an adjustment.

Schedule 1

In response to unexpected fluctuations in control, it may be necessary to alter the basal insulin requirement. This alteration (increase or decrease) is carried out by changing the total daily dose in stepwise increments of 2 U in the a.m. and 1 U in the p.m.

In this schedule the morning regular insulin covers breakfast and has its major action about 3 hr after injection, causing the need for a morning snack. The morning NPH covers lunch and las its major action about 8 hr after injection, causing the need for an afternoon snack. The evening regular will cover the food ingested at supper, and the evening NPH will maintain a normal blood glucose level throughout the night. The evening regular and NPH will overlap, causing the need for a bedtime snack. Use of this program called split-mix or conventional insulin therapy is described in Chapter 6 and is the regimen used in most patients. The morning and evening mixtures are usually two-thirds NPH and one-third regular, and about two-thirds of the total daily insulin is given before

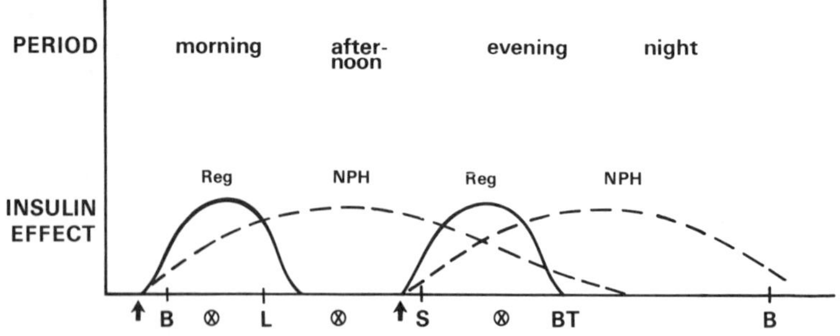

FIGURE 12.1 This shows the insulin effect of a two/daily injection schedule using NPH and regular. Symbols used above are: B = breakfast; L = lunch; S = supper; BT = bedtime; arrow = time of insulin injection 30 min before meal; * = meal plate; 0 = snack plate; REG = regular, short-acting insulin effect; and NPH = intermediate-acting insulin effect.

breakfast and one-third before supper. Alteration of this regimen is best carried out by modifying the food intake prior to the times of hyper- or hypoglycemia. Patterns of blood glucose changes are determined by the 24-hr profile with SBGM and changes are made in dietary intake to correct the problems found in the profile. Some authors (7) prefer to modify insulin dosages even with this regimen. A method of doing so is described in Table 12.5.

Schedule 2 (Figure 12.2)

In this schedule, the morning shot works as explained in Figure 12.1. Regular insulin is given to cover the food ingested for supper, and NPH is given to keep the blood glucose normal throughout the night. In some people NPH given with regular before supper will cause a low blood glucose in the early morning (2:00–3:00) with a high blood glucose upon awakening around 6:00 a.m. or later. This is called the "dawn phenomenon" (13, 14). This phenomenon is probably due to a declining or waning blood insulin level in the early morning hours as the presupper insulin dissipates and the serum cortisol and/or growth hormone rises. This early morning rise in

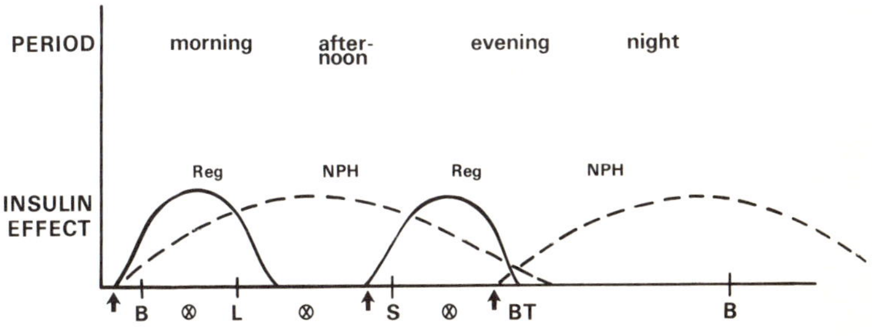

FIGURE 12.2 This shows the insulin effect of a 3/daily injection schedule using NPH with regular 30 min before breakfast, regular 30 min before supper, and NPH at bedtime.

Table 12.5 Two Daily Injections — Split-Mix Therapy

Assumptions

The morning short-acting regular insulin has major action between breakfast and lunch, and its effect is reflected in the blood glucose test results after breakfast and before lunch.

The morning intermediate-acting NPH insulin has major action between lunch and supper, and its effect is reflected in the blood glucose test results after lunch and before supper.

The evening short-acting regular insulin has major action between supper and bedtime, and its effect is reflected in the blood glucose test results after supper and at bedtime.

The evening or bedtime intermediate-acting NPH insulin has major action overnight, and its effect is reflected in the blood glucose test results on arising the next morning.

Hyperglycemia not explained by unusual diet/exercise/insulin.

If fasting blood glucose on arising is greater than 120 mg/dl for 2 days in a row, increase the evening NPH insulin by 1-2 U readings.* If using a premixed insulin (Mixtard or regular and NPH mixed), increase the evening mixture 1-2 U readings.*

If blood glucose 2 hr after breakfast is greater than 150 mg/dl OR if blood glucose before lunch is greater than 130 mg/dl for 2 days in a row, increase the morning regular insulin by 1-2 U readings.*

If blood glucose readings 2 hr after breakfast are greater than 150 mg/dl but less than 70 mg/dl before lunch, a change in amount or timing of the morning snack may be needed or more NPH insulin in the evening dose may be required.

If blood glucose 2 hr after lunch is greater than 150 mg/dl OR if blood glucose before supper is greater than 130 mg/dl for 2 days in a row, increase the morning NPH insulin by 1-2 U readings.* If using a premixed insulin (Mixtard or NPH and regular mixed), increase the morning mixture by 1-2 U readings.*

If blood glucose 2 hr after supper or at bedtime is greater than 150 mg/dl for 2 days in a row, increase the evening regular insulin by 1-2 U readings.* If using a premixed insulin (Mixtard or regular and NPH mixed), increase the evening mixture 1-2 U readings.*

If blood glucose readings 2 hr after lunch or supper are consistently greater than 150 mg/dl and values presupper or prebedtime are consistently below 70 mg/dl, a change in timing or amount of the meal or snack may be needed or supplemental regular insulin with lunch may be needed; a rebound phenomena may also be present.

Supplements

In addition, if blood glucose on arising OR before lunch or supper is greater than 130 mg/dl, take an extra 1-2 U readings* of regular insulin as a supplement at that time. If blood glucose on arising OR before supper is greater than 200 mg/dl, take an extra 2-4 U readings* of regular insulin as a supplement at that time. Have the patient *record the supplement separately so that they do not accidentally change the basal dose of regular insulin.*

Hypoglycemia not explained by unusual diet/exercise/insulin.

Prevent insulin reactions by eating meals and snacks on time.

If fasting blood glucose on arising is less than 60 mg/dl OR if there is evidence of hypoglycemic reactions occurring overnight, reduce the evening NPH insulin by 1-2 U readings.* If using a premixed insulin (Mixtard or regular and NPH mixed), decrease the evening mixture 1-2 U readings.*

If blood glucose after breakfast OR before lunch is less than 60 mg/dl OR if there are hypoglycemic reactions between breakfast and lunch, reduce the morning regular insulin by 1-2 U readings.*

If blood glucose after lunch OR before supper is less than 60 mg/dl OR if there are hypoglycemic reactions between lunch and supper, reduce the morning NPH insulin by 1-2 U readings.* If using a premixed insulin (Mixtard or regular and NPH mixed), decrease the morning mixture by 1-2 U readings.*

If blood glucose after supper OR at bedtime is less than 60 mg/dl OR if there are hypoglycemic reactions between supper and bedtime, reduce the evening regular insulin by 1-2 U readings.*

---

*The term unit readings rather than units is used throughout these tables to designate the numbers on a U100 syringe. If insulin is diluted to U50 or U25, as is often needed in small

Table 12.5 Two Daily Injections — Split-Mix Therapy (Cont'd)

children on low doses of insulin, then the syringe readings are the same but the change in actual insulin dosage will be different as follows: 1) using U50 insulin, the change would be one-half that of U100 or 0.5 U/1 U change; 2) using U25 insulin, the change would be one-fourth that of U100 or 0.25 U/1 U change.

blood glucose levels may carry over to the postbreakfast period causing postbreakfast hyperglycemia — a frequently recognized phenomenon. This regimen may help to correct not only an elevated fasting blood glucose level but also the postbreakfast hyperglycemia. The same snacks are required with this schedule as for Schedule 1 as are modifications and supplements. To alter this schedule use Table 12.5.

Schedule 3 (Figure 12.3)

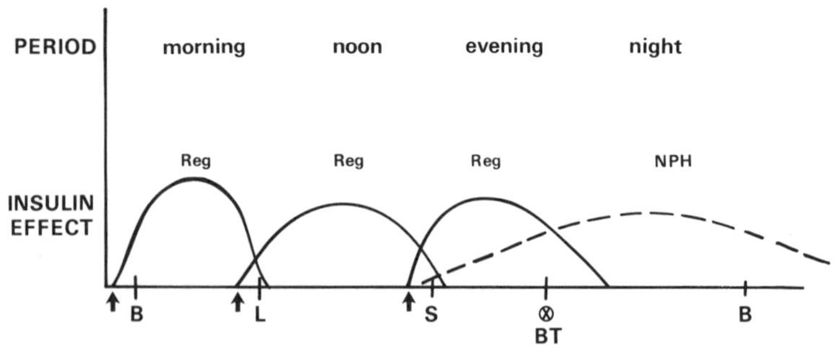

Figure 12.3 This shows the effect of a 3/daily injection schedule using regular before breakfast and lunch and a mixture of NPH and regular before supper.

This schedule is used when evening and fasting blood glucose values are controlled with a mixture in the evening, but control with a mixture is less than optimal during the day. With this schedule about one-third of the total daily insulin is given in the evening as a 2:1 NPH:regular mixture. The remaining two-thirds of the daily requirement is divided between the prebreakfast and prelunch doses according to the postprandial or premeal blood glucose levels. Usually the larger dose is needed before breakfast and the smaller dose before lunch. This schedule is usually used with three meals and a bedtime snack.

Schedule 4 (Figure 12.4)

In this schedule, the regular insulin covers food ingested at breakfast, lunch, and supper. The Ultralente insulin provides the basal need for insulin. Using this schedule no snacks are needed. Mealtime may be varied somewhat by giving the

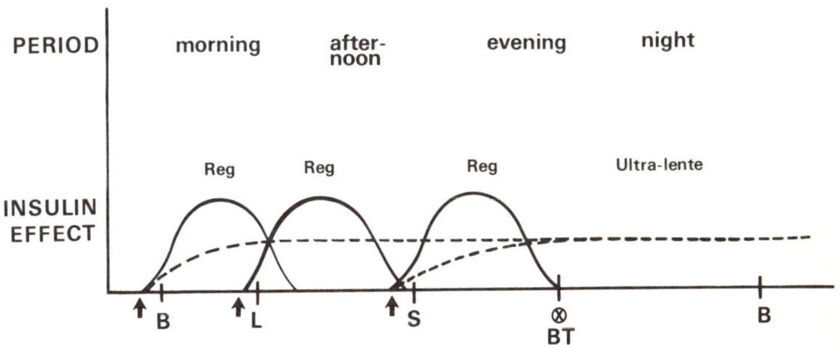

Figure 12.4 This shows the insulin effect of a 3/daily shot schedule using Ultralente mixed with regular 30 min before breakfast and supper, and regular alone 30 min before lunch.

corresponding shot 30 min before the meal. By increasing or decreasing the amount of regular given before a meal, the caloric intake may be increased or decreased. To alter this schedule, see Table 12.7. The Ultralente can be given as one dose in the morning optimally can be divided into two equal injections given with the morning and supper regular.

It is important to remember that when using the Ultralente regimen that the Ultralente should constitute about 40–50% of the total daily insulin. Also, because of the depot effect of Ultralente, some of the insulin remains in the pool to provide an equilibrium. Thus, the total insulin dose may need to go up by 20–30% over the dosage on other schedules. To alter this schedule, use Table 12.6.

Schedule 5 (Figure 12.5)

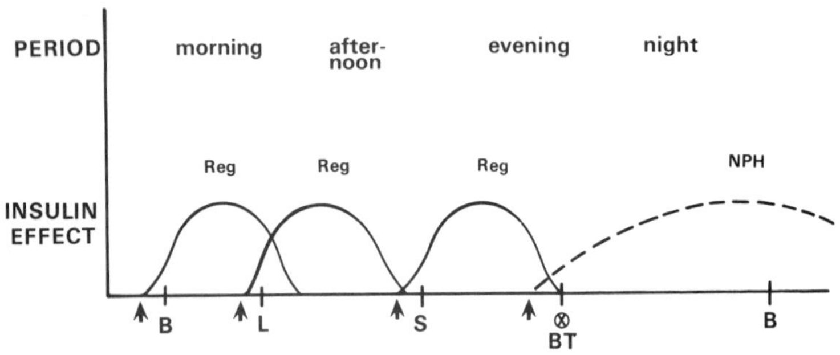

Figure 12.5 This shows the effect of a 4/daily shot schedule using regular 30 min before each meal and NPH at bedtime. To alter this schedule, see Table 12.5.

Table 12.6 Ultralente and Regular Insulin Schedule

Assumptions

The Ultralente insulin provides the background basal requirement of insulin and its effect is primarily reflected in the fasting blood glucose.

The morning regular insulin has major action between breakfast and lunch, and its effect is reflected in the blood glucose test results after breakfast and before lunch.

The prelunch regular insulin has major action between lunch and supper, and its effect is reflected in the blood glucose test results after lunch and before supper.

The presupper regular insulin has major action between supper and bedtime, and its effect is reflected in the blood glucose test results after supper and at bedtime.

Hyperglycemia not explained by unusual diet/exercise/insulin.

If fasting blood glucose on arising is greater than 120 mg/dl for 2 days in a row, increase the evening Ultralente insulin by 1-2 U readings.

If blood glucose 2 hr after breakfast is greater than 150 mg/dl OR if blood glucose before lunch is greater than 130 mg/dl for 2 days in a row, increase the morning regular insulin by 1-2 U readings.

If blood glucose 2 hr after lunch is greater than 150 mg/dl OR if blood glucose before supper is greater than 130 mg/dl for 2 days in a row, increase the prelunch regular insulin by 1-2 U readings.

If blood glucose 2 hr after supper or at bedtime is greater than 150 mg/dl, increase the presupper regular insulin by 1-2 U readings.

Hypoglycemia not explained by unusual diet/exercise/insulin.

Prevent insulin reactions by eating meals on time.

If fasting blood glucose on arising is less than 60 mg/dl OR if there is evidence of hypoglycemic reactions occurring overnight, reduce the evening Ultralente insulin by 1-2 U readings.

If blood glucose after breakfast OR before lunch is less than 60 mg/dl OR there are hypoglycemic reactions between breakfast and lunch, reduce the morning regular insulin by 1-2 U readings.

Table 12.6 Ultralente and Regular Insulin Schedule (Cont'd)

If blood glucose after lunch OR before supper is less than 60 mg/dl OR if there are hypoglycemic reactions between lunch and supper, reduce the prelunch regular insulin by 1-2 U readings.

If blood glucose after supper OR at bedtime is less than 60 mg/dl OR if there are hypoglycemic reactions between supper and bedtime, reduce the presupper regular insulin by 1-2 U readings.

If blood glucose values after each meal are greater than 150 mg/dl but values before the next meal are less than 70 mg/dl, an alteration in timing of the meal or injection or size or timing of the snack may be needed.

Supplements

In addition, if blood glucose on arising OR before lunch or supper is greater than 130 mg/dl give an extra 1-2 U readings of regular insulin as a supplement at that time. If blood glucose on arising OR before lunch or supper is greater than 200 mg/dl, give an extra 2-4 U readings of regular insulin as a supplement at that time. Record the supplement separately so that there is not an accidental change in the basal dose of regular insulin.

This schedule is useful during pregnancy or periods of chronic stress and has proved useful in some adolescents, in particular, adolescent girls with unstable diabetes on other regimens. This schedule is quite versatile in that each dosage can be modified both as to the time and amount in relation to changes in meal time and food intake, especially the latter. If the patient is diligent with SBGM and learns to match insulin changes to changes in food intake and activity, a very high degree of metabolic control can be achieved with this schedule. In addition, the schedule is flexible and allows adaptation to varying life-styles. We have found this schedule to be one of the most physiologic and flexible of all the available schedules and find it increasingly useful. To alter this schedule, use Table 12.5 with the following additions: 1) there is no morning NPH; 2) the lunch short-acting regular insulin has its major action between lunch and supper and its effect is reflected in the blood glucose measurements after lunch and before supper.

Schedule 6 (Figure 12.6)

Three meals are given at the usual time. The dosages are as follows: 35% of the total daily insulin before breakfast, 22% before lunch, 28% before supper, and 15% at 1:00 a.m. as described in Chapter 6. These percentages of total daily insulin were developed by modifying the respective doses in diabetic children as needed to restore normal diurinal blood glucose levels as defined in nondiabetic children on a similar activity and meal plan (Figure 12.7).

This insulin schedule is used during initial regulation of a newly diagnosed diabetic child, for reregulation of diabetes when control is less than optimal, during and after surgery, and during illness such as an infection. With this schedule, the percentages before each meal and at 1:00 a.m. are maintained as the total daily dose is modified each day until 24-hr euglycemia is established. Once stability of the blood glucose level and the insulin dosage is achieved, the total daily requirement is calculated by adding up the four doses. This

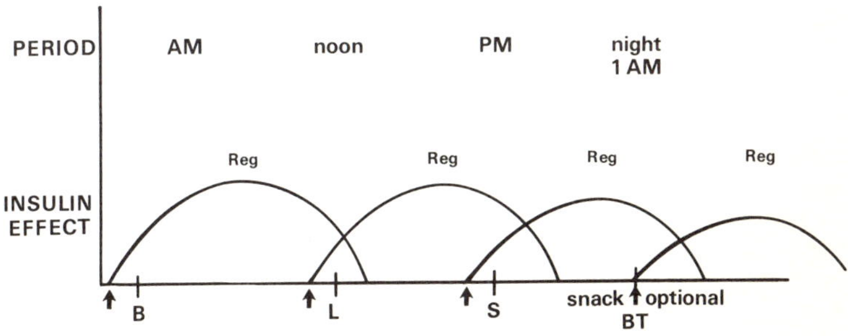

Figure 12.6 With this schedule, regular insulin is given before each meal and at 1:00 a.m. A snack at that time is optional.

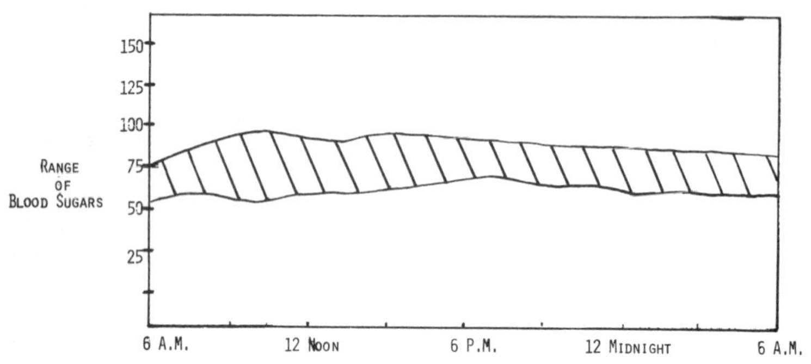

Figure 12.7

number is then used to calculate a two- or three-dose schedule for continuing care. Example: If an individual required 18 U in the morning, 11 U at noon, 14 U before supper, and 8 U at 1:00 a.m., the total requirement would be 51 U/day. If the desire was to convert to a split-mix schedule, then the daily dose would be converted as follows: 34 U morning (two-thirds of the total) as a 2:1 NPH:regular mix (or approximately 22 U of NPH and 11 U of regular) and 17 U evening (one-third of total) also as a 2:1 mix (or about 12 U NPH and 6 U of regular). Fractions of units are rounded off in these calculations. Premixing the regular and NPH avoids the fractional problems. The split-mix regimen can then be modified as per Table 12.6 or the food intake can be adjusted as in Chapter 6 to fine tune the control. With this type of program, we have been able to reregulate most persons with DMI in about 5 days. The four-dose schedule has also proven very useful for reregulation and for illness.

Illness

Table 12.7 contains algorithms for adjusting insulin with illness. Such schedules are given to the patient to use as needed

Table 12.7 Figuring Insulin Supplements for Illness

The insulin supplement is based upon body weight, blood glucose, and insulin concentration, (U100, U50, U25, U10). If you weigh 40 kg (88 lb) or more add 1-2 U readings per 30-50 mg/dl. If you weigh less than 40 kg (88 lb) add 0.5-1.0 U readings per 30-50 mg/dl unless your insulin concentration is less than U100 (e.g., U50, U25, U10).

FOR THE PERSON WEIGHING 40 KG (88 LB) OR MORE OR WEIGHING LESS THAN 40 KG (88 LB) BUT TAKING A LESS CONCENTRATED INSULIN (U50, U25, ETC.)

For blood glucose 150-200 mg/dl before meals or at bedtime, add 1-2 U readings of regular insulin.

For blood glucose 200-250 mg/dl before meals or at bedtime, add 2-3 U readings of regular insulin. If the patient is spilling ketones, add 3-4 U readings of regular insulin.

For blood glucose of 250-300 mg/dl, add 3-5 U readings of regular insulin every 4-6 hr. If the patient is spilling ketones, add 5-6 U readings of regular insulin every 4-6 hr.

For blood glucose of 300-350 mg/dl, add 5-7 U readings of regular insulin every 4-6 hr. If the patient is spilling ketones, add 7-8 U readings of regular insulin every 4-6 hr.

For blood glucose of 350-400 mg/dl, add 7-9 U readings of regular insulin every 4-6 hr. If the patient is spilling ketones, add 9-10 U readings of regular insulin every 4-6 hr.

After taking two or three supplements, the doctor or nurse should be informed that the patient is having problems. If the patient is unable to keep food down or are vomiting, call the doctor or nurse immediately.

The patient is told that when ill, be sure to drink plenty of fluids; more than is thought necessary.

As stated earlier, if the blood glucose is higher than the appropriate range and it is time to give one of the regularly scheduled shots, just add the correct number of insulin units to the shot. Be sure, however, to add these units in *regular* insulin, not the insulin *mixture*.

e.g., 25 U readings mixture -- normal shot
+ 5 U readings regular -- supplement
30 U readings total -- Mixed in the syringe

Table 12.7 Figuring Insulin Supplements for Illness (Cont'd)

FOR THE PERSON WEIGHING LESS THAN 40 KG (88 LB) WHO TAKES U100 INSULIN

For blood glucose 150–200 mg/dl before meals or at bedtime, add 0.5–1 U readings of regular insulin.

For blood glucose 200–250 mg/dl before meals or at bedtime, add 1–1.5 U readings of regular insulin.

For blood glucose of 250–300 mg/dl, add 1.5/2 U readings of regular insulin every 4–6 hr.

For blood glucose of 300–350 mg/dl, add 2–4 U readings of regular insulin every 4–6 hr.

For blood glucose of 350–400 mg/dl, add 4–5 U readings of regular insulin every 4–6 hr.

Check urines for ketones at the time of each blood glucose measurement. If urine ketones are large and blood glucose is 300 or more, double the amount of insulin to be taken.

Patients are told that after taking two or three supplements, they are to contact the doctor or nurse to let them know the patient is having problems. If the patient is unable to keep food down or is vomiting, the doctor or nurse is to be called immediately.

When ill, patients are to be sure to drink plenty of fluids; more than they think they need.

As stated earlier, if the blood glucose is higher than the appropriate range and it is time to give one of the regularly scheduled shots, just add the correct number of insulin units to the shot. Be sure, however, to add these units in *regular* insulin, not the insulin *mixture*.

e.g., 25 U readings mixture — Normal shot
+ 5 U readings regular — Supplement
30 U readings total — Mixed in your syringe

prior to calling the physician. Note that Table 12.7 also contains a table of the desirable blood glucose values which we hope to achieve by the appropriate use of the above insulin schedules and the adjustment of insulin for illness as contained in Table 12.7.

The following Table (Table 12.8) is a set of instructions

Table 12.8 The Following Instructions Are Given For Vomiting and Diarrhea*

WHAT SHOULD I DO WHEN I HAVE AN UPSET STOMACH OR DIARRHEA?

If you are vomiting and/or having diarrhea, you cannot retain or absorb all the food you eat. This is almost the only time that the insulin dosage needs to be decreased. If you are vomiting or have an upset stomach, take small quantities (1-2 oz) of a carbonated beverage such as ginger ale every 5-10 min. Alternate with 1-2 oz of fruit juice as soon as you are retaining foods. Popsicles, hard peppermint candy, or after-dinner mints may be used with small sips of water if you are unable to retain fluids. If you are vomiting and have diarrhea and the blood glucose test is 180 mg/dl or less, give about two-thirds of the usual dose of insulin.

Example: Usual morning insulin dose = 9 U readings regular + 18 U readings NPH (or 27 U readings 2:1 NPH:regular)

2/3 of 9 U readings = 6 U readings regular
2/3 of 18 U readings = 12 U readings NPH or
18 U readings 2:1 NPH:regular

If vomiting or diarrhea persists and the blood glucose test is 180 mg/dl or less, you will need to also decrease the evening dose to two-thirds of the usual evening dose.

Example: Usual evening insulin dose = 5 U readings regular + 9 U readings NPH (or 14 U readings 2:1 NPH:regular)

2/3 of 5 U readings = approximately 3 U readings regular
2/3 of 9 U readings = 6 U readings NPH or
9 U readings 2:1 NPH:regular

When the vomiting or diarrhea subsides, you should add solid foods gradually. Saltines or dry toast with honey or jelly may be given in small amounts. With stomach upset, sherbet is sometimes more palatable than ice cream. You may also use Jello (not diet Jello) as you will need simple sugars at this time.

Table 12.8 The Following Instructions Are Given For Vomiting and Diarrhea* (Cont'd)

If the blood glucose tests are greater than 180 mg/dl do not decrease the insulin dose, even though you are nauseated, vomiting, or having diarrhea. In this situation follow instructions for increasing insulin as outlined in the illness instructions in the home blood glucose monitoring section.*

*These tables were developed in the Department of Pediatrics, KUMC by Dr. Wayne Moore and Rachael Jorgensen, R.N., B.S.N., and are used with permission.

given to patients as instruction for illness. A version of Table 12.7 in patient language is also given for complete instruction for self management with illness and instruction as to when to call the medical team.

Guidelines for Adjustment to Correct Hyperglycemia

Before making an adjustment (longer lasting change) in the insulin dose due to high or low blood glucose, be sure the abnormal blood glucose is *not* due to illness, alterations in food or activity, or unusual stress.

Injection Timing

If the injection is taken immediately before the meal instead of 30 min prior to the meal, this will cause an increase in the blood glucose level, the reason being that the food is absorbed before the insulin has time to work, so the blood glucose rises in the absence of insulin. As a result of this, the high level of sugar in the blood may be filtered out through the kidneys and the calories from the food will be lost in the urine. In this instance, the patient may actually be taking enough insulin, but because it is not appropriately timed with food intake, there is a temporary blood glucose elevation. If the insulin is adjusted upward but still given immediately before the meal, the patient will probably begin to experience insulin reactions (hypoglycemia) prior to the next meal or snack and may still have hyperglycemia (high blood sugar) shortly after meals.

Correct the Early Morning Before Breakfast Blood Glucose

When adjusting the insulin dose, *correct only one blood glucose at a time, starting with the blood glucose done before breakfast.* After it is normalized, work with the lunch, supper, and bedtime blood glucose in sequence.

Number of Units for Adjustment

If the patient weighs 40 kg (88 lb) or more, adjust the dose 1 U for every 30–50 mg/dl the blood glucose is above the acceptable range (see Tables 5–7). For example, if the blood glucose done before supper is 160 mg/dl, the patient needs 1 extra U of insulin. Do not make an adjustment larger than 4 U per shot at one time. If the patient weighs less than 40 kg (88 lb), adjustments in the dosage should not be greater than 1 U per shot at one time, unless the patient is using an insulin concentration less than U100 (e.g., U50, U25, U10, etc.) that has been diluted as instructed. If the patient injects U50, U25, or U10 insulin, then the dose should be adjusted 1 U reading for every 30–50 mg/dl over the higher blood glucose in the acceptable range.

Rebound Hyperglycemia

Do not increase the basal insulin dose in response to hyperglycemia that may occur due to a rebound after a hypoglycemia reaction. This is most frequently seen in the fasting blood glucose. Rebound hyperglycemia may be suspected if the patient has a blood glucose greater than 120 and less than 250 mg/dl but has ketones in the urine. Bad dreams, nighttime sweating, fast heart rate (or pulse), and also morning "grumpiness" may be clues to rebound hypoglycemia. When nighttime hypoglycemia is suspected, do a blood glucose during the night. This could be done over several nights, at different times each night. For example, night one: 3:00 a.m.; night two: 2:00 a.m.; night three: 4:00 a.m. If any of these tests are 60 mg/dl or less, decrease the overnight insulin component.

Morning hyperglycemia may also be due to a *lack* of insulin coverage overnight; however, it is safer to assume the opposite. If the hyperglycemia is due to inadequate insulin coverage, the fasting blood glucose will rise even higher when the insulin dose is decreased (as previously explained). If this occurs, *increase* the next overnight insulin dose. High blood glucose values during the nighttime testing sequence also indicate inadequate nighttime insulin coverage.

Guidelines for Adjustments to Correct Hypoglycemia (Low Blood Glucose)

Whenever patients have symptoms of hypoglycemia (e.g., shaky, cold sweat, weak, dizzy, headache) have them check the blood glucose to determine if it is less than 60-70 mg/dl. This will accomplish two goals: 1) it will help them associate how they feel when the blood glucose is low; and 2) it will prevent them from eating something that will cause the blood glucose to go above the desired range, in the event that they are really *not* hypoglycemic.

If the blood glucose is 60-70 mg/dl or less, or if the patient cannot do a blood glucose test for some reason, treat the reaction with about 10 g of quick-acting (simple) sugar. This would be 2-3 Dextrosol tablets, sugar cubes, or some other small quantity of sweet food. If the next meal or snack is more than 1 hr away, follow the simple sugar with about two points or two exchanges of a complex carbohydrate food (e.g., bread, crackers, cereal) and/or a protein food (e.g., eggs, cheese, meat, peanut butter). If the hypoglycemic reactions cannot be explained by a change in food portions, food schedule, or activity, adjust the corresponding insulin dose downward (refer to tables).

Supplementing the Insulin Dose

Supplements of insulin may be given *to lower* an abnormally high blood glucose or to prevent the rise of the blood glucose due to an anticipated event (e.g., inactivity or a large meal). Supplemental insulin will always consist of regular insulin only. When the patient needs to supplement at a time when they normally take an insulin injection, just add the extra regular to the normal insulin mixture *in the syringe*. When giving the supplement be sure to use the same concentration of insulin (U100, U50, U25) used for the usual insulin dosage. Have the patients record the supplement of insulin separately from the usual insulin dose so they will not accidently take that amount later on and overdose themselves.

Two Types of Supplements

Anticipatory Supplements

This supplement is given in anticipation of an event that may cause blood glucose to rise (e.g., a large meal). The amount needed to supplement can be calculated initially by taking 5% of the total 24-hr insulin dose. This is then added to the normal dose. For example, in anticipation of a dinner party to supplement the p.m. dose of insulin:

The total 24-hr insulin dose is: Breakfast = 16 U NPH + 8 U regular = 24 U
Lunch = 00
Dinner = 8 U NPH + 4 U regular = 12 U

Total daily dose: 24 U + 12 U = 36 U/day

The *Supplement* is: 36 U x 5% or 36 U x 0.05 = 1.8 U (round up to 2 U)

So, the evening dose is:
12 U NPH & regular mix
+2 U regular *only* (determined in step 2)
= 14 U for dinner dose (NOT same as mix)

Another way to estimate the amount of supplement needed is to increase the dose 1 U of regular for every calorie point (75 calories) the patient plans to ingest in addition to the usual meal plan. As previously stated, this is the starting point for anticipatory supplementation. The patient and the medical team will have to discern the amount actually needed by trial and error through careful monitoring of blood glucose and careful recordkeeping.

Compensatory Supplements

As stated earlier, this type of supplement is given to decrease a blood glucose that has risen due to some *unanticipated* event (e.g., illness). If the patient weighs 40 kg (88 lb) or more, supplement 1-2 U of insulin for every 30-50 mg/dl the blood glucose reading is *greater* than the *upper* number of the appropriate blood glucose range (see Table 12.1). For people weighing less than 40 kg (88 lb) give 0.5-1.0 U of supplement per excess 30-50 mg/dl blood glucose. For further explanation see Table 12.7.

For example: The blood glucose reading before supper is 280 mg/dl. The upper number of the premeal blood glucose range is 130 mg/dl.

$$\begin{array}{r} 280 \text{ mg/dl} \\ -130 \text{ mg/dl} \\ \hline = 150 \text{ mg/dl} \end{array}$$

So, supplement 1 U of regular insulin for every 30-50 mg/dl the blood glucose is too high.

$$\begin{array}{r} = 3 \text{ U regular} \\ 50 \;\overline{)\,150 \text{ mg/dl}} \end{array}$$

Add an extra 3 U of regular insulin to the dosage normally taken before supper.

Blood Sugar Monitoring and Insulin Changes for Increases in Exercise

When the patient undertakes exercise that is greater than the usual daily activity, compensate with extra food consumption. Approximately 10-15 g of carbohydrate should be eaten for every 30-45 min of activity. See Table 12.9 for examples of foods in specific amounts that equal 10-15 g of carbohydrate. The blood glucose should be monitored before, during, and after exercise to determine how effective this food intake plan worked for the activities. The patient also may need to decrease the insulin dose before undertaking increased activity. Hypoglycemia may occur well after the patient stopped exercise (e.g., 12 hr *after* daytime jogging), so extra snacks may need to be taken before bedtime, especially

Table 12.9 Foods Equivalent to 10–15 g of Glucose*

Assumptions:

10 g carbohydrate = 40 calories (= 1/2 calorie point).
10 g carbohydrate will raise the blood glucose approximately 30–50 dl.
Liquid is absorbed more quickly. but is more difficult to carry with you.

Foods Equivalent to 10–15 g Carbohydrate

1 fruit exchange	5 small sugar lumps
4 oz orange juice	2 tsp. syrup
4 oz 7-Up	2 tsp. honey
4 oz Coke	6 Lifesavers
3 oz apple juice	7 jelly beans
2 oz grape juice	1 T. jelly
2 packets of sugar (2½ tsp.)	3 Dextrosol
2 large sugar lumps	2 B-D Glucose Tablets
3–4 lemon drops	2 butterscotch hard candies

*This table was developed by Rachael Jorgensen, R.N., B.S.N., KUMC, and is used with permission.

for afternoon activity such as football or basketball practice or similar heavy activities.

Guidelines for Adjusting Insulin for Individuals Who Take Only One Type of Insulin

Insulin adjustments for type I insulin-dependent diabetic individuals who take only one- or two-daily injections of an intermediate-acting insulin (NPH or Lente) are not described in this book; the authors of this book do not support this practice because research has demonstrated that a normal glycosylated hemoglobin (A_1C) cannot usually be attained in a type I diabetic individual who takes a single type of insulin one or two times daily. One exception to this rule is the individual who is newly diagnosed and still in the remission period. A similar exception occurs in some type II diabetic individuals who take insulin. These persons may be successfully controlled on just one two shots of NPH or Lente insulin in combination with meal planning and regular activity. One type of insulin may be all that is necessary because the individual still produces some endogenous insulin. Even in these individuals, however, the authors recommend small doses of insulin two times per day as a standard split-mix regimen in order to deliver the insulin in as physiologic a manner as possible.

Table 12.9 provides some information that has proved useful in treating hypoglycemia. Often this problem is overtreated with resulting hyperglycemia which must then be corrected later. To help calculate the amount of food needed to treat mild to moderate hypoglycemia use Table 12.9. This table is a useful guide to both the patient and the health care team to guide proper therapy for hypoglycemia.

For severe hypoglycemia (convulsions or unconsciousness), glucagon is recommended as the initial therapy by the parents while awaiting the arrival of the emergency team. Glucagon should be given when oral intake is not possible. The dosage is 0.5 mg for children under the age of 3 years and 1 mg for persons over age 3 years. The glucagon can be given intramuscularly. subcutaneously, or intravenously. It requires about 20 min for recovery after glucagon is administered, and posttreatment nausea is common. When the medical team is available (hospital, emergency room, ambulance medics, etc.) IV glucose is the preferred treatment for severe hypoglycemia. Ten to 20 cc of 50% glucose IV is usually sufficient to treat most hypoglycemia. Nausea and headache usually follow recovery.

After a severe hypoglycemic reaction, many patients may have a postictal state with some drowsiness and/or neurologic deficit (asphasia, paralysis, etc.). These deficits are temporary and usually subside in less than 24 hr, although they can persist for 36–48 hr. Supportive treatment to the patient and reassurance to the parents of eventual recovery is all that is usually needed. Adjustments in the diabetes program should be made after recovery to ensure that there is no recurrence of the problem.

Summary

All patients in our program begin with a conventional two-shot split-mix insulin schedule with three meals and three snacks. As long as control as measured by SBGM and HbA_1C

is maintained, their regimen is continued. When control cannot be maintained by conventional split-mix therapy, the patient is reregulated on an intensive insulin therapy schedule of three or four doses of insulin/day using schedules 2-6 to tailor the insulin schedule to the life-style of the patient. There is no preconceived notion of which regimen or schedule is best, but rather we attempt to fit the appropriate schedule to the needs of a given individual and stand ready to modify the schedules as needed if a person's needs or life-style changes.

For the small percent (about 5%) of patients who cannot achieve the desirable degree of metabolic control on one of the described schedules but who are compliant and perform regular SBGM, an insulin pump is the next step in the achievement of control.

Utilizing these schedules and/or an insulin infusion pump, it is possible in most individuals to attain and maintain physiologic control of diabetes mellitus and do so within a flexible life-style which is livable and acceptable to patients and their families.

MECHANICAL DEVICES

For many years investigators have dreamed of an implantable, mechanical insulin delivery device controlled by a glucose sensor and self-regulating computer. Such a device is called a closed-loop artificial beta cell. A closed-loop device has been developed and is now commercially available. Such a device is called a Biostator Glucose Controller-Monitor. The device is not implantable and must be a hospital-based device. The limiting factor in developing an implantable closed-loop device has not been miniaturization but has been the development of an implantable sensor which is stable for long periods of time. Chemical sensors lose sensitivity as the chemical is used up. Metallic sensors are walled off by fibrous tissue which is relatively avascular and does not reflect the true blood glucose level. Frequent replacement obviates their use, so the search for a sensor continues (see Chapter 13).

Biostator

The Biostator is a mechanical closed-loop artificial pancreas which can be used either as a continuous glucose monitor or as a controller to maintain normoglycemia by infusing insulin and/or glucose. Two models of the machine are available. A large research model of the Biostator which has two separately controlled pumps and a programmable computer sells for about $65,000. A smaller clinical model of the Biostator Glucose Controller-Monitor has only one pump and a less versatile computer; this model sells for about $38,000. The research model has greater flexibility in the research setting and can be used clinically. The clinical model can be used in a research setting but has greater applicability in a clinical setting.

The Biostator system requires placement of two IV catheters in separate extremities. One catheter must be an 18 gauge; the other may be of a smaller gauge. Approximately 2 ml of nonrecirculated blood is withdrawn from the patient every hour. Cannulae size and the amount of nonrecirculated blood that is withdrawn limit machine use to patients with appropriate body mass and blood volume. However, experience has shown that a 6-year-old child may use the Biostator without complications. A continuous flow of the patient's whole blood is passed across a membrane-bound enzymatic glucose sensor. A special double-lumen catheter dilutes and anticoagulates the blood as it leaves the patient. The blood glucose level is displayed continuously while six values per minute are averaged, with the average printed on a permanent record. A preprogrammed computer calculates a dose of dextrose and/or insulin according to the blood glucose level. This dosage is then administered intravenously to the patient via a peristaltic pump system, and is recorded each minute on the Biostator print-out. Use of the system has been reported in further detail in current literature (15-17).

The Biostator can be utilized for a number of purposes. The most practical use is that of reregulating the diabetic having poor blood glucose control. Biostator use can normalize the blood glucose of the diabetic experiencing ketoacidosis without the concern of causing a too-rapid drop in the blood glucose. It also provides a continuous feedback of the current blood glucose level for physician reference. A new insulin regimen can be computed for diabetic reregulation using the 24-hr, minute-by-minute Biostator print-out. The computed insulin regimen may be delivered by one of several multiple injection schedules or by continuous subcutaneous insulin infusion (CSII), better known as an insulin infusion pump. There are rules and protocols for determining the appropriate insulin need for individual diabetic patients; however, use of the Biostator provides a more rapid and scientific method. Using the Biostator as an adjunct, reregulation may take as little as 24-48 hr.

Another use for the Biostator occurs during surgery on the diabetic patient. Blood glucose regulation is often precarious at this time, and even the type II, nonketotic-prone diabetic may develop poor blood glucose control and ketosis prior to, during, or after surgery (18). The pregnant diabetic can greatly benefit from blood glucose control provided by the Biostator. Insulin requirements fluctuate at the initiation of labor and drop drastically during labor and delivery. Immediately after delivery exogenous insulin requirements return to the prepregnancy level (19). These fluctuations in insulin requirements require constant, vigilant supervision of the blood glucose level that can be provided easily by the Biostator. Jovanovic and Peterson (19) support the belief that normoglycemia is absolutely essential immediately prior to and continuously throughout the pregnancy to provide appropriate fetal growth, maturation, and prevention of neonatal hypoglycemia in the immediate postnatal period. In spite of normoglycemia throughout pregnancy, they document that hyperglycemia during labor and delivery definitely can increase the risk of postnatal fetal hypoglycemia. Use of the Biostator during labor and delivery totally eradicates this potential problem.

Biostator cost is approximately $40.00/hr of use, which is covered by Medicare and most insurance companies. Although machine use appears costly, it may decrease the hospital stay by several days, thus decreasing the overall hospitalization expense. In the stance of the pregnant diabetic undergoing Biostator glucose control during labor and delivery, hospitalization will probably be decreased for both mother and infant. Use of the Biostator can reduce hospitalization stay for diabetic regulation from 1-2 weeks to 1-2 days. This further decreases patient expense by preventing extended income loss from missed work days. The Biostator has been noted by these authors as being highly flexible, practical, and utilitarian.

Portable Insulin Infusion Pumps

While awaiting the dream of a closed-loop implantable infusion device, we have had to compromise to a portable, external, open-loop infusion system usually referred to as an insulin infusion pump. The device usually worn on the belt attaches to the patient by means of a small plastic tube tipped with a small needle which fits under the skin. The system is called CSII.

There are now many infusion devices on the market (Table 12.10) at a variety of prices and new devices are becoming available every few months. Some of the devices are more versatile than others, with a variety of programming and safety features.

Whatever the variations, all pumps have certain features in common. All consist of some type of reservoir for insulin (in most, it is a small syringe) and a pumping device (usually a syringe driver). There is usually a microprocessor which will control the syringe driver, infusing a very small bolus of insulin every few seconds for a more or less continuous infusion of insulin called basal. The microprocessor can also be programmed or the device controlled mechanically to infuse a large bolus of insulin at meal times to meet the postprandial needs. Some devices can be preprogrammed to change basal infusion rates or premeal boluses or give supplemental doses at various times. Some devices are very simple, giving only one fixed basal rate and a manual bolus. Other devices are very sophisticated with multiple basal rates, preprogrammed boluses, and supplemental features. The cost of the device is predicated by the features it contains. We have found the smaller, more expensive devices the most useful for children because of the small size and the preprogramming features. The latter are helpful in children in that the parents can preprogram the basal and bolus rates for the time the child is away from home and at school.

CSII is a valuable tool to facilitate physiologic control in a limited group of persons with unstable DMI. Since CSII administers insulin in a way which simulates normal physiology (i.e., a continuous basal infusion and a bolus with meals) it should have great benefit. Indeed, it does. There are, however, limitations to CSII therapy. There have been some 40

Table 12.10 Available Infusion Devices

NAME (Manufacturer)	SIZE (Ht x W x D = in)	WEIGHT (oz)	ALARM SYSTEM	POWER SOURCE	COST	COMMENTS
AS6C (Autosyringe, Inc. Flint Labs)	6.2 x 3.3 x 1.0	9.5	Yes (low battery, occlusion of tubing -- needle, runaway)	9 Volt NiCd Rechargeable (24 hr)	$1295	Insulin dilution required. Simple, one basal rate
AS6C-U100 (Autosyringe, Inc. Flint Labs)	6.2 x 3.3 x 1.0	9.5	Yes (low battery, occlusion of tubing -- needle, runaway)	9 Volt NiCd Rechargeable (24 hr)	$1295	Simple, one basal rate.
AS6MP (Autosyringe, Inc. Flint Labs)	6.3 x 3.4 x 1.1	10.1	Yes (low battery, occlusion of tubing -- needle, motor fault, microprocessor malfunction programming error)	9 Volt NiCd Rechargeable (24 hr)	$1795	Up to five programmable basal rates in a 24-hr period. Twenty-four hour clock used for programming basal rates
Beta I* (Orange Medical Instruments)	3.25 x 4.75 x 1.0	7	Yes (not programmed, low battery, motor fault, obstruction of tubing -- needle, empty syringe, pump malfunction)	9 Volt NiCd Rechargeable (24 hr)	$1500	Patient must initiate basal rate changes manually -- cannot be preprogrammed. Small.
CPI 9100 (Cardiac Pacemaker's, Inc.	3.25 x 5.5 x 1.3	13	Yes (Illegal entry, low battery, motor fault, microcomputer fault, occlusion of tubing -- needle, empty syringe)	CPI manufactured	$1500	Programmable basal rate and supplemental dose feature.

Table 12.10

NAME (Manufacturer)	SIZE (Ht x W x D = in)	WEIGHT (oz)	ALARM SYSTEM	POWER SOURCE	COST	COMMENTS
CPI 9200 Betatron II (Cardiac Pacemaker's Inc.)	3.9 x 2.6 x .9	5.8	Yes (unacceptable entry, low battery, motor fault, obstruction of needle -- tubing, empty empty reservoir, microcomputer fault, internal memory fault, dose limit, delay until hold)	CPI manufactured batteries and charger (24 hr) 3 Volt (6 months)	$2500	Two programmable basal rates allowing increase or decrease in insulin rate. Numerous alarms to enhance safety including dose limit and delay until hold. Delay until hold causes pump to go into hold if individual does not change program within a certain time (1-16 hr).
CPI 9205 Betatron I (Cardiac Pacemaker's Inc.	3.9 x 2.6 x .9	5.8	Yes (unacceptable entry, low battery, motor fault, obstruction of needle -- tubing, microcomputer fault, internal memory fault, delay until hold)	3 Volt (6 months) and CPI manufactured charger and batteries batteries (24 hr)	$2300	One programmable basal rate, simple, small, numerous safety feature. Delay until hold feature is set at 12 hr.
Medix 209-100 (Medix Corp)	4.25 x 2.56 x .87	5.3	Yes (low battery, motor fault, occlusion of tubing -- needle, empty syringe)	9 Volt NiCd Battery (1-3 weeks)	$995	Small, simple, one basal rate which is adjustable in increments of 2 units.

Minimed* (Pacesetter Systems, Inc.)	1.9 x 3.1 x .7	3.1	Yes (low battery, and depleted battery, motor fault microcomputer fault, occlusion of tubing -- needle, empty syringe, over delivery	3 Standard 1.5 V silver oxide watch cells (21 days)	$2600	Up to four programmable basal rates, operates on 24-hr clock.

*To be released in the near future.

deaths reported in persons on CSII, though most of these deaths were unrelated to the pumps. A few of the deaths, however, occurred in young persons and were sudden and unexpected. These deaths may have been due to complications related to the pumps and add a note of caution to their use.

There are many real and potential problems related to CSII, such as skin abscesses, DKA, and hypoglycemia. Skin abscesses are common and potentially quite dangerous (one death due to septicemia and subacute bacterial endocarditis secondary to a skin abscess has been reported). Scrupulous attention to skin hygiene is required to prevent this problem. When abscesses develop, rapid response with incision and drainage and antibiotics is needed. DKA is also a problem. Since there is no depot insulin with CSII, the patient can develop hyperglycemia, ketosis, or even DKA much more rapidly than persons taking injectable insulin. Any slight malfunction (such as pump failure; dead pump batteries; tubing breakage, leakage, or blockage; needle displacement; etc.) can result in DKA very quickly. (Hyperglycemia develops within minutes of insulin interruption, ketosis in 1-2 hr, and DKA in 3-6 hr.) Meticulous attention to detail and frequent blood glucose measurements are required to prevent these problems.

Hypoglycemia is a special problem with CSII therapy since the fall in blood glucose levels is often slow. The slow fall in glucose levels may not trigger the release of counterregulatory hormones, thus allowing the blood glucose level to fall to neuropenic levels. When neuropenic blood glucose levels are reached the patient may not be able to take action. Unless help is available there is danger of convulsions or death. The more vulnerable time for such problems is during the night when no food is available. Children are especially vulnerable to brain damage from nocturnal hypoglycemia and must be protected. Hypoglycemia with a pump is best prevented by frequent blood glucose measurements. Such monitoring should include some blood glucose measurements during the night until stability at a normal glucose level is reached. If nocturnal hypoglycemia is found during the monitoring, the nighttime basal should be decreased until the nighttime glucose levels are normal or even slightly above normal to ensure that no hypoglycemia develops throughout the night. A midnight and 3:00 a.m. as well as fasting blood glucose value in the morning are the preferred values to obtain to exclude nocturnal hypoglycemia.

Candidates must be carefully screened. The primary use for pumps in children is in persons whose diabetes is very unstable (i.e., metabolic instability). Children whose instability is due to psychosocial problems are not good candidates for pumps. We screen every candidate with a thorough psychosocial evaluation utilizing all members of the health care team. If the diabetes cannot be well controlled with multiple-dose insulin therapy in children from psychosocially stable families, we will initiate CSII. Insulin pumps do inhibit activity somewhat, so they are not indicated for children who are very active, particularly in athletic boys. Of our 96 persons currently on pumps, five are under 13 years and seven are adolescent. Only one of these is a boy. This number represents 2% of our total patient population in this age group. Thus, while very beneficial in some patients (indeed the pumps have been lifesaving in some), at our present state of technology their use in children is limited. Furthermore, the pumps should be initiated and managed only by experts in the field who can provide a team of people for support. The team must be able to provide a 24-hr hot line for patient consultation and support since problems develop quickly and usually not during the working day.

We Anticipate improved technology in the future (see Chapter 13) which should increase the usefulness of insulin infusion pumps in children. For the present their usefulness is limited to a few select children under the care of a few experts in the field.

SUMMARY

The future holds the promise of a prevention or a cure for DMI (see Chapter 13). For the present, it is possible to slow or prevent and possibly reverse the long-term complications of the disease by attaining and maintaining nearly physiologic control of the metabolic parameters. Such control is possible with the tools presently available to us for insulin administration and feedback (monitoring of blood glucose levels). Though present techniques of control are not yet perfect or even as yet completely physiologic, we can now approximate normal metabolism and do so without harm to the child, assisting the child and the family to a productive and useful life.

REFERENCES

1. Reeves, M., Forhan, S. E., Skyler, J. S., and Peterson, C. M.: Comparison of methods for blood glucose monitoring. *Diabetes Care* 4:404, 1981.

2. Skyler, J. S., O'Sullivan, M. J. et al: Blood glucose control during pregnancy. *Diabetes Care* 3:69, 1980.

3. Ohlsen, P., Panowski, T. S. et al: Discrepancies between glycosuria and home estimates of blood glucose in insulin-treated diabetes mellitus. *Diabetes Care* 3:178, 1980.

4. Peterson, C. M., Jones, R. L., Dupuis, A., Berstein, R. O., and O'Shea, M.: Feasibility of improved control of patients with juvenile onset diabetes mellitus through exercise and patient monitored glucose determinations. *Diabetes Care* 2:329, 1979.

5. Guthrie, R. A., Guthrie, D. W., Tatpati, O. A., Hinnen, D., and Childs, L.: Unpublished data, Kansas Regional Diabetes Center, 1984.

6. Symposium of home blood glucose monitoring. *Diabetes Care* 3:57-186, 1980.

7. Skyler, J. S., Skyler, D. L., Seigler, D. E., and O'Sullivan, M. J.: Algorithms for adjustment of insulin dosage by patients who monitor blood glucose. *Diabets Care* 4: 311, 1981.

8. Shapiro, B., Savage, P. J. et al: A comparison of accuracy and estimated cost of methods for home blood glucose monitoring. *Diabetes Care* 4:396, 1981.

9. Sonksen, P. H., Judd, S. L., Gole, E. A. M., and Tattersall, R.: Home monitoring of blood glucose: Methods for improving diabetic control. *Lancet* 1:729, 1978.

10. Hinnen, D., Conley, K., and Childs, L.: Assessment of accuracy of 11 glucose machines for home use. *Diabetes* 33(Suppl. 1):131A, 1984.

11. Blanc, M. H., Barnett, D. M., et al: Hemoglobin A_1c compared with three conventional measures of diabetes control. *Diabetes Care* 4:349, 1981.

12. Goldstein, D. E., Parker, K. M., England, J. E. et al: Clinical application of glycosylated hemoglobin measurements. *Diabetes* 31(Suppl. 3):70, 1982.

13. Schmidt, M. I. et al: The dawn phenomenon, an early morning glucose rise: Implications for diabetic introday blood glucose variation. *Diabetic Care* 4:574, 1981.

14. O'Schmidt, M. I. et al: A fasting hyperglycemia and associated free insulin and cortisol changes in "somogyilike" patients. *Diabetes Care* 2:457, 1979.

15. Clark, W. L., Thomas, L., and Santiago, J. V.: Clinical evaluations and preliminary studies on the use of an artificial pancreatic beta cell in juvenile diabetes mellitus. *J. Ped.* 91:590, 1977.

16. Clemens, A. H., Chang, P. H., and Myers, R. W.: The development of Biostator, a glucose-controlled insulin infusion system (GCIIS). *Horm. Metab. Res.* 7(Suppl.): 23, 1976.

17. Pieffer, E. F., Thum, C., and Clemens, A. H.: The artificial beta cell: A continuous control of blood sugar by external regulation of insulin infusion (glucose-controlled insulin infusion system). *Horm. Metab. Res.* 487:339, 1974.

18. George, K., Alberti, M. M., Gill, G. V., and Elliott, M. J.: Insulin delivery during surgery in the diabetic patient. *Diabetes Care* 5(Suppl.):65-77, 1982.

19. Jovanovic L., and Peterson, C. M.: Optimal insulin delivery for the pregnant diabetic patient. *Diabetes Care* 5(Suppl.):65-77, 1982.

Chapter 13

RESEARCH – HOPE FOR THE FUTURE

Richard A. Guthrie, M.D.

Research in diabetes mellitus has followed a tortuous course. After its initial description many centuries ago, little was done to understand it or to treat it. Major changes began in the nineteenth century with the description of the islets of Langerhans and the discovery that the islets contained a hormone, named insulin even before its discovery, that was responsible for the disease. Nothing more of importance occurred until that fateful summer of 1921 when insulin was isolated by Banting and Best. Insulin was then thought to be the answer, and diabetes research began to languish. Insulin was not the answer, however, and problems began to surface in later years. In those years between 1921 and the 1960s, very little money was available for research in diabetes and very few developments occurred. Some of the notable achievements were the crystallization of insulin and its subsequent purification and concentration; the production of longer-acting insulins with the introduction of PZI, globin, NPH, and the Lente series; the introduction of oral hypoglycemic agents for type II diabetes; the better understanding of nutrition and growth in children with diabetes; recognition of the interrelationship of retinopathy to the metabolic control of diabetes in children and the need for multiple dose insulin therapy; and the development of the radioimmunoassay for diabetes. Some negative developments of this era were the marketing of the intermediate-acting insulin as a once-a-day drug, and the data suggesting that vascular disease was genetic and was not related to control of blood glucose.

Two factors which stimulated a renewal of research in diabetes was the recognition of the vascular and neurologic problems associated with diabetes (insulin was not a cure, since those children saved from certain death by insulin went on to develop the complications little known in 1921) and the development of the assay for insulin. The latter development has allowed the detailed study of insulin secretion and insulin levels and has resulted in the classification of diabetes into the various types. We can now define diabetes not as a disease but as a syndrome of altered metabolism characterized by inappropriate hyperglycemia and vascular and neurologic complications.

Research began to accelerate in the 1960s, but funding was still limited for diabetes. In 1972, a movement began to increase the funding for diabetes research. This was a grass-roots movement sponsored by the volunteer health organizations involved in diabetes, and resulted in the creation by Congress of the National Diabetes Commission by the National Diabetes Act of 1974. Through the work of the Commission [now the National Diabetes Advisory Board (NDAB)], funding for diabetes research has increased significantly. The result has been an upsurge of new interest in diabetes and major changes in management techniques. The last 5 years have been exciting times in diabetes research, and the view on the horizon is even more exciting. Medical personnel caring for the young person with diabetes should be conversant with the new developments in order to convey a feeling of hope, not despair, to these young people and their parents. The pace of biomedical research aimed at a prevention, a cure, and improved medical management is accelerating and will continue to accelerate more rapidly in the near future. This is perhaps the most exciting era to be involved in diabetes since that fateful summer of 1921. Important findings lie just over the horizon. A prevention and a cure now, for the first time in many years, seems possible.

A cure and prevention of diabetes remain elusive. Although they remain the only ultimately acceptable solutions to the diabetes problem, and we are more optimistic for a cure in the foreseeable future than at any time since 1921. In the meantime, treatment must be carried out, and the search for better methods of treatment (including health care delivery and education) must also continue. Although some treatment programs seem to achieve better results than others, the people involved in the health care of individuals with diabetes must be innovative and willing to submit all ideas, treatments, delivery systems, and educational approaches to careful clinical investigation to validate their effectiveness and establish their possible effect on complications.

The current status of biomedical and clinical research is discussed in this chapter, as are the major controversies in the field, to introduce some of the questions that remain to be answered. We are aware that this chapter may well be obsolete by the time of publication, and we sincerely hope that the pace of the accumulation of new knowledge is such that the research developments presented here have been surpassed. However, we include this chapter as the latest available knowledge, which the health care team should know and impart to the children and families of children with diabetes mellitus.

As pediatricians, we especially hope that increased knowledge will lead to the prevention to overt IDDM by interruption of the pathogenic sequence, and that application of improved methods of maintaining metabolic control will prevent or delay the development of the serious vascular complications.

RADIOIMMUNOASSAY

With the development of the radioimmunoassay in the early 1960s by Berson and Yalow (1), it became possible for the first time to measure circulating insulin levels directly. (Dr. Yalow received the Nobel prize for the discovery in 1977.) This led to a whole new understanding of insulin secretion and action, and made possible many additional findings. Using the electron microscope, radioimmunoassay, and radioactive labeling techniques, Lacy (2) and Milner and Hales (3) have added greatly to our understanding of the synthetic steps in insulin production. More recently, Orci and others (4), using freeze etching and the scanning electron microscope, have greatly enhanced our knowledge of insulin release. The studies of Steiner and associates (5), and Chance and others (6), have supplemented the work of Lacy and Orci with development of the biochemical concepts of synthesis. These authors developed the concept of proinsulin, a precursor of insulin, and the need for degradation of proinsulin before secretion. A spin-off of their research has been the development of an assay for the connecting peptide, or C peptide, the fragment broken off from proinsulin, to make the finished insulin molecule. Proinsulin and C peptide can now be made biosynthetically by recombinant DNA technology, and they are now being tested for various therapeutic uses.

The assay for C peptide now makes possible the study of beta-cell function in the individual receiving insulin. C peptide is secreted in a molar relationship to insulin. The levels of C peptide in the blood then give a measure of the insulin-secreting ability of the beta cell in an individual in whom insulin cannot be measured directly because of interfering antibodies or because the assay cannot distinguish between endogenous and exogenous insulin. As a result of this development, we have learned that after initial treatment, the beta cell may temporarily recover some insulin-secreting ability. The declining insulin requirements and stability of the so-called honeymoon period (often seen in children with type I diabetes soon after treatment) are accompanied by rising C-peptide levels. This indicates recovery of endogenous insulin secretion. The obvious implication of this remarkable finding is that we should be attempting to design therapeutic regimen to preserve and protect beta-cell function. Recent studies indicate that early, vigorous treatment of the person with newly diagnosed diabetes may preserve beta-cell functions, as measured by C peptide, for a much longer period of time than conventional therapy.

GENETICS

The cause of diabetes remains unknown. New research, however, is leading us to the concept that there may be many causes of diabetes. Indeed, diabetes is a syndrome, not a disease. Diabetes is not one disease but the common pathway for many diseases that ultimately cause beta-cell failure.

Diabetes has always been thought of as a genetic or inherited disease, although the mode of inheritance has not been characterized. This is largely true because a genetic marker for the disease in nondiabetic relatives of diabetic persons has not been found. Data are now beginning to emerge to indicate that diabetes is an inherited disease, but that there are many modes of inheritance. These modes of inheritance vary in different families; moreover, the different environmental factors that determine (at least partially) the manifestations of the inheritance may vary for the different inheritance patterns.

Evidence for a genetic predisposition for IDDM comes from studies that show that the concordance rate for diabetes is higher in monzygotic twins than in dyzygotic twins. The genetic predisposition is probably conferred by genes which reside on the short arm of the number six chromosome, closely associated with the HLA (human leukocyte antigen) gene system (7). The HLA system (also known as the major histocompatibility complex), originally described as important in organ transplants, is assuming more and more importance in the understanding of the control of the immune system. Several autoimmune diseases have now been described which have associated HLA genes. When certain genes are present (and/or certain other genes are absent), then abnormalities in the control of the T- and B-lymphocyte systems occur. Study of the relationship of the genes of the sixth chromosome that are involved in immunity and autoimmunity are just beginning, and some of the findings are very interesting not only to those interested in diabetes, but to those interested in other immune-related diseases.

Racial differences also occur, leading researchers to suggest that multiple genes may be able to confer the immune defect. The exact locus of the "diabetogenic" gene os not known, but its position can be approximated by the association of other locus and the occurrence of clinical IDDM. In Caucasian children, the DR3 and DR4 genes are associated with the development of IDDM. Recent studies in Japan indicate that the DR4 gene is present in Japanese children, but not the DR3 gene. In these children, the DR9 and perhaps that DW52 and 35 genes substitute for the DR3 gene seen in Caucasian children (8). By contrast, recent studies in China indicate that Chinese children with IDDM have the DR3 gene, but not the DR4 or DR9 (9). Within families, there is clearly linkage between IDDM and the HLA system, regardless of what HLA alleles are manifest in any given family. And as shown previously, across populations, there is clearly an association between IDDM and certain HLA alleles, although the alleles involved may vary in different groups. This suggests that more than one gene may confer the defect. In Caucasian children with the heterozygotic state of HLA DR3/DR4, there is the highest degree of susceptibility.

Ultimately, the IDDM-HLA association will be refined to the DNA level with the goal of identification and characterization of the specific diabetic genes. Recent studies using DNA restriction enzymes and radiolabeled cDNA probes have been used to probe for the DR gene (10,11). These studies show that the DR4 gene is polymorphic, and only some subtypes of that gene are associated with a susceptibility to IDDM (10). Much remains to be learned about the subtypes and linkages of these genes, but progress has been rapid and should eventually result in the identification of specific diabetogenic genes and their gene products. This should lead to tissue typing on cord blood at birth and the identification of the susceptibles for intervention therapy.

ENVIRONMENTAL FACTORS IN THE ETIOLOGY OF IDDM

Genetic predisposition is necessary for the development of IDDM. Environmental factors or triggers are, however, also necessary for the development of the disease. Evidence for this belief are the studies of identical twins. Although identical twins have a higher con cordance rate for IDDM than nonidentical twins, the concordance rate is only about 50%. If the disease was entirely genetic, the concordance rate would be nearly 100%. What is inherited then is disease susceptibility. An environmental trigger is needed to bring about the disease in the susceptible individual. Since the protective mechanism for environmental insults is in the immune system, and since the inherited defect is in the immune system, this observation is consistent. The inherited defect is a vulnerability to certain pancreatotoxic viruses, or chemical toxins and/or immune over- or underreaction to these insults with resultant beta cell damage. The damage may be from underreaction of the immune system with direct insult to the pancreas or may be an overreaction with a chronic autoimmune destruction of the beta cells. The final result is the same beta-cell destruction and insulinopenia.

VIRUSES

Evidence is accumulating that a number of viruses can infect and damage beta cells in experimental animals (12). Review of these studies is included in Chapter 3. With some viruses and some animal species, genetic factors control susceptibility and species specificity. The role of these viruses in humans remains problematic. Of most importance, perhaps, is the observation that certain forms of virus-induced diabetes in animals can be prevented by immunosuppression. This observation illustrates the role of altered immunity in mediating the viral effects and offers promise for the future in the developing of immune intervention therapy in the prevention of IDDM.

Limited clinical observations suggest (13) that breast-feeding might alter the immunological response of genetically susceptible infants and protect them from the diabetogenic effect of certain viruses. If this observation were to prove to be true, breast-feeding could be a simple, pleasurable, and beneficial way to prevent or delay the onset of IDDM.

CHEMICAL TOXINS

A variety of chemical toxins have been shown to have the potential of inducing beta-cell damage. Researchers have long used various drugs, including an antibiotic (streptozocin) to cause beta-cell damage and induce diabetes in animals. Recently, other toxins have been identified which can cause beta-cell damage; among these are the nitrosurea compounds (12). These compounds are ubiquitous in our environment and represent only one class of chemical compounds which may have the potential of leading to IDDM.

The identification of environmental triggers such as viruses and chemical toxins should, in theory, permit the development of vaccines, use of interferon therapy, use of other antiviral drugs and the development of antidotes to chemical toxins. Perhaps, more practically, the knowledge of toxins could lead to their removal from the environment. The problem with this theory is that the large array of potential viruses and chemicals with a potential diabetogenesis may preclude the development of specific counteracting measures. Indeed, it may be that the insults to the beta cells are not one-time events susceptible to specific treatment, but rather are cumulative insults (both viral and chemical) which may progressively lead to beta-cell destruction to the susceptible individual. Such environmental exposure may be quite remote in time (even in utero) from the time of development of the IDDM. If this is the case, environmental manipulation may be less effective that we had hoped. Nonetheless, research in this area goes on and offers promise for the eventual prevention of IDDM.

AUTOIMMUNITY

The immune system is vitally important since it determines the host response to most of the environmental factors. Exposure to environmental factors initiates an immune reaction which, if all works right, results in elimination of the triggering antigen. When there are defects in the immune system, as seems to be the case in diabetes, exposure to the trigger results not in elimination of the antigen, but rather the triggering of an immune reaction directed at certain cells of the body such as the beta cells of the pancrease. According to this theory, "autoimmune" destruction of the beta cells is the final common pathway leading to hypoinsulinemia, hyperglycemia, and IDDM. There may be varying degrees of beta-cell distruction by insulting agents, or autoimmunity may be the primary factor including islet-cell damage. This hypothesis remains to be proven; however, evidence is accumulating that autoimmunity mediated through both humoral (antibody) and cell-mediated (lymphocyte) abnormalities is a significant factor in the etiology of IDDM (14,15). These findings are similar to the findings in several other autoimmune diseases such as lupus erythematosus and other collagen diseases, and involves defects in antibody production and T lymphocytes.

The most recent data on this subject were presented by Dr. Jorn Nerup as part of his Banting address to the American Diabetes Association, June, 1985 in Baltimore, Maryland (16). Dr. Nerup presented an exciting new hypothesis:

In genetically susceptible individuals exposed to specific antigen (a virus particle), a series of events occur leading to beta-cell destruction. Step one is the incorporation of the antigen into a genetically activated macrophage where the antigen is "processed" and passes on to a T lymphocyte, probably a T-helper cell. This lymphocyte is also "activated" by the genetic determinent. When it receives the processed antigen, the T cell produces a variety of immune substances (lymphakines), including Interleukin I. This substance, Interleukin I, then interacts with various cells including immune cells to enhance the immune reaction. Dr. Nerup hypothesizes that B cells of the pancreas contain receptors to Interleukin I with a receptor on the B cell that damages the B cell or sets up the cell for destruction by cells of the immune system. Dr. Nerup presented new data to support the hypothesis.

If this hypothesis is true, then the Interleukin-I receptor can be blocked by chemicals or by monoclonal antibodies to the receptor, thus preventing damage to the B cell and preventing IDDM.

IMMUNE INTERVENTION

Evidence that an immune mechanism may be important in the etiology of IDDM, as well as the demonstration of prevention or reversal of the disease in animal models such as the NOD (nonobese diabetic) mouse (17,18) by immune intervention, has led to clinical trials of various immune therapies in humans. Elliot, et al. (19), Jackson, et al. (20), and Ludvigsson, et al. (21) have used glucocorticoids. Eisenbarth (22) has used antilymphocyte globulin. Leslie and Pyne (23) have used a combination of glucocorticoids - azathioprine-antilymphocyte globulin with or without plasmaphoresis. Plasmaphoresis alone has been used (21,24-25), as has inosiplex (24), monoclonal antibody T-12 (26), and cycloprine-A (27,28). Most of these studies were carried out in persons with newly diagnosed IDDM, and although the results have indicated some beta-cell preservation in some patients, the results have not been dramatic. Indeed the results of most of these studies have not exceeded the beta-cell recovery achieved with intensive insulin therapy by Jackson, as outlined in Chapter 4B.

Stiller, Dupre, and colleagues in Canada (27,28) initiated cyclosporine therapy within 6 weeks of inset of overt IDDM. They observed that a few postpubescent children so treated remained in remission without insulin replacement for over a year. No control groups of subjects maintained in excellent control were reported. These human studies are somewhat hazardous because of the toxity of cyclosporine, but are of considerable interest as they may confirm or refute the immune theory of the etiology of IDDM and possible lead to the identification of less toxic preventative agents. Dr. Nerup believes that the mechanism of action by cyclosporin in blocking the immune system is to block the Interleukin-I receptor. Better and less toxic receptor blockers may be possible in the future.

It is our belief that immune intervention has greater potential for the prevention of diabetes than does immunization and other such specific strategies, since it is less specific and can be applied to a broader group of antigenic triggers. We are optimistic that this form of therapy will, in a generation or two, lead to the total prevention of IDDM in children, and we feel that families should have this information as a part of their education and genetic counseling. The optimism should be controlled and not lead to raising false hope; nonetheless, hope in such a life-threatening process, is important and should be imparted firmly, but with caution.

Dr. Jay Skyler of the University of Miami has postulated the following: "As the pathogenic sequence is clarified, it is possible to postulate the following sequence: at birth we could routinely screen the population for diabetogenic genes or gene products; having identified individuals with the potential of developing IDDM, we could follow the children longitudinally by seeking evidence of the initiation of beta-cell damage by measuring islet cell antibodies; in such individuals, evidence of altered or diminishing beta-cell function would be sought; if identified, such individuals would become candidates for intervention therapy designed to abort the pathogenic sequence. Such an approach may become a reality in the next decade"(29).

PREVENTION OF COMPLICATIONS

Since we do not yet have a prevention, and in all probability will not have one for many years, we will continue to have to deal with the disease on a day-to-day basis. Though we hope for the future, we must deal with the reality of today. That reality is that many children with diabetes will develop the acute complications of hyper- and hypoglycemia, the intermediate complications of infections and psychologic problems, and the long-term complications of vascular disease and neuropathy. The tragedy of these complications is that they are, for the most part, preventable with proper therapy of the disease and patient education.

Practice and experience over many years and with many patients by the authors has proved the practicality and efficacy of the following approach: by the principles of good preventive pediatrics make an early diagnosis of IDDM before complete beta-cell destruction has occurred; at the first evidence of sustained hyperglycemia, hospitalize the child, and initiate insulin therapy and adequately insulinize the child using the principles and dosages found in Chapters 5 and 6. Adequately replenish lost body nutritional stores as rapidly as possible by replacing calories as needed; attain and maintain optimal glycemic control as soon as possible and continue optimal glycemic control after hospitalization by supplying insulin and calories in a physiologic way. After hospitalization, see the child often and adjust the diabetes program as often as necessary to maintain normal or near normal glycemic control as evidenced by home monitoring of urine and/or glucose and by office monitoring of glycosylated hemoglobin. Educate and reeducate the family, and the child when old enough, in the principles of diabetes and especially in the principles of self-management. Evaluate and reevaluate the program as often as necessary to support the family in their needs and to adjust the program to meet the changing needs of the growing child and the changing life style of the family and the individual with the disease. Referral to a specialist with a team of people to support the family is highly desirable. Such a program of preventive and prophylactic medicine has been successful in our hands, as evidenced by the many children we have observed into late adulthood who are free of the chronic complications of the disease. These individuals, the majority of our large patient population, live healthy and productive lives, making significant contributions to their families and to society - the ultimate goal of any therapeutic program.

IMPROVING GLUCOSE CONTROL

In keeping with the goals stated previously and the principles regarding the pathogenesis of complication, there are emerging improved strategies for attaining glucose control. The strategy outlined previously and in Chapter 12 of this book is effective in the majority of patients. Some patients need and want an alternative. All patients ultimately want a cure and to be free from the "needle." So the search for better methods of control and for a cure continue. Current research centers on four areas: new forms of insulin; mechanical insulin delivery; islet cell transplantation; and islet cell regeneration.

NEW FORMS OF INSULIN

The development of the new purified insulins and human insulin has been documented in Chapter 6. Other strategies for the delivery of insulin by modifying the insulin are being developed. A preparation of insulin conjugated with bile salts has been developed and is being tested as a nasal insufflation or as a rectal suppository. Both of these methods of insulin delivery have the defect of being unable to deliver both the 24-hour basal insulin and the meal boluses. In all probability, injectable insulin in the form of a long-acting insulin, such as Ultralent to provide basal insulin, will be needed. The nasal or rectal insulin could then be used before each meal for the meal boluses.

Another strategy for insulin delivery is the development of an oral insulin. Though there have been many attempts to do this, none have been successful. The search for a coating agent that will protect the insulin from stomach acid and intestinal digestion and still allow absorption has had only limited success. The most promising strategy for coating insulin for either oral use or implantation is the use of a plastic, or similar material, semipermeable membrane. Such membranes can be so constructed to permit the slow leakage of insulin through the membrane. Beads of encapsulated insulin can be ingested or implanted and can provide at least basal insulin. Perhaps a combination of encapsulated insulin for basal effect and insulin by nasal insufflation before meals may be a treatment of the future.

Recently, the Eli Lilly Company has developed a new technique for producing insulin by recombinant DNA technology. In this process, the bacteria make proinsulin. The connecting peptide (C peptide) can then be enzymatically split out to make regular insulin and combined with protomine to make NPH insulin. These insulins are being tested. Animal studies have shown that the proinsulin itself has biologic activity which may be similar to that of NPH insulin. If so, the step of production of NPH could be eliminated, thus reducing the cost of insulin production. If proinsulin can be substituted for NPH and Lente insulin, then the future therapy of diabetes could be treatment with a combination of regular insulin made from proinsulin and proinsulin itself both made by recombinant DNA technology.

MECHANICAL DEVICES FOR INSULIN DELIVERY

The Biostator

The idealized insulin delivery system would consist of a device containing or connected to a continuing glucose sensor which sould feed information to a microprocessor programmed to control a pumping device connected to an insulin-containing reservoir. Ideally, such a device would also contain a reservoir for a counterregulatory hormone or glucose and should be sufficiently miniaturized to be implantable.

Except for the counterregulatory reservoir and miniaturization, such a device now exists. There are two forms commercially available of the artificial insulin pancreas. These devices are called Biostators and are marketed by Life Science Instruments, a division of Miles Laboratories. The larger model is the Biostator GCIIS and costs approximately $65,000. It is primarily a research instrument and has great versatility for controlling insulin delivery, especially for sophisticated research studies.

The smaller model of the Biostator is the Glucose Monitor Controller (Figure 13.1). This instrument is a clinical model of the Biostator but can also be in research, though it is less flexible and versatile. The clinical Biostator costs about $42,000 and can be used in the hospital for a variety of clinical purposes. The instrument is about the size of an EKG machine and is mounted on wheels for portability. A

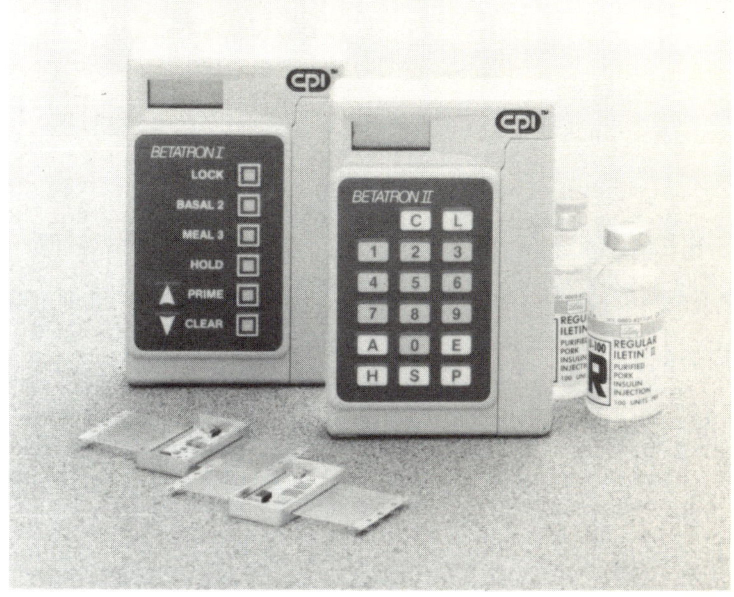

FIGURE 13.1 The Glucose Monitor Controller.

battery pack can be connected to the instrument, allowing it to be wheeled to the operating room, delivery room, intensive care unit, etc., or allowing the patient to exercise by pushing the machine in the hall. The Biostator, in addition to a myriad of research uses, can be used in a variety of clinical settings such as during surgery, labor and delivery, managing diabetic ketoacidosis, reregulation of diabetes, and programming insulin pumps. The machine is especially useful in maintaining euglycemia before, during, and after surgery. The Biostator draws 2 cc of blood/hr (negligible in the older child or adult but significant in a small child) and is able to monitor the blood glucose level with a 90-sec delay arm to readout. There are few, if any, dangers or complications associated with the machines, but they are expensive to purchase and operate and require constant attendance by trained medical personnel. Nonetheless, we have found the Biostator clinically useful in many patients and many situations.

Insulin Pumps

No satisfactory, implantable, miniaturized, self-controlled insulin pump has as yet become commercially available. The limiting factor in the development of such a device (a miniature, implantable Biostator) is the development of an internal glucose-sensing device. Several devices utilizing a variety of chemical reactions which generate an electrical current have been tried. None of the devices tested so far have maintained long-term linearity due to utilization of chemical and walling off in fibrous tissue by the body. However, progress is being made, and while a permanent implantable sensor may yet be a long way off, a temporary, changeable sensor may be very close. Several investigators and commercial companies are testing temporary electrodes in needle form, which can be implanted in the subcutaneous tissue and changed every 7-14 days. Such devices usually contain glucose oxidase, an enzyme which, when it reacts with glucose, liberates an electron that can be picked up by a standard silver-platinum electrode. The needle is connected to a telemetry device outside the skin which can relay the electrical signal to a variety of pickup or recording devices. The reagent device could be a wrist watch-sized microprocessor which could be read visually or could be the microprocessor of an internal or external insulin pump. Such devices are on the horizon and may have important implications in diabetes management apart from their connection to a pump.

The frequent or nearly continuous glucose reading can be used to regulate frequent doses of short-acting insulin and/or food intake to more closely regulate the diabetes. Even the person with type II diabetes may find the device useful, as it would give instant and nearly continuous feedback on the effects of dietary intake, dietary indiscretions, exercise, stress, and emotions on diabetes control. The sensor may therefore be a marvelous teacher of the consequences of our actions, and can result in much finer control of blood glucose with less likelihood of hypoglycemia. The telemetry device of the sensor can even relay a signal to an audible device which the parents keep at their bedside, set to awaken them in case of impending nocturnal hypoglycemia in the child. Such a device would give great peace of mind and a better night's sleep to many parents of small children.

The development of an implantable insulin pump has been slowed awaiting the development of a sensor. Several devices have been tested in animals and a few in a small number of humans. Probably the most widely used implantable device is the Infusaid, a device originally developed to infuse intrahepatic chemotherapy agents in cancer patients. The device looks something like a hockey puck and consists of two round envelopes - the outer one a hard material and the inner one of elastic material. The inner envelope or balloon is filled with insulin through an access port and, when it expands, it compresses a gas, such as freon, contained between the inner balloon and the outer hard shell. When implanted, body heat expands the gas, compressing the inner balloon, forcing the insulin out through portals whose sizes have been scaled to the rate of insulin delivery desired. The insulin can be delivered either intravenously or intraperitoneally. The defect to the system is that the insulin can be delivered at only one rate (basal insulin). No meal boluses or differing basals for exercise or night can be delivered. The Infusaid may have most use in the type II diabetic, although some persons with IDDM may be able to use it alone or in conjunction with injectable boluses of insulin for meals.

External insulin pumps are currently in widespread use. Continuous Subcutaneous Insulin Infusion (CSII) with an external pump is now an established form of insulin delivery. There are a variety of external insulin pumps on the market today, ranging from very simple, nonprogrammable devices to more complex (and more versatile) programmable pumps (Figure 13.2). These devices are becoming progressively smaller and are now quite small and light-weight. Most are about the size of a deck of playing cards or a pack of cigarettes; one pump is as small as a cigarette lighter. The smallest devices, while cosmetically desirable, are less versatile since some degree of programmability is usually lost with decreasing size.

CSII is now an established therapy and is no longer experimental. It has limited usefulness, however, in children because of the limitations it places on activity. The devices are external, so are subject to breakage in contact sports, in "rough and ready" children, and in water activities. During

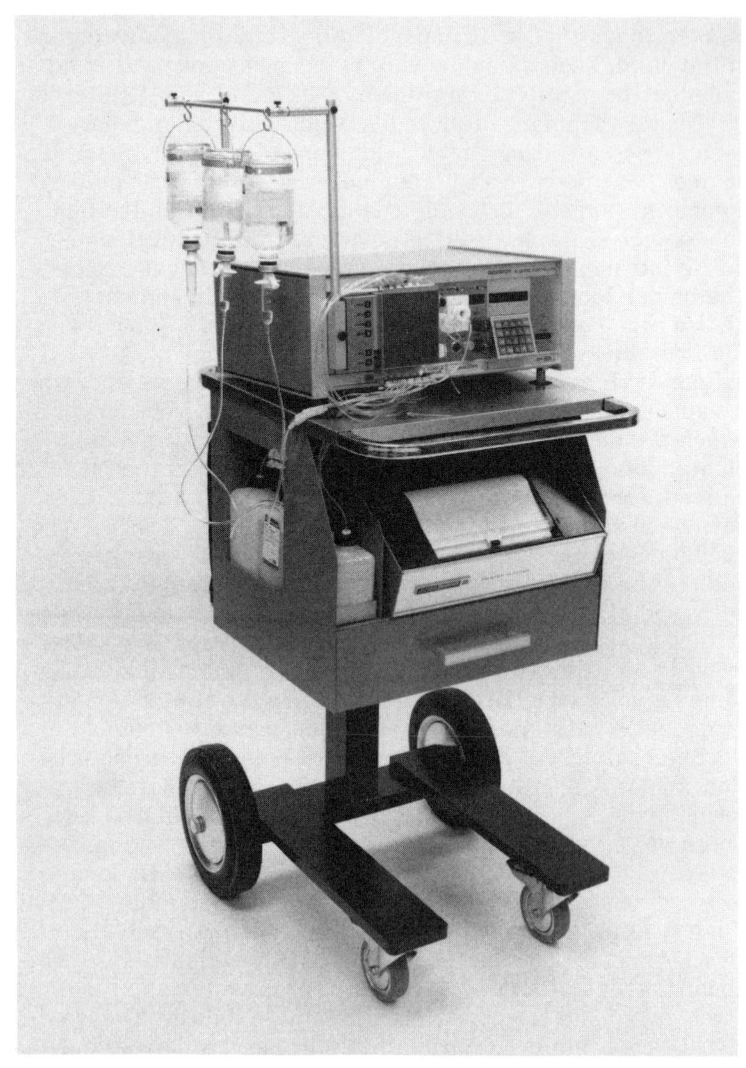

FIGURE 13.2

swimming and water sports, the device can be temporarily removed, however, so that this limitation in their use can be minimized. The Kansas Regional Diabetes Center has had experience with 150 people on CSII therapy. Of these, four or five have been children and 15-20 have been adolescents. The therapy has been highly successful and satisfactory, with significant improvement in glucose control (in many instances, normalization of glycosylated hemoglobin levels) and with improvement in a feeling of well-being and self-confidence. In many of these children and adolescents, there was an important improvement in school performance with better glucose control.

In carefully selected individuals, with proper diabetes and pump education and under careful medical supervision by a well trained pump team, CSII can significantly improve the quality and perhaps the quantity of life. There are, however, problems peculiar to pump therapy (hypoglycemia, and increased possibility of DKA with interruption of insulin flow, abscess formation at the needle site, etc.) so that the patients must be carefully selected and supervised. Experience has taught us that CSII is an important tool for insulin delivery and for improvement in diabetes control, but patients must be carefully selected and trained and CSII should only be initiated by a well trained and constantly available medical team. The therapy has important but limited usefulness in children. It is most useful in adolescents and young adults with IDDM.

ISLET CELL TRANSPLANTATION

Organ transplantation, including transplantation of the pancreas, is an established medical procedure. Whole pancreas transplantation has, however, been nearly completely abandoned because of the difficult surgical procedure involved. The tail of the pancreas can be more easily transplanted and is more successful. However, both procedures require immunosuppression, which carries the inherent danger of uncontrollable infection. Such procedures are not recommended in children.

Investigators are now beginning to work in the field of islet cell transplantation. The signal for rejection of donor tissue by the recipient is proteins on the cell surface of the donor cells. These proteins or antigens (called class II antigens) are genetically different in each individual, thus triggering the immune system of the recipient. It has been shown that pancreatic islet tissue, like most indocrine tissue, does not have class II antigens on their cell surfaces. Thus, islet tissue can be transplanted without immunosuppression. By transplanting individual cell masses, rather than organs, no vascular anastomosis is needed when the tissue is transplanted to a vascular area (liver, spleen, kidney capsule, omentum, etc.). Thus, islets should be amenable to transplant. The problem is purification of the islets. All tissue containing class II antigens (pancreatic tissue, fibrous connective tissue, vascular endothelium, passenger leukocytes, and dendrite cells) must be removed. The purification of the islet cells without injuring the cells is a difficult, laborous, and costly process and currently limits the clinical usefulness of the process.

A number of laboratories in this country, as well as in Candda, Europe, and Austrailia, have been pursuing a variety of strategies to alter islet cell immunity or eliminate contaminating cells. Low yields of viable cells persist, but research continues to increase the efficacy of the pancreas and viability of the cells.

Human islet cell transplantation using fetal islet cells began in Austrailia in 1984. Experiments using both human fetal and adult cells began in the United States in early 1985 in several centers. Results as of this writing have been only marginal, and much work remains to be done. Nonetheless, we are optimistic that this work will be successful, and we will be transplanting islet cells without tissue rejection and without immunosuppression within the next decades.

ISLET CELL REJUVENATION

Islet cells of the pancreas form in the fetus from buds of tissue from the pancreatic ducts. These ducts remain viable in the adult and even in persons with diabetes. Evidently some chemical agent or agents causes them to bud and form islet tissue in the fetus, and stops the process after birth or in infancy. If these substances could be applied to tissue cultures of pancreatic ducts or perhaps given to a living patient, there might be the formation of new islets and a cure of the diabetes. If islets are not totally destroyed in early diabetes, perhaps the remaining ones could be rejuvenated by the above or similar substances. Work is beginning in several centers to identify the mechanisms of islet-cell formation in the fetus, with the hope that this process can be duplicated in the child or adult with IDDM and that a cure can be found. Much work remains to be done, but we are optimistic for the future of our young people with diabetes as we:

1. Improve treatment methods to better control hyperglycemia and prevent complications
2. Develop methods to prevent diabetes in the next generation
3. Develop a cure for those with this disease today

SUMMARY

Therapy of IDDM has changed dramatically in the last decade with the introduction of self-monitoring of blood glucose, and the recognition of the need for physiologic insulin delivery and glucose control for the prevention of the chronic complications of the disease. The concept of the need for maintaining a normal blood glucose level has been established, and new methods of doing so have evolved rapidly.

We can anticipate further dramatic changes in the therapy of IDDM in the next few years. Emphasis will be away from the need to treat complications to the ability to prevent complications. Emphasis will be on methods to prevent diabetes and to better control the disease, with less trauma to the person with the disease. We will see the use of immune intervention to prevent diabetes and reverse the diabetic process. Ultimately, this type of intervention will be applied earlier in the pathogenic sequence during a stage which we do not yet recognize as clinical diabetes. New delivery systems, mechanical devices, computerized devices, sensors, transplants, and preventative strategies will alter the face of diabetes as we know it in the next decade. It will be difficult for us as medical people to keep up with these developments, but it will make life infinitely better for the children of the world with, or destined to develop, diabetes mellitus. The outlook for the future is good and getting better, and important fact to transmit to our children. Hope for a better future will make the present more endurable.

REFERENCES

1. Berson, S.A. and Yalow, R.S.: Diagnosis, radioimmunoassay of plasma insulin. Diabetes mellitus: diagnosis and treatment. Vol. 1. *American Diabetes Association, Inc.* 1:47-54, 1964.

2. Lacy, P.E.: Beta cell secretion from the standpoint of a pathobiologist. Banting Memorial Lecture. *Diabetes* 19(12):895, 1970.

3. Milner, R.D. and Hales, G.W.: The role of calcium and magnesium in insulin secretion from rabbit pancreas studied in vitro. *Diabetologia* 3:47, 1967.

4. Malaisse-Lagae, F., Ravazzola, M., and Orci, L.: Electron Microscope Cytochemical Demonstration of the External Coast of Islet Cells. *Excerpta Medica,* 7th Congress of the International Diabetic Federation, 1973, p. 4.

5. Steiner, D.F., et al.: Isolation and properties of proinsulin, intermediate forms and other minor components from crystalline bovine insulin. *Diabetes* 17:725, 1968.

6. Chance, R.E., Ellis, R.M., and Bromer, W.W.: Porcine proinsulin characterization and amino acid sequence. *Science* 161:165, 1968.

7. Cudworth, A.G. and Wolf, E.: The genetic susceptibility to type I (insulin dependent) diabetes. *Clin. in Endocrinol. and Metab.* 11:389-408, 1982.

8. Presentations from Japanese delegation at 2nd Asian Conference on Diabetes in Children. Okinawa, November, 1984.

9. Presentations from Chinese delegation at 2nd Asian Conference on Diabetes in Children. Okinawa, November, 1984.

10. Owerback, D., Lernmark, A., Platyz, P., Ryder, L. P., Rask, L., Peterson, P.A., and Ludvigsson, J.: HLA-DR region beta chain DNA endonuclease fragments differ between HLA-DR identical healthy and insulin dependent

diabetic individuals. *Nature* 303:815-817, 1983.

11. Cohen, D., Cohen, O., Marcadet, A., Massart, C., Lathrop, M., Deschamp, I., Hors, J., Schuller, E., and Dausett, J.: Class II HLA-DC beta chain DNA restriction fragments differentiate among HLA-DR2 individuals in insulin-dependent diabetes and multiple sclerosis. *Proc. Natl. Acad. Sci. USA.* 81:1774-1778, 1984.

12. Mordes, J. P. and Rossini, A. A.: Animal models of diabetes. *Am. J. Med.* 70:353-360, 1981.

13. Borch-Johnsen, K., Mandrup-Poulsen, T., Zachau-Christiansen, B., Joner, G., Christy, M., Kastrup, K., and Nerup, J.: Relationship between breast-feeding and incidence rates of insulin-dependent diabetes mellitus - a hypothesis. *Lancet* November:1083-1086, 1984.

14. Andreani, D., DeMario, U., Federlin, K.F., and Heding, L.G. (eds.): *Immunology in Diabetes.* Kimpton Medical Publications, London, 1984.

15. Gupta, S. (ed.): *Immunology of Clinical and Experimental Diabetes.* Plenum Press, New York, 1984.

16. Nerup, J.: The Banting Award Address, A.D.A. Annual Scientific Convention, Baltimore, Maryland, 1985.

17. Tochino, Y., Kanaya, T., and Makino, S.: Studies on spontaneously nonobese diabetic mice. *J. Jap. Diab. Soc.* 21:295, 1978.

18. Yamada, K., Nonaka, K., Hanafusa, T., Miyazaki, A., Toyoshima, H., and Tarui, S.: Preventive and therapeutic effects of large-dose nicotinamide injections on diabetes associated with insulitis. An observation in nonobese diabetic (NOD) mice. *Diabetes* 31:749-753, 1982.

19. Elliott, R.B., Crossley, J.R., Berryman, C.C., and James, A.G.: Partial preservation of pancreatic B-cell function in children with diabetes. *Lancet* ii:1-4, 1981.

20. Jackson, R., Dolinar, R., Srikanta, S., Morris, M.A., and Eisenbarth, G.S.: Prednisone therapy in early type I

diabetes: Immunologic effects. *Diabetes* 31(suppl. 2): 48A, 1982.

21. Ludvigsson, J., Heding, L., Lermark, A., and Lieden, G.: An attempt to break the autoimmune process at the onset of IDDM by the use of plasmapheresis or high doses of prednisone. *Bulletin of the International Study Group of Diabetes in Children and Adolescents* 6:11-12, 1982.

22. Eisenbarth, G.: Anti-lymphocyte Globulin as an Immunosuppressant in Diabetes Mellitus. Presented to the International Study Group on Children and Adolescents at a Symposium in St. George, Utah, August, 1984.

23. Leslie, R. D. G. and Pyke, D. A.: Immunosuppression of Acute Insulin-Dependent Diabetics. In: *Immunology of Diabetes,* Irvine, W. J. (ed.). Edinburgh, Teviot Scientific Publications, Ltd., 1980, pp. 345-347.

24. Ludvigsson, J., Heding, L., Lieden, G., Marner, B., and Lernmark, A.: Plasmapheresis in the initial treatment of insulin-dependent diabetes mellitus in children. *Brit. Med. J.* :176-178, 1983.

25. Rabinovitch, A., MacKay, P., Ludvigsson, J., and Lermark, A.: A prospective analysis of islet cell cytotoxic antibodies in insulin-dependent diabetic children: Transient effects of plasmapheresis. *Diabetes* 33:224-228, 1984.

26. Greulich, B., Lander, T., Standl, E., Kolb, H., Gerbitz, K-D., Kuschak, D., and Gries, F. A.: Immune intervention trial in newly diagnosed type I (insulin-dependent) diabetes. *Diabetologia* 25:158, 1983.

27. Stiller, C.R., Laupacis, A., Dupre, J., Jenner, M.R., Keown, P.A., Rodger, W., and Wolfe, B. M. J.: Cyclosporin for treatment of early type I diabetes: Preliminary results. *N. Engl. J. Med.* 308:1226-1227, 1983.

28. Stiller, C. R., Dupre, J., Gent, M., Jenner, M. R. , Keown, P. A., Laupacis, A., Martell, R., Rodger, N. W., Graffenried, B. V., and Wolfe, B. M. J.: effects of cyclosporin immunosuppression in insulin-dependent diabetes mellitus of recent onset. *Science* 223:1362-1367, 1984.

29. Skyler, J.: Personal Communication, 1985.

INDEX